Fetal Cardiology

SIMPLIFIED

A PRACTICAL MANUAL

Gurleen Sharland

i

tfm Publishing Limited, Castle Hill Barns, Harley, Nr Shrewsbury, SY5 6LX, UK
Tel: +44 (0)1952 510061; Fax: +44 (0)1952 510192
E-mail: info@tfmpublishing.com;
Web site: www.tfmpublishing.com

Design & Typesetting: Nikki Bramhill BSc Hons Dip Law
First Edition: © 2013
ISBN: 978 1 903378 55 7

Printed by Gutenberg Press Ltd.,
Gudja Road, Tarxien, PLA 19, Malta
Tel: +356 21897037; Fax: +356 21800069

Contents

Foreword

This handbook is designed to be an aid to those involved in the detection, diagnosis and management of fetal heart abnormalities. This will include obstetric sonographers, obstetricians, fetal medicine specialists, cardiac technicians/physiologists and paediatric cardiologists training in fetal cardiology, as well as paediatric cardiology consultants with less experience of fetal cardiology. This book will also be useful as a teaching tool for anyone involved in scanning the fetal heart.

It is assumed that the reader will be familiar with scanning the fetus and the fetal heart and it is not the aim of this book to teach the practicalities of fetal cardiac scanning, as there are many publications already available to help with this. The purpose of this book is to help interpret cardiac findings and aid in making a correct cardiac diagnosis. The focus of this book is on structural cardiac malformations, though a section on arrhythmias is also included. It is envisaged that many of those using this manual will not have a background in paediatric cardiology. For this reason, the abnormalities have been grouped depending on whether the four-chamber view is likely to be abnormal or not. However, paediatric cardiologists will examine the heart by initially examining the cardiac connections and then looking for further associated abnormalities. This concept has been maintained, both in descriptions of the normal heart and in discussions of abnormal heart anatomy.

Whilst some information is included regarding management and outcome, this is not a textbook of paediatric cardiology and further information can be sought in larger textbooks or publications and by consulting paediatric cardiology colleagues, who have wider in-depth knowledge and experience in managing congenital heart disease. It is well recognised that the outcome and associations documented from fetal life may differ from those reported in postnatal series. Therefore the outcomes and associations noted in a large fetal series are referred to here. This information is based on a single-centre experience of fetal cardiac abnormalities seen between 1980 and 2010 at the Evelina Children's Hospital, which is part of Guy's and St Thomas' NHS Foundation Trust, in London, UK.

Gurleen Sharland BSc MD FRCP
Reader/Consultant in Fetal Cardiology
Fetal Cardiology Unit
Evelina Children's Hospital
Guy's & St Thomas' NHS Foundation Trust
London, UK

Acknowledgements

I would like to thank all my family and dear friends for endless encouragement and support.

I would also like to thank and acknowledge my colleagues and all members of the fetal cardiology team at Evelina Children's Hospital, London. Their continuing dedication and professionalism has enabled the development of a first class service providing high standards of care for patients and their families.

Dedication

To

Mike, Peter and Emma

with all my love and much more

and

with love and thanks to my very dear parents,

Mani and Puran

Abbreviations

A	atrial
Abs PV	absent pulmonary valve syndrome
ALSCA	aberrant left subclavian artery
Ao	aorta
AoA	aortic arch
AoAt VSD	aortic atresia with a ventricular septal defect
AoV	aortic valve
ARSCA	aberrant right subclavian artery
AS	aortic stenosis
Asc Ao	ascending aorta
AVSD	atrioventricular septal defect
AV valve	atrioventricular valve
AVVR	atrioventricular valve regurgitation
CAT	common arterial trunk
CCAML	congenital cystic adenomatoid malformation of the lung
CCTGA	congenitally corrected transposition of the great arteries
CHB	congenital heart block
CHD	congenital heart disease
Coarct	coarctation of the aorta
Coll	a collateral vessel
CS	coronary sinus
DAo	descending aorta
Diabetic	maternal diabetes
DIV	double-inlet ventricle
DORV	double-outlet right ventricle
Ebstein's	Ebstein's anomaly
ECG	electrocardiogram
Fabn	fetal abnormality
Farr	fetal arrhythmia
FH	family history
Fhyd	fetal hydrops
FO	foramen ovale
HLH	hypoplastic left heart syndrome
INFD	death in infancy
Int AA	interrupted aortic arch
IUD	intrauterine death
IVC	inferior vena cava
LA	left atrium
LAI	left atrial isomerism
LAVV	left atrioventricular valve

LCA	left coronary artery
LPA	left pulmonary artery
LSVC	left superior vena cava
LTFU	lost to follow-up
LV	left ventricle
LVDD	left ventricular diastolic dimension
LVSD	left ventricular systolic dimension
MAT	mitral atresia
MPA	main pulmonary artery
MR	mitral regurgitation
MV	mitral valve
NND	death in neonatal period
NT	nuchal translucency
PA	pulmonary artery
PAPVD	partial anomalous pulmonary venous connection
PAT IVS	pulmonary atresia with an intact ventricular septum
PAT VSD	pulmonary atresia with a ventricular septal defect
PE	pericardial effusion
PV	pulmonary valve
PS	pulmonary stenosis
RA	right atrium
RAI	right atrial isomerism
RAVV	right atrioventricular valve
RCA	right coronary artery
RPA	right pulmonary artery
RSVC	right superior vena cava
RV	right ventricle
SVC	superior vena cava
SVT	supraventricular tachycardia
T	trachea
TAPVD	total anomalous pulmonary venous connection or drainage
TAT	tricuspid atresia
Tetralogy	tetralogy of Fallot
TGA	transposition of the great arteries
ToF	tetralogy of Fallot
TOP	termination of pregnancy
TR	tricuspid regurgitation
TV	tricuspid valve
TVD	tricuspid valve dysplasia
UV	umbilical vein
V	ventricle or ventricular
VSD	ventricular septal defect

Chapter 1

Screening for congenital heart disease

Summary

- **Introduction**
- **Prenatal detection of congenital heart disease**
  - **Screening for fetal congenital heart disease**
  - **Factors influencing screening of low-risk populations**
  - **Spectrum of abnormality detected prenatally**
- **Referral reasons for fetal echocardiography**
- **Gestational age at diagnosis**

Introduction

Cardiac abnormalities are the commonest form of congenital malformation, with moderate and severe forms affecting about 0.3-0.6% of live births. One of the main reasons for making an antenatal diagnosis is to detect major forms of cardiac abnormality early. Diagnosis of anomalies associated with significant morbidity and mortality in early pregnancy allows parents to consider all available options. Prenatal diagnosis also gives time to prepare families for the likely course of events after delivery and to optimise care for the baby at birth. Where appropriate, delivery can be planned at or near a centre with paediatric cardiology and paediatric cardiac surgical facilities. While treatment for the vast majority of cases will take place after birth, prenatal treatment may be considered in a few select cases. Additionally, the value of confirming normality and providing reassurance to anxious parents, particularly if they have already had an affected child, should not be underestimated.

Antenatal diagnosis of congenital heart disease has become well established over the last 30 years and a high degree of diagnostic accuracy is available and expected in tertiary centres dealing with the diagnosis and management of fetal cardiac abnormalities. Virtually all major forms of congenital heart disease, as well as some of the minor forms, can be detected during fetal life, in experienced centres. There are, however, some lesions that cannot be predicted before birth, even in experienced hands, and this should be acknowledged. These include a secundum type of atrial septal defect and a persistent arterial duct, as all fetuses should have a patent foramen ovale and an arterial duct as part of the fetal circulation. In addition, some types of ventricular septal defect may be difficult to detect, either because of their size or position. The milder forms of obstructive lesions of the aorta and pulmonary artery can develop later in life with no signs of obstruction during fetal life.

Prenatal detection of congenital heart disease

Screening for fetal congenital heart disease

A two-tier system has developed for the examination of the fetal heart. Pregnancies at increased risk for fetal congenital heart disease are generally referred to tertiary centres for detailed fetal echocardiography, though the expected rate of cardiac abnormality is relatively low in these groups. Table 1.1 shows the indications for fetal echocardiography and the common groups considered to be at increased risk. The majority of cases of congenital heart disease, however, will occur in low-risk groups and these will only be detected prenatally if examination of the fetal heart is incorporated as part of routine obstetric ultrasound screening. Whilst four-chamber view examination is an effective method of detecting some of the severe forms of cardiac malformation before birth, some major lesions, such as transposition of the great vessels and tetralogy of Fallot, are often associated with a normal four-chamber view. Therefore, including examination of the arterial outflow tracts would greatly improve the prenatal detection rates of major life-threatening forms of congenital heart disease. Current national guidelines recommend examination of the outflow tracts in addition to the four-chamber view at the time of the fetal anomaly scan (Table 1.2).

Factors influencing antenatal screening for heart defects

Antenatal screening for major forms of heart abnormality is possible though there are many issues relating to its success. Detection of cardiac abnormalities is mainly dependent on the skill of sonographers performing routine obstetric ultrasound scans. A formal programme for education and training regarding the fetal heart is necessary to ensure that sonographers are taught the skills of fetal heart examination. As well as learning to obtain the correct views of the heart, sonographers must learn to interpret the views correctly. It is also very important that they maintain these skills. In order to detect anomalies, obstetric ultrasound units need to have appropriate and adequate ultrasound equipment. The time allowed for the obstetric anomaly scan will also influence how long can be spent examining the fetal heart and, thus, the detection rates of abnormalities. A very important aspect of antenatal screening is audit of activity, including monitoring and feedback of both false positive and false negative cases, as well as the true positives.

Spectrum of abnormality detected in the fetus

The cardiac diagnoses in most large fetal cardiac series are generally skewed towards the severe end of the spectrum of cardiac abnormality, with the majority of abnormalities being

Table 1.1. Pregnancies at increased risk for fetal cardiac abnormality and indications for detailed fetal echocardiography.

Maternal and familial factors identified at booking

1) Family history of congenital heart disease

  - Sibling
    - one affected child – recurrence risk 2-3%
    - two affected children – recurrence risk 10%
    - three affected children – recurrence risk 50%
  - Parent
    - either parent affected – risk in the baby between 2-6%

2) Family history of gene disorders or syndromes with congenital heart disease or cardiomyopathy

3) Maternal metabolic disorders, especially if poor control in early pregnancy

  - Diabetes – risk 2-3%
  - Phenylketonuria – risk 8-10%

4) Exposure to cardiac teratogens in early pregnancy such as lithium, phenytoin or steroids

  - Risk 2%

5) Maternal viral infections

  - Rubella, CMV, coxsackie, parvovirus, toxoplasma

6) Maternal collagen disease with anti-Ro and/or anti-La antibodies

  - Risk 2-3% of congenital heart block in baby

7) Maternal medication with non-steroidal anti-inflammatory drugs

Fetal high-risk factors

1) Suspicion of cardiac malformation or disease during an obstetric anomaly scan

  - This is the most important and effective way in which fetal cardiac abnormalities are detected

2) Fetal arrhythmias

  - Sustained bradycardia – heart rate <120 beats per minute
  - Tachycardia – heart rate >180 beats per minute

Continued

Table 1.1 *continued.* **Pregnancies at increased risk for fetal cardiac abnormality and indications for detailed fetal echocardiography.**

3) Increased nuchal translucency in the first trimester

    * 6-7% risk when nuchal translucency (NT) >99th centile for crown rump length (= or >3.5mm) even when the fetal karyotype is normal
    * The risk increases with increasing NT measurement
    * A nuchal translucency >95th centile is also associated with an increased risk of congenital heart disease but with lower risk and due to the workload involved, local policies will determine whether this group should be offered a detailed cardiac scan

4) Structural extracardiac fetal anomaly present on ultrasound

    * For example, exomphalos, diaphragmatic hernia, duodenal atresia, tracheo-oesophageal fistula, cystic hygroma
    * Abnormalities in more than one system in the fetus should raise the suspicion of a chromosome defect

5) Chromosomal abnormalities

6) Genetic syndromes

7) Pericardial effusion

8) Pleural effusion

9) Non-immune fetal hydrops

    * May be caused by structural heart disease or fetal arrhythmia

10) Monochorionic twins

    * Risk 7-8%

11) Other states with known risk for fetal heart failure:

    * Tumours with a large vascular supply
    * Arteriovenous fistulas
    * Absence of ductus venosus
    * Acardiac twin
    * Feto-fetal transfusion syndrome
    * Fetal anaemia

Initial assessment of some of the above cases could be made by a fetal medicine specialist or by an experienced sonographer who have had appropriate training in fetal heart scanning. Cases with a suspected cardiac abnormality can then be referred to a fetal cardiology specialist for further assessment.

Table 1.2. Screening of low-risk pregnancies – cardiac evaluation during the 18-20+6-week anomaly scan.

National guidelines are now available in the UK regarding cardiac examination during the obstetric anomaly scan. The following is an outline which, if incorporated into all anomaly scans, would significantly help to improve prenatal detection rates of congenital heart disease.

1) Stomach and heart on the left side of the fetus

2) Normal heart rate 120-180 beats per minute

3) A normal four-chamber view

- Size
  - about one-third of the thorax
- Position
  - septum at an angle of about 45° to the midline
- Structure
  - two atria of approximately equal size
  - two ventricles of approximately equal size and thickness
  - two opening atrioventricular valves of equal size
  - intact crux of heart with offsetting of atrioventricular valves
  - intact ventricular septum from apex to crux
- Function
  - equally contracting ventricles

4) Examination of both great arteries

- Aorta arises from LV, with anterior wall of aorta being continuous with the ventricular septum
- PA arises from RV
- PA equal to or slightly bigger than aorta in size
- Cross-over of great arteries at their origin

5) Three-vessel and tracheal view

- Aorta and pulmonary artery of approximately equal size
- The aortic arch descends to the left of the trachea

LV = left ventricle; RV = right ventricle; PA = pulmonary artery

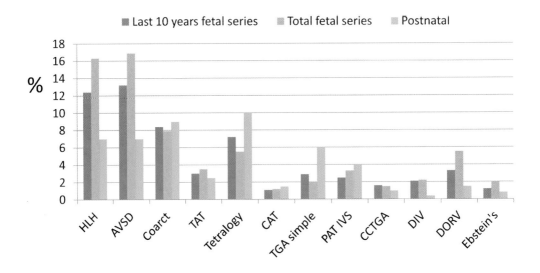

■ Last 10 years fetal series   ■ Total fetal series   ■ Postnatal

Figure 1.1. The prevalence of 12 cardiac defects in the fetal cardiac series seen between 1980 and 2010 at Evelina Children's Hospital is compared to expected prevalence of the same lesions in postnatal series. The prevalence of the same defects in the last 10 years from 2000-2010 is also shown. HLH = hypoplastic left heart syndrome; AVSD = atrioventricular septal defect; Coarct = coarctation of the aorta; TAT = tricuspid atresia; Tetralogy = tetralogy of Fallot; CAT = common arterial trunk; TGA = transposition of the great arteries; PAT IVS = pulmonary atresia with intact interventricular septum; CCTGA = congenitally corrected transposition of the great arteries; DIV = double-inlet ventricle; DORV = double-outlet right ventricle; Ebstein's = Ebstein's anomaly.

associated with an abnormal four-chamber view. This bias is a reflection of four-chamber view screening which has been used in routine obstetric anomaly scanning for over 25 years. As a result there has been a predisposition towards lesions that will result in single-ventricle palliation rather than a corrective procedure. However, with the increasing inclusion of great artery examination at the time of the fetal anomaly scan there has been some improvement in the proportion of great artery abnormalities being detected by screening, though further improvement could still be made. Figure 1.1 shows the prevalence of 12 cardiac defects in the large fetal series seen between 1980 and 2010 at Evelina Children's Hospital compared to expected prevalence of the same lesions in postnatal series. Also shown is the prevalence of the same cardiac defects in the last 10 years of the fetal series. It can be noted that there has been an improvement in the detection of some great artery abnormalities, such as transposition of the great arteries and tetralogy of Fallot, so that the prevalence in the fetal series in latter years more closely approximates postnatal series, though a difference still remains.

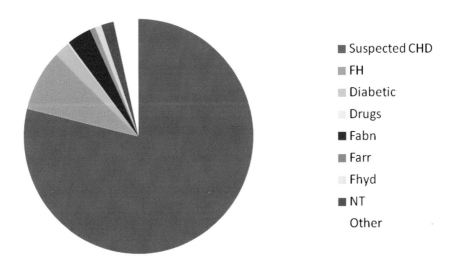

■ Suspected CHD
▨ FH
▨ Diabetic
▨ Drugs
■ Fabn
▨ Farr
▨ Fhyd
■ NT
Other

Figure 1.2. The referral reasons for fetal echocardiography in over 4000 cardiac abnormalities detected in the Evelina fetal series between 1980 and 2010. CHD = congenital heart disease; FH = family history; Diabetic = maternal diabetes; Fabn = fetal abnormality; Farr = fetal arrhythmia; Fhyd = fetal hydrops; NT = increased nuchal translucency.

Referral reasons in cases of fetal congenital heart disease in large fetal series

The referral reasons in over 4000 cardiac abnormalities in the fetal series seen between 1980 and 2010 at Evelina Children's Hospital is shown in Figure 1.2. Nearly 80% of all fetal cardiac abnormalities were diagnosed following referral because of a suspected abnormality at the time of the obstetric anomaly scan.

Gestation age at diagnosis in a large fetal series

The gestational age at time of diagnosis of fetal congenital heart disease seen between 1980 and 2010 is shown in Figure 1.3. In the last 10 years of the series there has been an increase in the number of cases diagnosed below 16 weeks of gestation, with the largest number of diagnoses being made between 17-24 weeks. In the last 10 years the majority have been seen between 21-24 weeks of gestation. This is a reflection of abnormalities being picked up during the screening fetal anomaly scan at 18-22 weeks of gestation. In the first

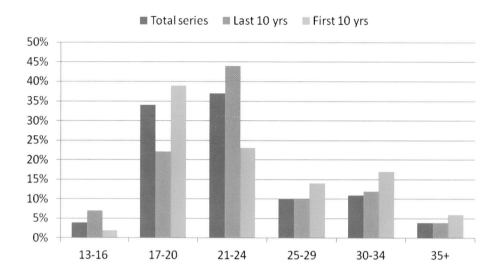

Figure 1.3. The gestational age at time of diagnosis of fetal congenital heart disease in the Evelina fetal series between 1980 and 2010. The gestational age is shown for the total series in this time frame, as well as for the first 10 years and the last 10 years of the series.

10 years the majority were seen at 17-20 weeks as the anomaly scans were often performed at 16 weeks in that era, to fit in with the timing of amniocentesis.

Chapter 2

The normal fetal heart

Summary

- Normal connections of the heart
- Establishing normality
  - Position of the heart
  - Abdominal situs
  - Four-chamber views
  - Great artery views
    - aorta from left ventricle
    - pulmonary artery from right ventricle
  - Arch views
    - aortic arch
    - ductal arch
  - Three-vessel view/three-vessel tracheal view
  - Normal cardiac Dopplers
  - Normal heart at different gestations
    - 13 weeks
    - 15 weeks
    - 18 weeks
    - 28 weeks
- Variations of normal
  - Asymmetry in later gestation
  - Normal rim of fluid
  - Echogenic foci
  - Normal heart with other fetal abnormality

The normal fetal heart

A systematic approach to the examination of the fetal heart will enable the confirmation of normality easily and will ensure an accurate diagnosis in cases with congenital heart malformations. How well the heart can be imaged will depend on several factors, which include the gestational age and position of the fetus, the maternal habitus and the type of ultrasound scanner and the transducers being used. Other abnormalities in the baby, such as a large exomphalos or diaphragmatic hernia, can distort the appearance of the heart, making it more difficult to confirm normality, or accurately diagnose an abnormality. The presence of other conditions, such as oligohydramnios or polyhydramnios, can also make imaging the fetal heart more challenging.

Normal cardiac structure and cardiac connections

The best approach to confirm cardiac normality and to diagnose malformations of the heart is to start by checking the connections of the heart. There are six cardiac connections to consider, three on each side. These are the venous-atrial connections, the atrioventricular connections and the ventriculo-arterial connections. On the right side, the superior vena cava and the inferior vena cava connect to the right atrium (venous-atrial connection on right). The right atrium is connected to the right ventricle via the tricuspid valve (atrioventricular connection on right). The right ventricle is connected to the pulmonary artery via the pulmonary valve (ventriculo-arterial connection on right). On the left side, four pulmonary veins connect to the left atrium (venous-atrial connection on left). The left atrium is connected to the left ventricle via the mitral valve (atrioventricular connection on left). The left ventricle is connected to the aorta via the aortic valve (ventriculo-arterial connection on left). In the fetal circulation there are two cardiac communications present that will close after birth. These are the foramen ovale in the atrial septum between the right and left atria and the arterial duct, which is a communication between the aorta and pulmonary artery.

Summary of normal connections.		
	Left	**Right**
Veno-atrial	Pulmonary veins to left atrium	Superior and inferior vena cava to right atrium
Atrioventricular	Left atrium to left ventricle via mitral valve	Right atrium to right ventricle via tricuspid valve
Ventriculo-arterial	Left ventricle to aorta via aortic valve	Right ventricle to pulmonary artery via pulmonary valve

Additional cardiac anomalies, such as defects in the interventricular septum or abnormalities of the atrioventricular valves, for example, Ebstein's anomaly, can be excluded once the major connections have been checked.

Approach for scanning the fetal heart

The starting point of all fetal heart scans should be to establish the fetal position in the maternal abdomen and to determine the left and right side of the baby. The position of the heart and stomach can then be established and both these structures normally lie on the left side of the body. After noting the abdominal situs and cardiac position, the simplest and easiest method to examine the structure of the heart in the fetus, is firstly to obtain and analyse the four-chamber view and then proceed to examine views of the great vessels. The function of the heart, the heart rate and heart rhythm should also be observed as part of the cardiac examination. Further evaluation, as described in Chapters 10 and 13, will be required if any functional or rhythm disturbances are noted.

Abdominal/atrial situs

The abdominal situs can be checked in a transverse section of the abdomen as shown in Figure 2.1. This view demonstrates the position of the stomach and the relative positions of

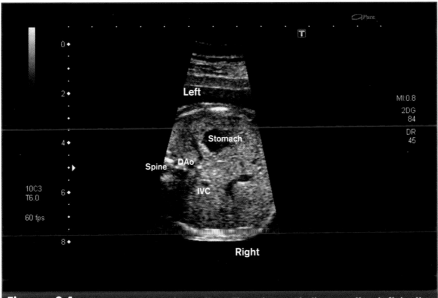

Figure 2.1. Normal abdominal situs. The stomach lies on the left in the abdomen. The descending aorta normally lies anterior and to the left of the spine. The inferior vena cava lies to the right of the spine, lying anterior and to the right of the descending aorta.

the descending aorta and inferior vena cava in the abdomen. The stomach lies on the left in the abdomen. The descending aorta normally lies anterior and to the left of the spine. The inferior vena cava lies to the right of the spine, lying anterior and to the right of the descending aorta. This normal arrangement is termed situs solitus. From this arrangement it is usually inferred that the morphologically right atrium is right-sided and the morphologically left atrium is left-sided.

Cardiac position and size

The normal fetal heart lies in the left chest with the apex pointing to the left. The angle of the ventricular septum to the midline of the thorax is usually between 30-60° (Figures 2.2a and 2.3a). The size of the fetal heart is about one-third of the thorax and this can be measured using the circumference ratio of the heart to the thorax.

The four-chamber view
(Venous atrial connection on left and atrioventricular connections on right and left)

Examination of the four-chamber view can demonstrate three of the six cardiac connections. These are the venous-atrial connection on the left (pulmonary veins draining to left atrium) and both the atrioventricular connections (mitral and tricuspid valves connecting the corresponding atrium and ventricle). The interventricular septum can also be examined in this view, as can the atrioventricular septum and differential insertion of the two atrioventricular valves. The sizes of the cardiac chambers can be compared and the function of the ventricles can be noted. An initial assessment of heart rhythm can also be made.

The fetal heart lies in a horizontal position in the thorax with the right ventricle lying directly anterior to the left ventricle. The four-chamber view is achieved in a horizontal section of the fetal thorax just above the diaphragm. The appearance of the four chambers will vary depending on whether it is imaged in apical or lateral projections of the heart. In the former, the ultrasound beam will be parallel to the ventricular septum (Figure 2.2a) and in the latter the ultrasound beam will be perpendicular to the septum (Figure 2.3a). Although the appearance of the four-chamber view varies in the different projections (Figures 2.2-2.5), the same cardiac structures and features outlined below can still be identified, though some are more easily recognised in certain projections. For example, the differential insertion (see below) of the atrioventricular valves is more easily seen in Figure 2.2a and the foramen ovale is more easily seen in Figures 2.3a-b and 2.4a. An example where the differential insertion of the atrioventricular valves was very difficult to demonstrate is shown in Figure 2.6. Using different views, however, minimal differential insertion could be identified and this proved to be normal after birth.

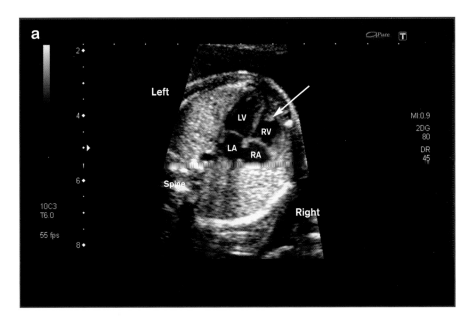

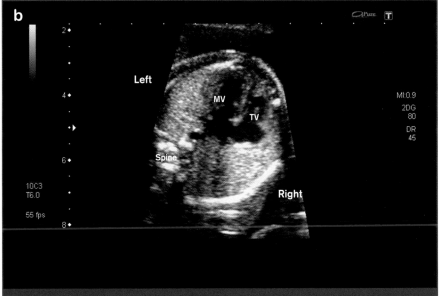

Figure 2.2. a) An apical four-chamber view. The moderator band can be seen clearly in this view (arrow). b) View with both atrioventricular valves open. Both mitral and tricuspid valves should open equally.

Figure continued overleaf.

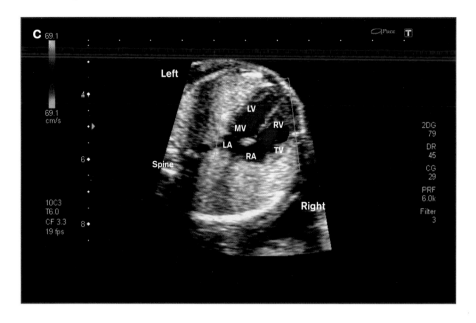

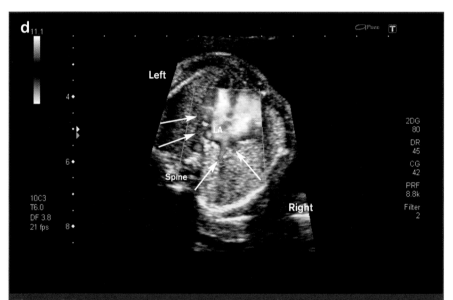

Figure 2.2 *continued.* c) The inflow across the mitral and tricuspid valves is seen with colour flow (shown in red). d) The pulmonary veins (arrows) can be seen entering the back of the left atrium.

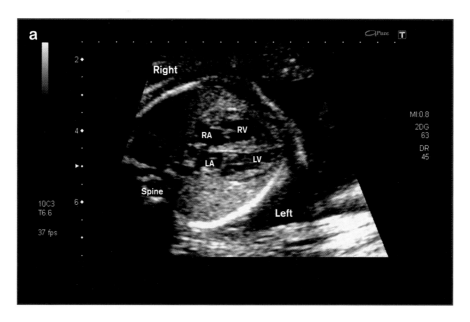

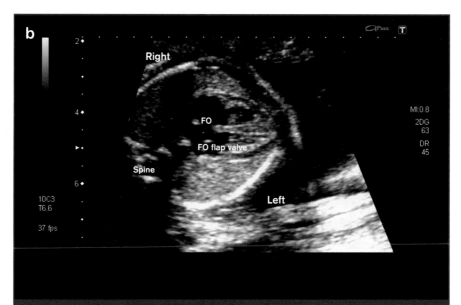

Figure 2.3. a) A four-chamber view with the ultrasound beam perpendicular to the ventricular septum. b) In this projection the foramen ovale and foramen ovale flap are easily seen.

Important features to note in the four-chamber view.

- Heart position
  - the apex points out of the left anterior thorax
- Heart size
  - the heart should occupy approximately a third of the thorax
- Right atrium and left atrium of approximately equal size
- Right ventricle and left ventricle of approximately equal size and thickness. Both show equal contraction. The right ventricular apex has the moderator band of muscle (Figures 2.2a and 2.5). Note that in the third trimester, the right heart can appear dilated compared to the left and this can be a normal feature in some babies (see below)
- Two patent atrioventricular valves (mitral and tricuspid) which open equally and are of approximately equal size (Figure 2.2b)
- The atrial and ventricular septa meet the two atrioventricular valves (mitral and tricuspid) at the crux of the heart forming an offset cross (differential insertion). In the normal heart, the septal insertion of the tricuspid valve is slightly lower or more apical, than that of the mitral valve, resulting in the normal differential insertion (see Figure 2.2a)
  Occasionally the differential insertion is minimal making it very difficult to exclude an atrioventricular septal defect (Figure 2.6)
- There is an interatrial communication, the foramen ovale. This is usually guarded by the foramen ovale flap valve, which can usually be seen flickering in the left atrium (Figure 2.3b)
- The interventricular septum should appear intact
- The pulmonary venous connections to the back of the left atrium should be identified. It is vital to ensure that pulmonary flow can be demonstrated entering the left atrium using colour flow (Figures 2.2c and 2.4b)

Features of the four-chamber view when the ultrasound beam is parallel to the septum (apical four-chamber view)

- Crux of the heart seen well
- Differential insertion of the atrioventricular valves demonstrated
- Opening of the mitral and tricuspid valves seen well
- Moderator band of the right ventricle seen clearly
- May get dropout in the ventricular septum at the crux of the heart making it difficult to exclude a ventricular septal defect (see Chapter 5)

Features of the four-chamber view when the ultrasound beam is perpendicular to the septum.

- Wall and septal thickness are more clearly defined
- Ventricles may appear more thickened in this view
- Margins of the foramen ovale are better defined
- May see a normal rim of fluid around the ventricles (see below)

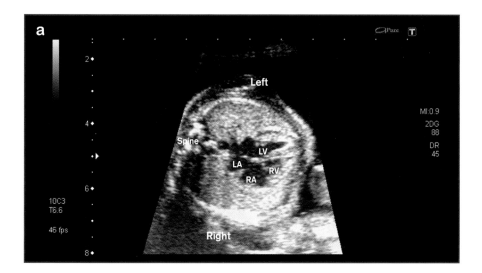

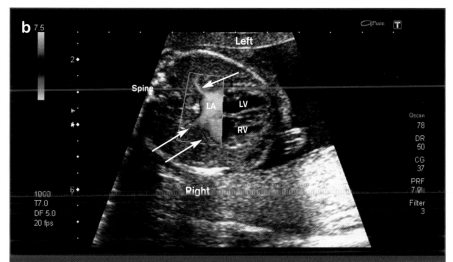

Figure 2.4. a) Another four-chamber view. The ventricular walls and septum often appear more thickened in this projection. b) The pulmonary veins (arrows) can be seen entering the back of the left atrium.

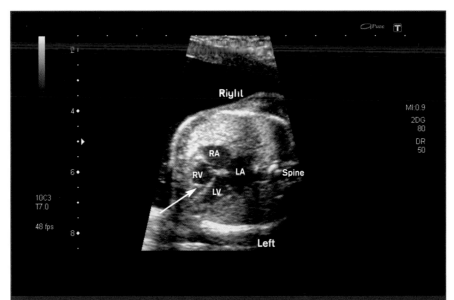

Figure 2.5. A four-chamber view shown in a different projection. The moderator band can be seen clearly in this view (arrow).

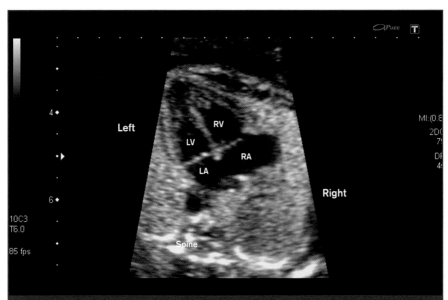

Figure 2.6. In this example the differential insertion of the atrioventricular valves was very difficult to demonstrate, but this proved to be normal after birth.

The venous-atrial connection on the right

The superior and inferior vena cavae connect to the right atrium. Both vessels can be viewed in transverse or longitudinal planes. Figures 2.7a-b show a longitudinal section

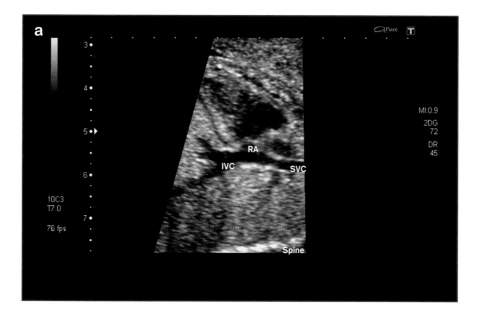

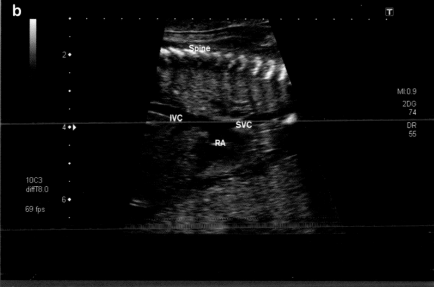

Figure 2.7. a) A longitudinal section demonstrating both vena cavae entering the right atrium. This view is sometimes referred to as the bicaval view. b) Another view showing both vena cava entering the right atrium.

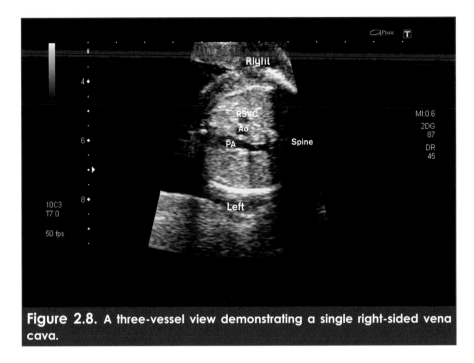

Figure 2.8. A three-vessel view demonstrating a single right-sided vena cava.

demonstrating both vena cavae entering the right atrium. This view is sometimes referred to as the bicaval view. The superior vena cava enters the roof of the right atrium and the inferior vena cava passes through the diaphragm to enter the floor of the right atrium. There is usually a single right-sided superior vena cava, which can also be viewed in the three-vessel view and tracheal views (Figures 2.8 and 2.9a, and see section below). A left-sided superior vena cava in isolation is regarded as a normal variant, but it can be also associated with cardiac malformations. Bilateral superior vena cavae (Figure 2.10) may also be a normal variation or associated with other malformations. The inferior vena cava lies anterior and to the right of the descending aorta in the abdomen (Figure 2.1).

The coronary sinus

The coronary sinus is the venous drainage of the heart itself. This structure crosses behind the left atrium to enter the floor of the right atrium. It can be dilated in the presence of a left-sided superior vena cava (Figures 2.11a-b). A dilated coronary sinus should not be mistaken for a partial atrioventricular septal defect (see Chapter 4).

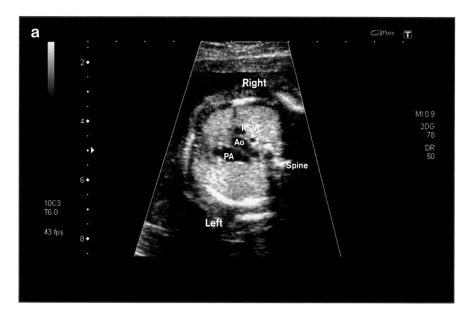

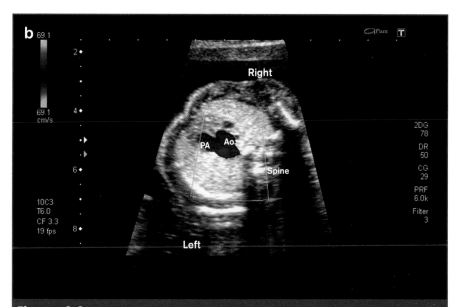

Figure 2.9. a) A three-vessel view/tracheal view showing the aorta as it heads towards the descending aorta. The aorta lies to the left of the trachea. The sizes of the aorta and pulmonary artery are better compared in this view and isthmal narrowing is more likely to be detected (see also Chapter 9). b) Colour flow in both great arteries (shown in blue) is in the same direction towards the descending aorta.

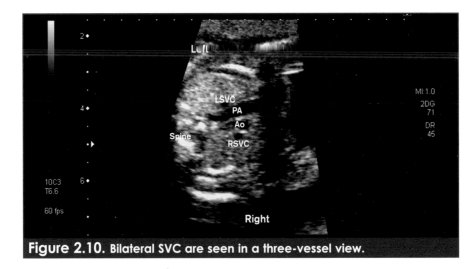

Figure 2.10. Bilateral SVC are seen in a three-vessel view.

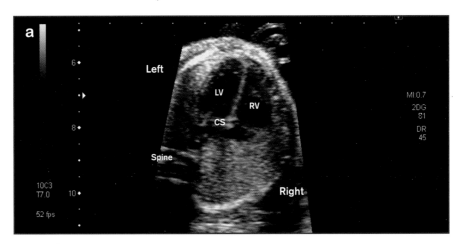

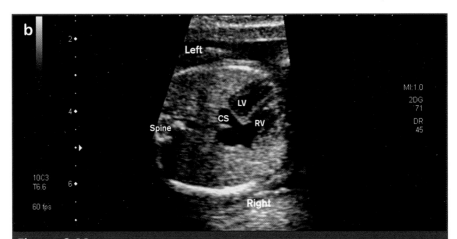

Figure 2.11. a) The coronary sinus is seen in a view just inferior to the four-chamber view. b) A dilated coronary sinus. This should not be mistaken for an atrioventricular septal defect.

Ventriculo-arterial connections

The connections and relationships of the two great arteries (aorta and pulmonary artery) can be imaged in both horizontal and longitudinal projections.

Aorta from left ventricle (normal ventriculo-arterial connection on left)
The aorta arises in the centre of the chest, with the aortic valve being wedged between the two atrioventricular valves. After leaving the heart, the aorta sweeps cranially and crosses the midline towards the right shoulder, forms an arch which then takes a leftward and posterior direction to cross the midline again, to descend to the left of the trachea (see section below on three-vessel/tracheal views).

The origin of the aorta and aortic valve arising from the left ventricle can be seen in a horizontal section just cranial to the four-chamber view. This view is often referred to as the five-chamber view and is illustrated in Figures 2.12a-b. This view can be opened out, by angling the ultrasound beam cranially from the four-chamber view towards the right shoulder, to demonstrate the long axis view of the left ventricle, which will show the aorta arising from the left ventricle and its initial course towards the right shoulder (Figures 2.13a-c). In the long axis view, the anterior wall of the aorta should be seen to be continuous with the ventricular septum. The posterior wall of the aorta is continuous with the anterior leaflet of the mitral valve. Note that the first vessel to be visualised when moving cranially from the four-chamber view in the normal heart is the aorta.

Pulmonary artery from right ventricle (normal ventriculo-arterial connection on right)
The pulmonary artery arises more anterior to the aorta, close to the anterior chest wall and is directed straight back towards the spine. The pulmonary valve is anterior and more cranial than the aortic valve. A horizontal section, more cranial from the four-chamber view and the origin of the aorta, will demonstrate the pulmonary valve and pulmonary artery (Figures 2.14a-d). The pulmonary artery can also be viewed in a more longitudinal view showing all the right heart structures (Figure 2.15). This vessel branches, giving rise to the right and left pulmonary arteries and the arterial duct, which joins the descending aorta forming the ductal arch (see below). Both the right and left pulmonary arteries can be identified in the fetus, though both pulmonary arteries are not usually seen together in the same plane as the duct (Figures 2.14c and 2.16e). The right pulmonary artery is usually more easily seen in transverse views along with the duct (Figure 2.14b). The left pulmonary artery is more easily visualised in more longitudinal views imaging the right heart structures and long axis of the duct (Figure 2.15), though can also be seen in transverse views (Figures 2.14c and 2.16c).

Cross-over of the great arteries
In the normal fetal heart, the aorta arises from the centre of the heart and courses superiorly towards the right shoulder. The pulmonary artery arises more anteriorly and cranially and takes a straight course towards the spine. Thus, there is a cross-over of the

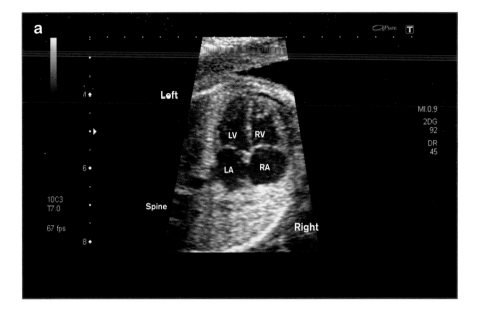

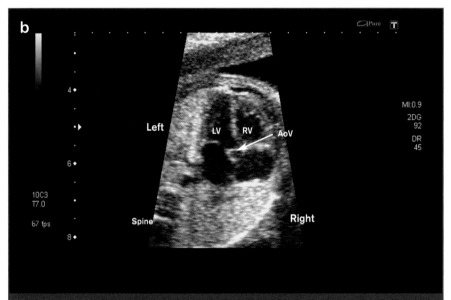

Figure 2.12. a) A normal four-chamber view. b) A view angling cranially from the four-chamber view showing the aortic root at its origin from the left ventricle. This view has been termed the five-chamber view.

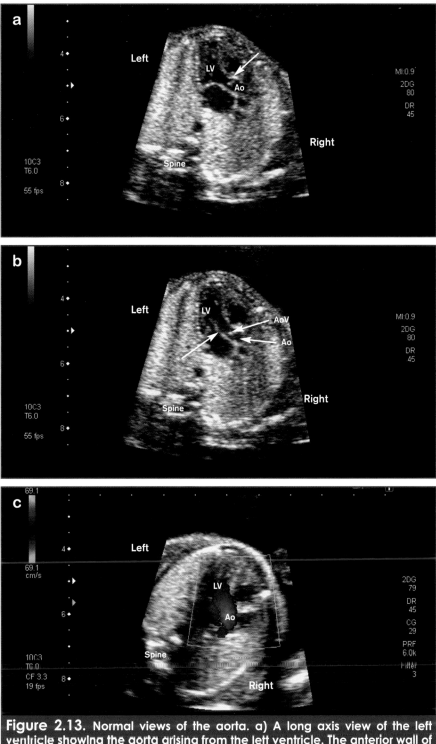

Figure 2.13. Normal views of the aorta. a) A long axis view of the left ventricle showing the aorta arising from the left ventricle. The anterior wall of the aorta (arrow) should be seen to be continuous with the ventricular septum. b) The posterior wall of the aorta is continuous with the anterior leaflet of the mitral valve (arrow). c) Colour flow shows normal forward flow in the aorta (shown in blue).

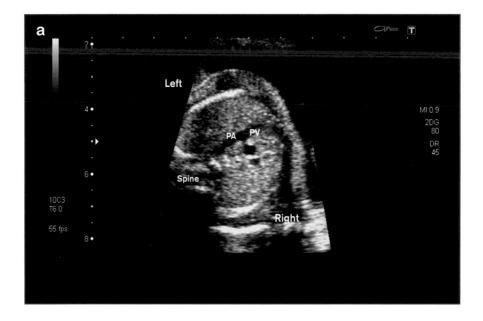

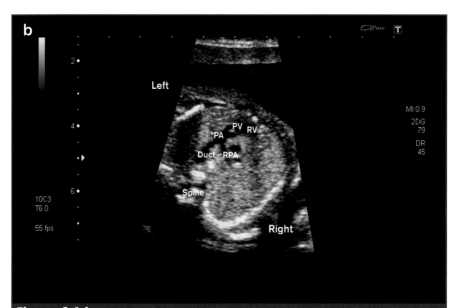

Figure 2.14. Normal views of the pulmonary artery. a) A horizontal section, more cranial from the four-chamber view and the origin of the aorta, will demonstrate the pulmonary valve and pulmonary artery. b) The pulmonary artery branches, giving rise to the right and left pulmonary arteries and the arterial duct. The right pulmonary artery and duct are seen in this view.

Figure continued overleaf.

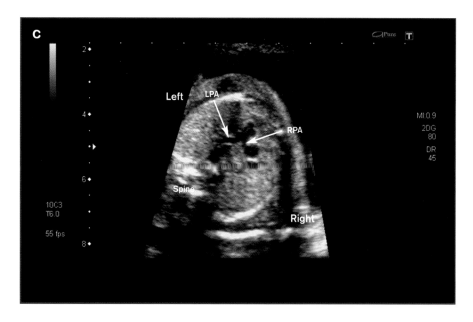

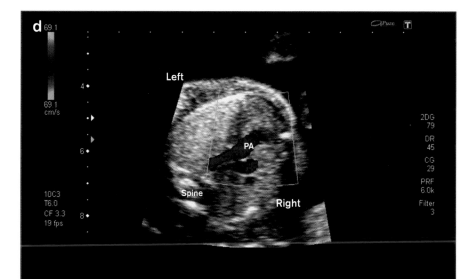

Figure 2.14 *continued.* **Normal views of the pulmonary artery. c) Both branch pulmonary arteries are seen in this view and the left pulmonary artery is clearly seen. d) Colour flow showing forward flow in the pulmonary artery (shown in blue).**

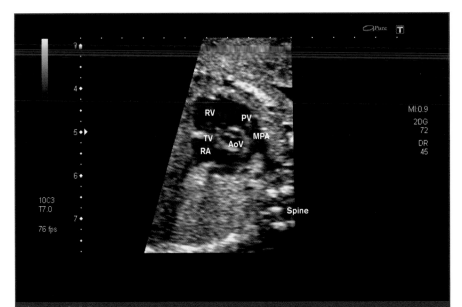

Figure 2.15. A short axis view of the right heart structures showing the right atrium, tricuspid valve, the right ventricle, the pulmonary valve and the main pulmonary artery branching. The aorta and aortic valve are seen in short axis in this view.

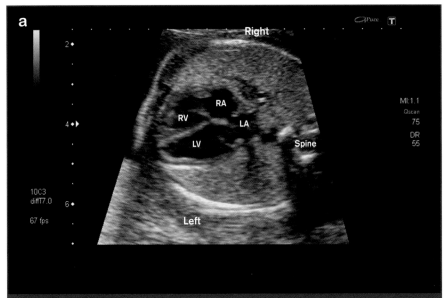

Figure 2.16. Views showing a sweep from the four chambers to the great arteries. The cross-over of the great arteries is demonstrated in the direction they leave the heart. This is also seen with the direction of flow seen with colour flow. a) Four-chamber view.

Figure continued overleaf.

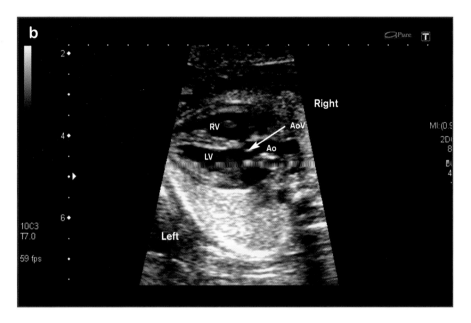

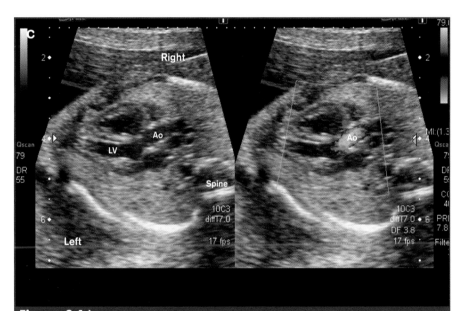

Figure 2.16 *continued*. Views showing a sweep from the four chambers to the great arteries. The cross-over of the great arteries is demonstrated in the direction they leave the heart. This is also seen with the direction of flow seen with colour flow. b) Long axis view of the left ventricle showing the aorta arising from the left ventricle. c) Colour flow shows forward flow in the aorta (seen in red).

Figure continued overleaf.

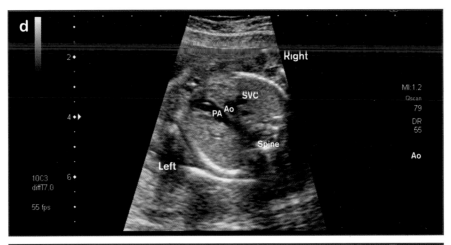

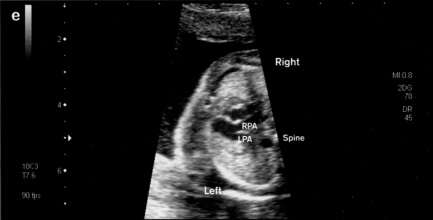

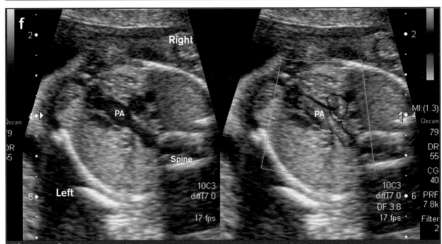

Figure 2.16 *continued.* Views showing a sweep from the four chambers to the great arteries. The cross-over of the great arteries is demonstrated in the direction they leave the heart. This is also seen with the direction of flow seen with colour flow. d) A view of the pulmonary artery in the three-vessel view. e) Both the branch pulmonary arteries are seen. f) Colour flow shows forward flow in the pulmonary artery (seen in blue).

direction the two vessels take from their origin. Figures 2.16a-f illustrate a sweep from the four chambers to the great arteries. In these views, the direction of the aorta and aortic flow can be compared with the direction of the pulmonary artery and the pulmonary artery flow. There is a cross-over of the direction the vessels take as they leave the heart. Note that the first vessel and arterial valve that should normally be visualised when moving cranially from the four-chamber view is the aorta and the aortic valve.

The three-vessel view, the aortic arch and the ductal arch

The three-vessel and tracheal views

The three-vessel view is obtained in a horizontal section similar to that used to image the pulmonary artery and duct described above. The three vessels seen in this view are the pulmonary artery and duct to the left, the aorta in the middle and the superior vena cava on the right (Figures 2.8 and 2.9a-b). In this view, the pulmonary artery and aorta should appear of approximately equal size, though the pulmonary artery can appear slightly bigger. The views shown in Figures 2.9a-b and 2.17a-b, known as the three-vessel tracheal view, allow better comparison of the sizes of the aorta and pulmonary artery, and isthmal narrowing is more likely to be detected (see also Chapter 9). In this view, the pulmonary artery and duct meet the aorta and aortic isthmus to the left of the trachea, to join the descending aorta in a 'V' shape.

The aortic arch and ductal arch

A horizontal section more cranial to the three-vessel view will demonstrate the crest of the aortic arch (Figure 2.18). The aortic arch is the most superior arch and lies superior to the transverse view of the duct. The vessel forms a curve from the right thorax to the left thorax, crossing the midline in front of the spine. The vessel then descends anterior and slightly to the left of the spine.

The aortic and ductal arches can be imaged in longitudinal sections of the fetus. In a longitudinal view the aortic arch is imaged by angling the transducer towards the right shoulder. The aortic arch arises in the centre of the chest; a tight hooked arch that gives rise to the head and neck vessels (Figures 2.19 and 2.20a-b). The ductal arch and right heart connections can be demonstrated in a long axis projection by angling the transducer towards the left shoulder (Figures 2.21a-b). In this view, the aorta is seen as a circular structure in short axis. The ductal arch is a wide sweeping arch, formed by the pulmonary artery and duct joining the descending aorta. In contrast to the aortic arch, this arch arises close to the anterior chest wall and is a branching vessel.

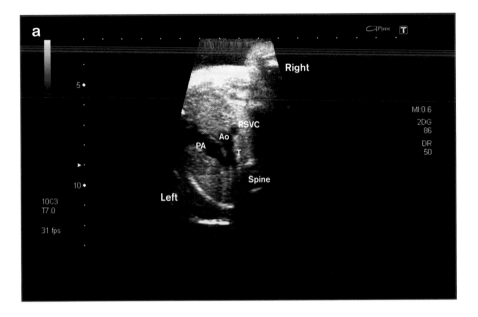

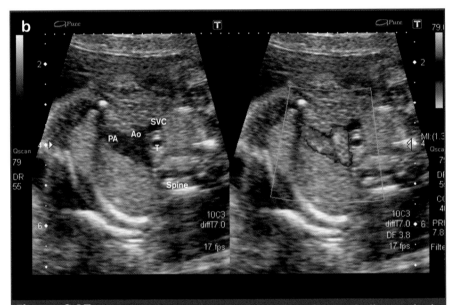

Figure 2.17. a) A three-vessel 'V' tracheal view demonstrating a single right-sided vena cava. b) The direction of flow in both the aorta and pulmonary artery is in the same direction towards the descending aorta (shown in blue).

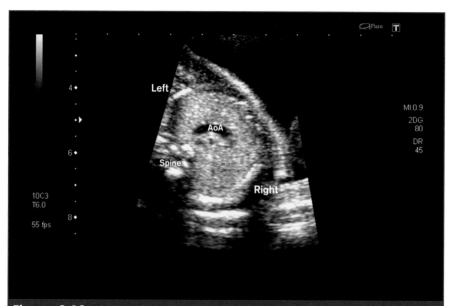

Figure 2.18. The crest of the aortic arch is seen in this view. This is the most superior arch.

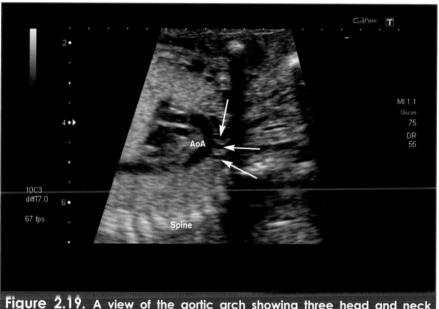

Figure 2.19. A view of the aortic arch showing three head and neck vessels (arrows) arising from it.

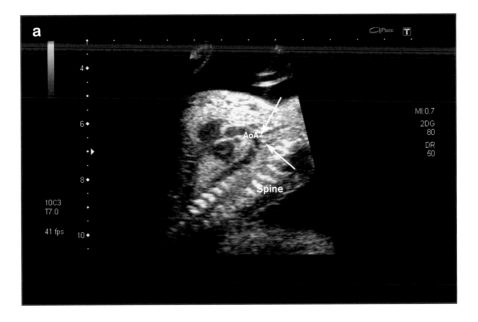

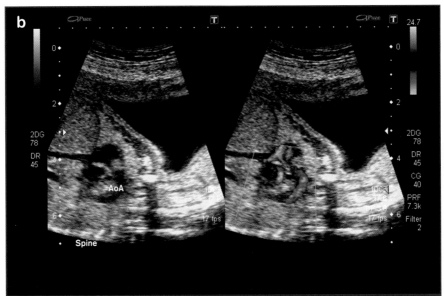

Figure 2.20. a) The aortic arch is seen in a longitudinal view. The aorta arises centrally in the chest and forms a tight hooked arch. Head and neck vessels can be seen arising from the aortic arch (arrows). b) There is normal forward flow around the aortic arch (shown in blue).

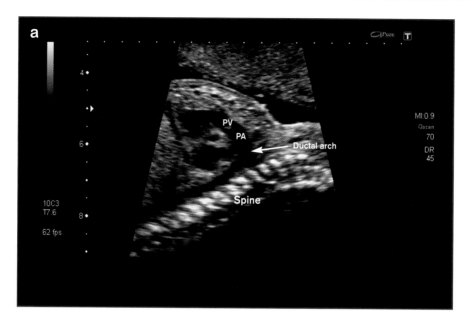

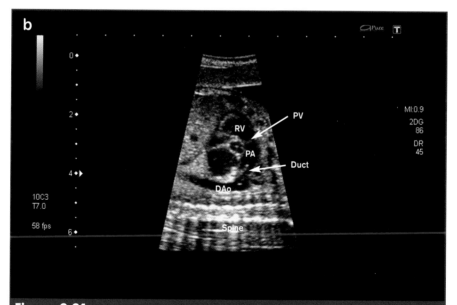

Figure 2.21. a) The pulmonary artery and ductal arch are seen in this view. The ductal arch is a wide sweeping arch and arises nearer to the anterior chest wall than the aortic arch. b) Another view of a ductal arch where the duct can be seen joining the descending aorta.

> **Important features to note regarding the great arteries and arterial connections.**
>
> - Two vessels with two separate arterial valves should be identified
> - The aorta arises from the centre of the chest and is committed to the left ventricle. The anterior wall of the aorta is continuous with the ventricular septum and the posterior wall is continuous with the anterior leaflet of the mitral valve
> - The aorta gives rise to the aortic arch, which can be identified by head and neck vessels
> - The pulmonary artery arises from the right ventricle and is directed towards the spine. This is a branching vessel, which gives rise to the branch pulmonary arteries and the arterial duct
> - The pulmonary artery connects to the descending aorta via the arterial duct. This forms the ductal arch
> - The great arteries are similar in size
> - The pulmonary valve is anterior and cranial to the aortic valve
> - The great arteries cross over at their origin

Colour flow and the normal fetal heart

Although most structural abnormalities of the fetal heart can be detected by careful examination of the two-dimensional ultrasound image, colour flow is an integral part of fetal heart examination. It can be used to examine the flow through the normal connections of the heart, to check the patency of all four cardiac valves and to ensure the direction of flow is correct. It can also be used to make sure there is no evidence of regurgitation across any of the cardiac valves, or of turbulent flow across the valves. In addition, colour flow can be used to ensure that there is no flow across the ventricular septum and to check the flow pattern across the foramen ovale. In some instances, when vessels or structures are not easily seen, colour flow can help to identify the structure.

The superior and inferior vena cavae can be demonstrated draining to the right atrium in longitudinal views (Figure 2.22). In the four-chamber view of the fetal heart, colour flow can be used to demonstrate the pulmonary veins entering the left atrium (Figures 2.2d and 2.4b). To examine the venous flow to the heart the colour velocity scale should be lowered, as the velocity of flow is low in these vessels. In the four-chamber view, the flow through both atrioventricular valves should be equal and in the same direction (Figure 2.2c). There should be no atrioventricular valve regurgitation. The ventricular septum should be intact with no flow demonstrated across it. The interatrial shunt across the foramen ovale should normally be right to left (Figure 2.23). In views of the great arteries, flow should be demonstrated from the ventricle, across the arterial valve into the great artery. Thus, flow should be seen from the left ventricle, across the aortic valve into the ascending aorta and arch (Figures 2.13c, 2.16c and 2.20b). Flow from the right ventricle should be demonstrated across the pulmonary valve into

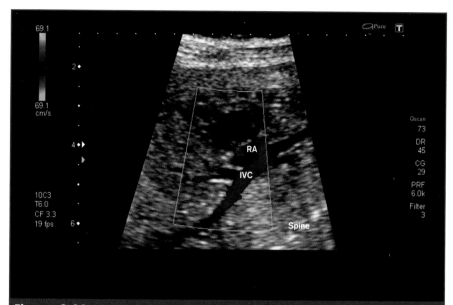

Figure 2.22. Colour flow showing flow from the inferior vena cava entering the right atrium (shown in red).

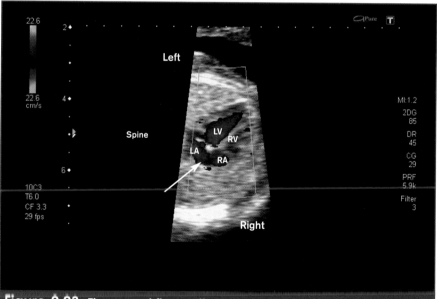

Figure 2.23. The normal flow pattern across the foramen ovale is usually predominantly right to left (shown in red and arrow).

the main pulmonary artery and duct (Figures 2.14d and 2.16f). The flow across both arterial valves should be laminar, with no turbulent flow, provided the velocity scale is set to fall in the normal range for the gestation. In the three-vessel and transverse arch views, flow in the transverse aortic arch and duct should be in the same direction, directed towards the spine and descending aorta (Figures 2.17b).

Pulsed-wave Doppler and the normal fetal heart

Pulsed-wave Doppler is used in conjunction with colour flow for a complete fetal cardiac assessment. Pulsed-wave Doppler can be used to evaluate the direction of blood flow, the pattern of blood flow and the velocity of blood flow. The Doppler sample volume can be positioned anywhere within the cardiovascular system for examination. Most commonly this is used to measure the Doppler velocities across both arterial valves. It is also used to examine pulmonary venous flow entering the left atrium, the flow patterns across both atrioventricular valves, flow patterns in the arterial duct and aortic isthmus, branch pulmonary arteries and flow patterns across the foramen ovale.

Pulmonary venous Doppler

To obtain a pulmonary venous Doppler trace the sample volume is positioned at the junction of the pulmonary vein entering the left atrium, in a position where the flow is parallel to the Doppler sample volume. An example of a normal pulmonary venous Doppler trace is shown in Figure 2.24. The pulmonary venous flow pattern reflects left atrial haemodynamics. Usually there is forward flow in systole and diastole, with cessation of flow or a small reversal of flow during atrial contraction in late diastole. The velocities of flows in the systolic and diastolic peaks are similar, increasing from about 10cm/second at 16 weeks of gestation to between 30-40cm/second at term. The reversal wave is usually less than 10cm/second.

Atrioventricular valve Doppler

For interrogation of the atrioventricular valves the Doppler cursor is placed on the ventricular side of the valve to establish the inflow pattern. However, it should be placed across the valve or, on the atrial side of the valve, to detect regurgitation. The atrioventricular inflow traces normally show a biphasic pattern during diastole (Figure 2.25). The initial E wave represents the passive filling as the atrioventricular valve opens at the end of systole and then the active A wave represents the flow through the valve in atrial contraction. The mitral valve E wave increases from 25cm/second at 16 weeks to about 45cm/second at term. The A wave is relatively constant at around 45cm/second, though can increase slightly. The velocity of flow across the tricuspid valve is slightly higher than that through the mitral valve. The tricuspid valve E wave increases from 30cm/second at 16 weeks to about 50cm/second at term. The tricuspid valve A wave is relatively constant at 50cm/second, though can increase slightly. Thus, the E/A ratio across the atrioventricular valves increases as pregnancy advances from about 0.5 to 1. The E/A ratio is about 1.5 after birth.

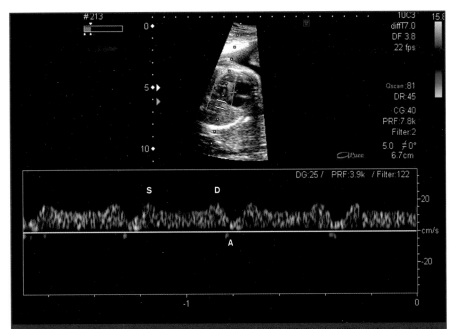

Figure 2.24. A normal pulmonary venous Doppler trace. There are equal peaks in systole (S) and diastole (D), and absent or little flow during atrial contraction (A).

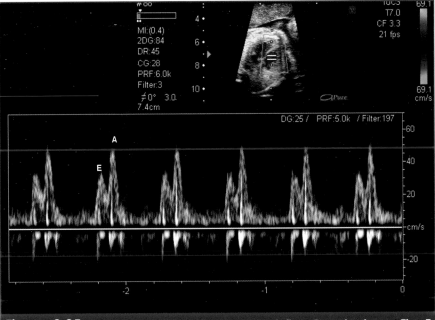

Figure 2.25. A normal atrioventricular valve inflow Doppler trace. The E and A waves can be seen.

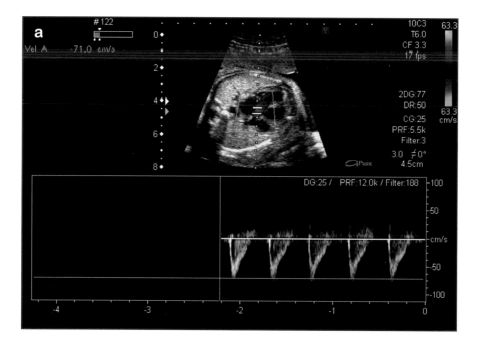

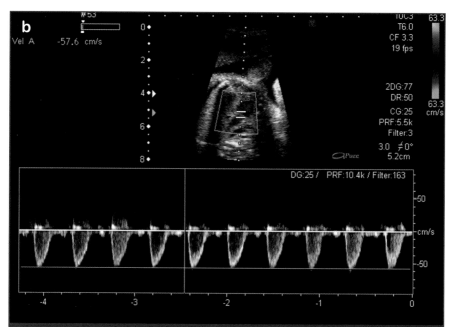

Figure 2.26. Doppler traces across arterial valves. a) A normal Doppler trace and velocity across the aortic valve. b) A normal Doppler trace and velocity across the pulmonary valve.

Arterial valve Doppler

The Doppler sample volume should be positioned in the great artery just distal to the arterial valve. The Doppler trace across the aortic and pulmonary valves is normally a single peak of forward flow in systole, with a short time to peak (Figures 2.26a-b). The peak velocity increases as gestation advances from around 30-40cm/second at 14 weeks to 1m/second at term. Occasionally traces just above 1m/second can be found in normal fetuses in late gestation. The peak velocity in the aorta is usually slightly higher than that in the pulmonary artery.

Simultaneous measurement of atrioventricular valve and arterial valve Doppler

Placing the Doppler curser in the left ventricle to capture the left ventricular inflow and outflow allows simultaneous measurement of the atrioventricular valve and arterial valve Doppler. This allows measurement of the atrioventricular (AV) time interval which can be helpful in the assessment of arrhythmias (Figure 2.27 and see Chapter 13).

Arterial duct

The arterial duct has the highest cardiac velocity which increases as gestation advances. This can range from 50cm/second at 16 weeks to 1.8m/second at term. The time to peak velocity is longer in the duct than in the aorta or pulmonary artery. A normal Doppler trace from the arterial duct is shown in Figure 2.28. In contrast to the Doppler traces across the arterial valves, there is usually some forward flow in the arterial duct during diastole, making the appearance of the ductal Doppler trace different to the traces obtained across the arterial valves.

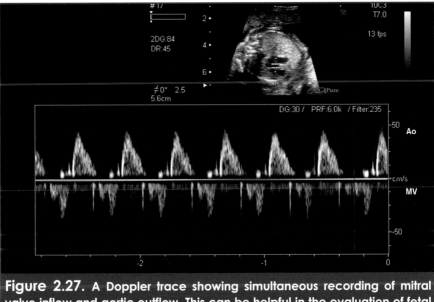

Figure 2.27. A Doppler trace showing simultaneous recording of mitral valve inflow and aortic outflow. This can be helpful in the evaluation of fetal arrhythmias (see Chapter 13).

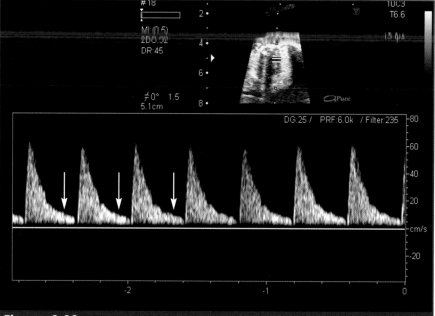

Figure 2.28. A Doppler trace from the arterial duct. The velocity in the arterial duct is higher than that in the pulmonary artery. The appearance of the ductal trace is different from the trace across arterial valves, as there is usually forward flow in the arterial duct during diastole (arrows).

M-mode and the normal fetal heart

The main use of M-mode echocardiography in fetal cardiology assessment in the current era is for the evaluation of fetal arrhythmias, as it allows interrogation of atrial and ventricular contractions at the same time. M-mode can also be used to assess ventricular function and to make measurements of cardiac chambers and structures.

In the evaluation of cardiac rhythm and arrhythmias (see Chapter 13), the M-mode line is positioned to go through the atrial and ventricular wall, or, the left atrial wall and the aortic valve. Normal traces should demonstrate that each atrial contraction is followed by a ventricular contraction with a fixed and regular time relationship between them (Figure 2.29). The time interval between the atrial and ventricular contraction is similar to the PR interval seen on an electrocardiogram (ECG).

Traditional positions for measuring the ventricular sizes and the septal and free wall thickness of the left ventricle include a short axis view of the left ventricle (Figure 2.30) or a long axis view of the left ventricle. These views can also be used to assess the systolic function of the left ventricle by measuring the distance from the ventricular surface of the septum to the inner surface of the posterior free wall of the left ventricle. The largest dimension (end diastole) and smallest dimension (end systole) are measured and the shortening fraction (SF), which is an estimate of systolic function, is calculated by the formula

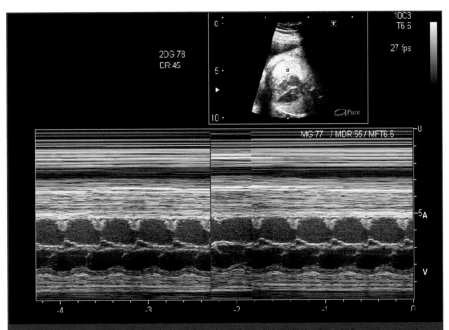

Figure 2.29. A normal M-mode showing atrial and ventricular contractions. Every atrial beat is followed by a ventricular beat with a fixed time relationship between them.

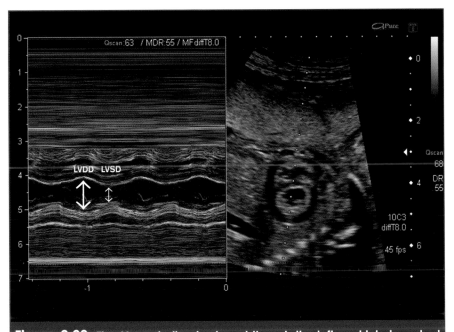

Figure 2.30. The M-mode line is placed though the left ventricle in a short axis view. This can be used to measure the left ventricle shortening fraction. As there is no ECG trace to relate the timing of cardiac events in the fetus, the left ventricular diastolic dimension (LVDD) is taken as the maximum dimension and the systolic dimension (LVSD) is taken as the smallest dimension.

SF = EDD - ESD/EDD (where EDD is the end-diastolic dimension and ESD is the end-systolic dimension). The shortening fraction of the left ventricle is usually between 28-40%. Assessment of right ventricular function is more difficult as this is not a cylindrical structure.

Imaging the heart at different gestations

The main structure of the fetal heart is usually formed by the 12th week of pregnancy, though obstructive lesions can develop with advancing gestation. Although normality can be confirmed from an early stage, imaging the heart can be challenging until the mid-trimester. The fetal heart approximates the size of a pea at 13-14 weeks of gestation, the size of a grape at 18-22 weeks and the size of a plum near term. The echocardiographic appearances of a normal fetal heart at 13 weeks of gestation is shown in Figures 2.31a-c, at 15 weeks in Figures 2.32a-c, at 18 weeks in Figures 2.33a-d and at 28 weeks in Figures 2.34a-c.

Variations of normal

Asymmetry in late gestation

The right and left heart structures should be of approximately equal size up until 24 weeks of gestation. However, after this time and particularly after 30 weeks, the right heart structures may appear dilated compared to the left, in the absence of any cardiac abnormality. Though this finding is often normal in late gestation, there is no clear boundary between what is normal and what may be signs of a problem, such as coarctation of the aorta (see Chapter 9). Thus, if cardiac asymmetry is noted when evaluating a fetus for the first time in later gestation, it can sometimes prove impossible to categorically decide if there is a problem or not. The sizes of the great arteries, particularly in the three-vessel/tracheal view are more important indicators of a possible arch problem, rather than asymmetry seen in the four-chamber view (Figures 2.35a-b).

Normal rim of fluid

There is usually a small rim of fluid around the ventricles of the fetal heart, which can sometimes appear quite prominent (Figures 2.36 and 2.37) and be mistaken for a pericardial effusion. The normal rim is usually symmetrical, mainly around the ventricles and measures less than 2mm.

Echogenic foci (golf balls)

These bright echogenic specks can occur as single or multiple lesions and can be found in either ventricle, but more commonly in the left ventricle (Figures 2.38). They are of no consequence from a cardiac perspective, regardless of whether seen as a single or multiple entities. The concern has been the possible association with other abnormalities, in particular

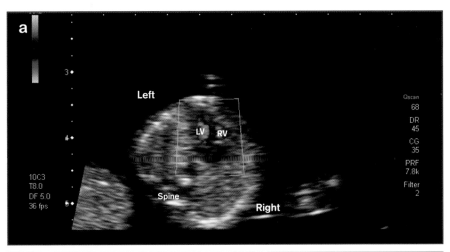

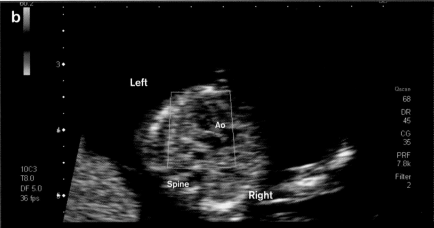

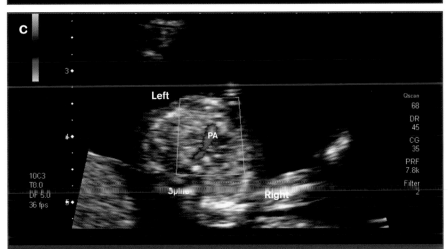

Figure 2.31. A normal heart at 13 weeks. a) Inflow across both atrioventricular valves into the ventricular chambers is seen (seen in red). b) Normal outflow from the left ventricle into the aorta (seen in blue). c) Normal flow in the pulmonary artery (seen in blue).

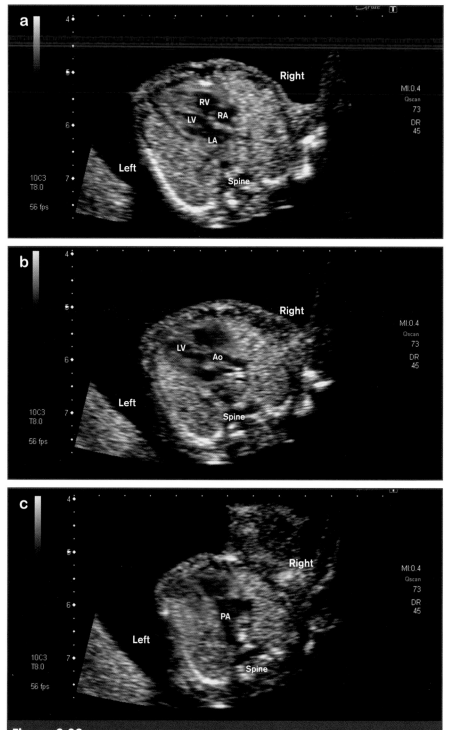

Figure 2.32. A normal heart at 15 weeks. a) A normal four-chamber view. b) The aorta arises normally from the left ventricle. c) The pulmonary artery arises normally.

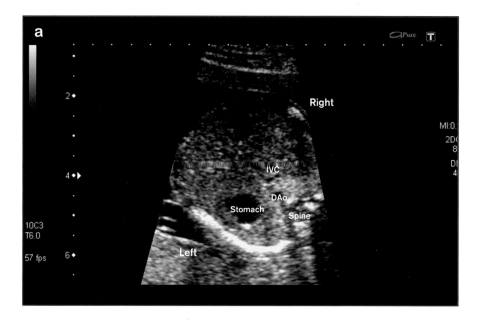

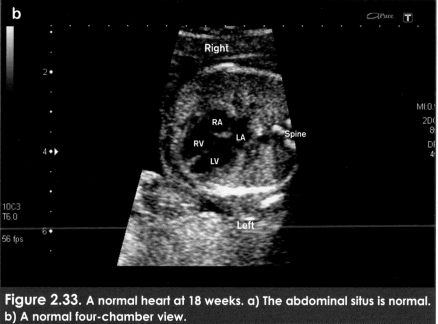

Figure 2.33. A normal heart at 18 weeks. a) The abdominal situs is normal. b) A normal four-chamber view.

Figure continued overleaf.

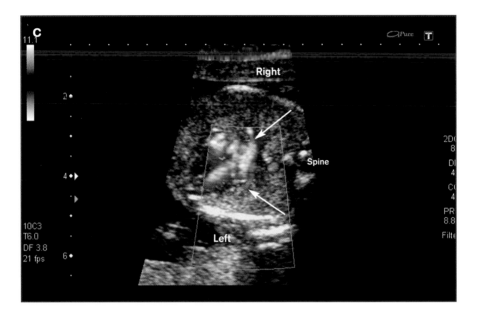

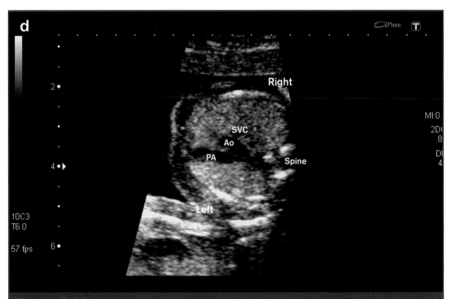

Figure 2.33 *continued.* A normal heart at 18 weeks. c) The pulmonary veins (arrows) drain normally to the left atrium. d) A normal three-vessel/tracheal view.

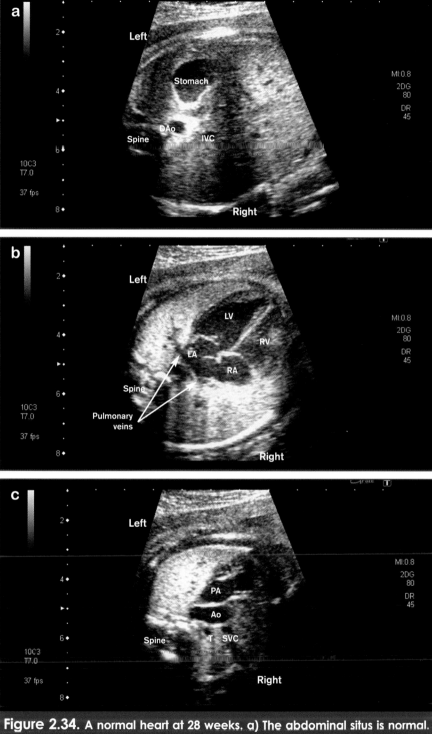

Figure 2.34. A normal heart at 28 weeks. a) The abdominal situs is normal. b) A normal four-chamber view. All the cardiac structures including the pulmonary veins are more easily seen. c) A normal three-vessel/tracheal view.

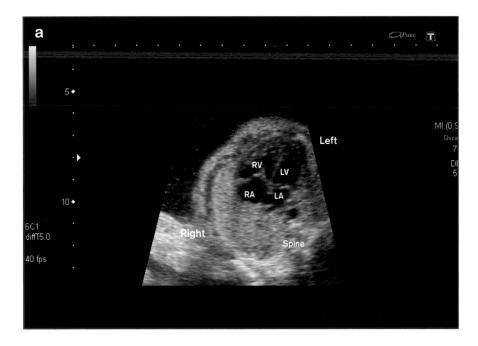

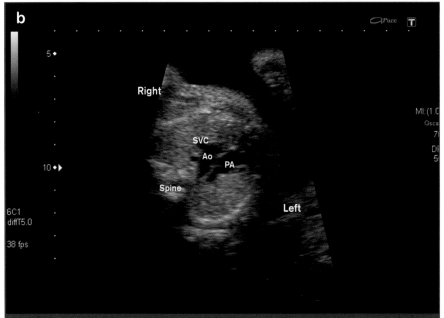

Figure 2.35. a) In this example of a normal heart, the right heart structures appear slightly dilated compared to the left heart structures in the four-chamber view in later gestation. b) The aorta and pulmonary artery are, however, of approximately equal size.

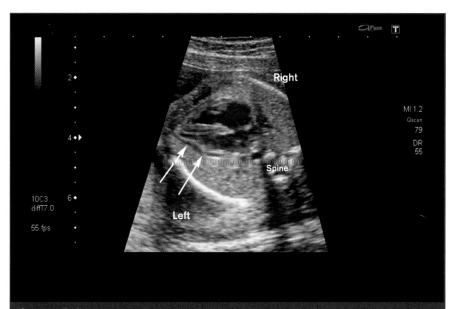

Figure 2.36. A normal rim of fluid around the heart (arrows). This is often seen, particularly in this orientation and can sometimes appear quite prominent.

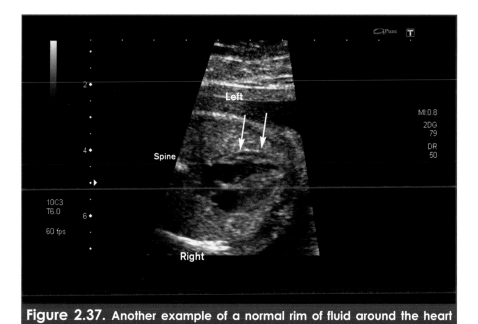

Figure 2.37. Another example of a normal rim of fluid around the heart (arrows).

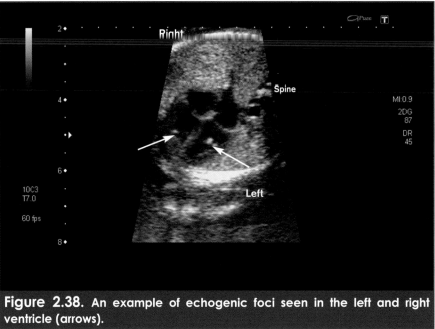

Figure 2.38. An example of echogenic foci seen in the left and right ventricle (arrows).

chromosomal abnormalities and there remains controversy about their significance in this light. Echogenic foci are regarded to be a soft marker for chromosomal abnormalities by some centres, but are ignored in others. In general it is important to make sure a detailed anomaly scan has been performed to exclude any other features or markers of chromosomal abnormality.

Aneurysmal foramen ovale flap

The flap valve of the foramen ovale can sometimes appear aneurysmal though flow can be demonstrated across the foramen (Figures 2.39a-b). In the absence of any other abnormality this is unlikely to cause any problems and is generally regarded as a normal variant.

Persistent left superior vena cava or bilateral superior vena cava with structurally normal heart

See section above on the venous-atrial connection on the right and Chapter 4.

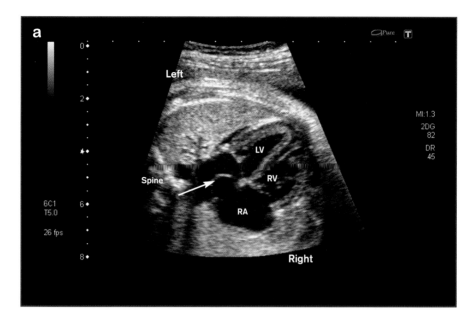

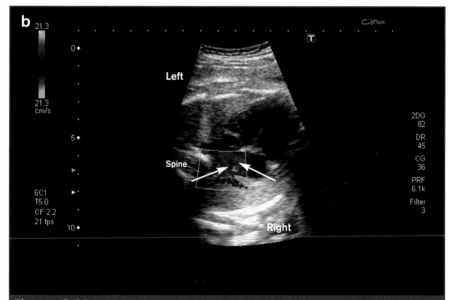

Figure 2.39. a) An example of an aneurysmal atrial septum (arrow). b) Colour flow shows flow across the foramen ovale (arrows). There was no cardiac abnormality associated with this and no cardiac abnormality was evident after birth.

Appearance of a normal heart when distorted by extracardiac abnormality

Extracardiac abnormalities such as a diaphragmatic hernia or an oxomphalos can distort the appearance of the heart, making it more difficult to confirm normality, even when the cardiac structure is normal. However, a systematic approach to examining the heart will help determine whether the heart structure is normal or not.

Chapter 3

Abnormalities of cardiac size, position and situs

Summary

- **Abnormalities of cardiac size**
  - Cardiomegaly
  - Small heart
- **Abnormalities of cardiac position**
  - Dextrocardia
  - Dextroposition
  - Levoposition
- **Abnormalities of cardiac situs**
  - Situs inversus or mirror image
  - Left atrial isomerism
  - Right atrial isomerism

Abnormalities of cardiac size

Cardiomegaly

An increase in cardiac size, or cardiomegaly, may be global or may be the result of enlargement of one of the cardiac chambers. Cardiomegaly can occur as a result of a cardiac abnormality or can be associated with extracardiac abnormalities. Occasionally, slight cardiomegaly can be noted in the absence of any other abnormalities.

Cardiac causes of cardiomegaly affecting the whole heart include cardiomyopathy (see Chapter 10) and complete congenital heart block (see Chapter 10). Non-cardiac causes include high output states such as an arteriovenous malformation, fetal anaemia, sacrococcygeal teratoma and twin to twin transfusion syndrome.

A dilated right atrium resulting in cardiomegaly can be seen when there is significant tricuspid regurgitation, as seen in tricuspid valve abnormalities such as Ebstein's anomaly or tricuspid valve dysplasia (see Chapter 5). A coronary artery fistula draining into the right atrium can also cause right atrial dilatation (see Chapter 12). Other causes include an absent ductus venosus with the umbilical vein draining directly into the right atrium (see Chapter 12).

A dilated left atrium may be seen in association with significant mitral regurgitation. This may also be seen in association with critical aortic stenosis, particularly if the atrial septum is restrictive (see Chapter 6). A coronary artery fistula draining to the left atrium can cause left atrial dilatation, as can an umbilical vein draining directly to the left atrium in association with an absent ductus venosus.

The right ventricle can appear dilated in some cases of critical pulmonary stenosis, absent pulmonary valve syndrome, a right ventricular aneurysm, a coronary artery fistula draining to the right ventricle and a right ventricular cardiomyopathy (see Chapters 6, 8, 10 and 12).

The left ventricle can appear dilated in some cases of critical aortic stenosis, an aortico-left ventricular tunnel, a left ventricular aneurysm, a coronary artery fistula draining to the left ventricle and a left ventricular cardiomyopathy (see Chapters 6, 10 and 12).

A small heart

The heart may appear small in the chest in cases of tracheal atresia, some cases of diaphragmatic hernia and in cases with pleural effusions (Figure 3.1).

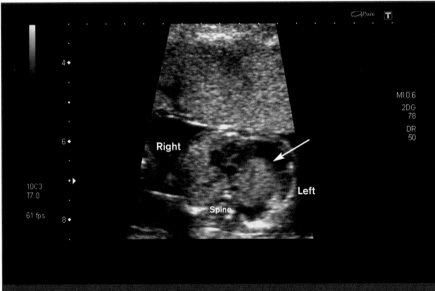

Figure 3.1. An example of a left-sided pleural effusion (arrow) causing mediastinal shift to the right. The heart structure was normal but the heart appears slightly small in the chest.

A small right atrium can be seen in some cases of tricuspid atresia (see Chapter 4). A small left atrium may be seen in association with hypoplastic left heart syndrome, coarctation of the aorta, and total anomalous pulmonary venous drainage (see Chapters 4, 5, 6 and 9).

A small right ventricle can be seen in tricuspid atresia, pulmonary atresia with an intact interventricular septum, some cases of critical pulmonary stenosis, an unbalanced atrioventricular septal defect with a small right side, a double-inlet left ventricle and some types of cardiomyopathy (see Chapters 4, 6 and 10). A small left ventricle can be seen with hypoplastic left heart syndrome (mitral atresia and aortic atresia), mitral atresia with a double-outlet right ventricle, coarctation of the aorta, some cases of critical aortic stenosis, an unbalanced atrioventricular septal defect with a small left side, and a double-inlet right ventricle (see Chapters 4, 6 and 9).

Abnormalities of cardiac position

Abnormalities of cardiac position are associated with a range of abnormalities and it is important in all cases to evaluate the fetal heart as well as the rest of the baby to identify the extent of associated abnormality.

Dextrocardia

The term dextrocardia implies that the heart lies in the right chest with the cardiac axis pointing to the right. The heart is usually 'flipped' over. Dextrocardia can occur with situs solitis, situs inversus or situs ambiguous (atrial isomerism). Dextrocardia may be associated with a structurally normal heart but it is also associated with structural heart disease, which is often complex. In cases where the heart structure is normal, the appearance of the four chambers in the chest will appear normal, though the heart will lie in the right chest with the apex pointing to the right. These cases, particularly if associated with situs inversus, will only be evident if the left and right of the baby are established during the scan. Cases of dextrocardia associated with other forms of congenital heart disease will often be detected in association with the other cardiac abnormalities. Again, the left and right of the baby must be established to make the diagnosis of dextrocardia. An example of mitral atresia with a double-outlet right ventricle associated with dextrocardia is shown in Chapter 4.

Dextroposition

In dextroposition the heart appears displaced or pushed to the right. This can occur if the contents of the left chest push the heart to the right, for example, in cases of left-sided diaphragmatic hernia (Figure 3.2) or congenital cystic adenomatoid malformation of the left lung (Figure 3.3). Or, this can occur when if the contents of the right chest are reduced, for example, if there is a hypoplastic right lung. In this situation there may be associated Scimitar syndrome where there is also partial anomalous pulmonary venous drainage.

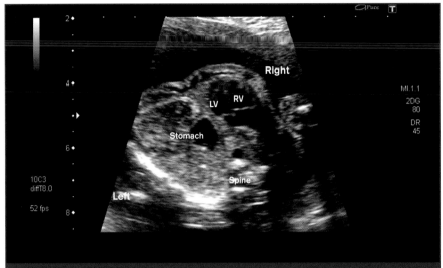

Figure 3.2. An example of a diaphragmatic hernia resulting in dextroposition. There is mediastinal shift to the right with the heart lying against the right chest wall.

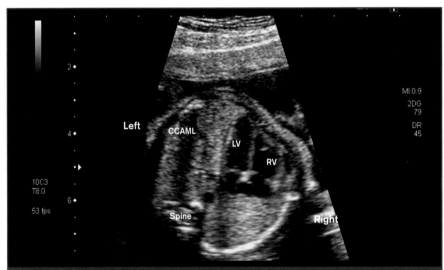

Figure 3.3. An example of congenital cystic adenomatoid malformation (CCAML) of the left lung resulting in dextroposition. There is a mediastinal shift to the right.

The apex of the heart can point to the right or to the left, even though the heart lies in the right chest (Figure 3.3). There may be mesocardia with the apex pointing in the midline, though the heart is diplaced towards the right (Figures 3.4). Although dextroposition can occur with a structurally normal heart, it is important to look for congenital heart abnormalities, as dextroposition is often associated with complex congenital heart abnormalities and isomerism (see below).

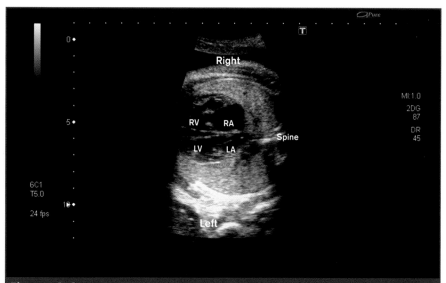

Figure 3.4. There is mesocardia with the heart lying centrally in the chest. There is cardiomegaly but the heart structure is normal.

Levoposition

The heart can lie more in the left chest than normal or the apex can point more towards the left axilla. This can be seen in cases of a right-sided diaphragmatic hernia or congenital cystic adenomatoid malformation of the right lung (Figure 3.5). This can also occasionally be seen

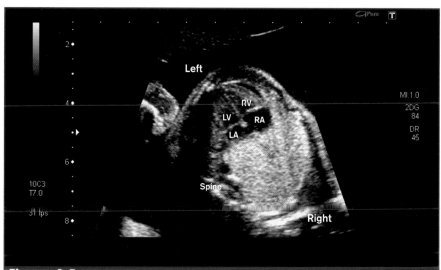

Figure 3.5. An example of congenital cystic adenomatoid malformation (CCAML) of the right lung resulting in levoposition. There is a mediastinal shift to the left in this example, with the cardiac apex pointing towards the left axilla.

in association with structural heart disease, such as tetralogy of Fallot, common arterial trunk and pulmonary atresia with a ventricular septal defect (see Chapter 8).

Abnormalities of situs and atrial isomerism

Situs is a term used to describe the position of the cardiac atria and viscera. Abdominal and thoracic structures normally develop with well-defined right- and left-sided structures, which have defined positions in the body. Hallmarks of left-sidedness include the stomach, the spleen, the left atrium with its atrial appendage and a bi-lobed lung, with a hyparterial bronchus (gives off its first branch below the pulmonary artery). Those of right-sidedness include the liver, the right atrium with its atrial appendage, and a tri-lobed lung, with an eparterial bronchus (gives off its first branch above the pulmonary artery). The right main bronchus is wider, shorter and more vertical than the left main bronchus.

Normal situs

The normal arrangement of the two cardiac atria and the viscera is termed situs solitus, where the morphological left atrium is on the left and the morphological right atrium is on the right. In the normal situation the left lung is bi-lobed and the right lung is tri-lobed, the liver and gall bladder are on the right, with the spleen and stomach being on the left.

Situs inversus or mirror image

A mirror image arrangement of the cardiac atria and viscera is termed situs inversus, where the morphological left atrium is on the right and the morphological right atrium is on the left. In these cases, the lung anatomy is also reversed, so the left-sided lung is tri-lobed and the right-sided lung is bi-lobed. The liver and gall bladder are on the left, with the spleen and stomach on the right. Situs inversus with dextrocardia is known as complete situs inversus, or situs inversus totalis.

Situs inversus can be associated with structural congenital heart abnormalities. It is also associated with Kartagener syndrome, an abnormality of primary ciliary dyskinesia characterised by bronchiectesis.

Situs ambiguous and isomerism

Any other arrangement, whereby the relationship between the cardiac atria and viscera is inconsistent, is termed situs ambiguous. This group consists of syndromes involving abnormalities of lateralisation, where structures with normally distinct right and left forms, mainly the cardiac atrial appendages, the lungs and the bronchi, do not lateralise normally to right- and left-sided structures. This can result in duplicate forms of some structures, with the other form being absent. The terms left and right atrial isomerism or isomerism of the atrial appendages are used to describe this group of abnormalities in relation to the cardiac atrial appendages. Other names for this group of abnormalities include heterotaxy, asplenia, polysplenia and Ivemark syndrome. Syndromes involving abnormalities of lateralisation of this type are commonly associated with structural cardiac abnormalities.

Prevalence

The prevalence of this group of conditions is difficult to establish as there have been many classifications and names. Isomerism may also be undiagnosed in cases with no significant cardiac abnormality. The reported prevalence in postnatal series varies from 2.3-4%. In the Evelina fetal series, isomerism was associated in 6.6% in the total series and 4.3% of cases seen in the last 10 years. Of all cases of isomerism, 61% had left atrial isomerism and 39% had right atrial isomerism.

Left atrial isomerism (LAI)

Definition

Left atrial isomerism is situs ambiguous with bilateral left-handedness. Thus, bilateral structures show features of the normal left-sided structure and the right-sided structure is likely to be absent. The cardiac atrial appendages will both be of left-type morphology, both lungs will be left type (bi-lobed) and the distance from the carina to the first bronchial division will be long in both lungs, as in a normal left lung. An interrupted inferior vena cava is typical of left atrial isomerism and the hepatic veins drain directly to the atria. Left atrial isomerism is also known as heterotaxy, Ivemark or polysplenia syndrome.

Spectrum

A wide spectrum of cardiac abnormalities is found in left atrial isomerism, though occasionally there may be no structural cardiac abnormality. The most commonly associated structural cardiac lesions are atrioventricular septal defects. The sinus node is usually found in the morphological right atrium, so that bradycardia is often associated in left isomerism. This may be a sinus bradycardia or, in some cases, may be complete congenital heart block.

Fetal echocardiographic features

When the inferior vena cava is interrupted, the normal arrangement of the descending aorta and inferior vena cava in the abdomen cannot be seen. Instead of the inferior vena cava, a vessel is seen posterior to the descending aorta both in cross-sectional and longitudinal views. This is the azygos or hemi-azygos vein, which carries the venous drainage of the lower body in the absence of the inferior vena cava. The azygos continuation of the inferior vena cava can be clearly seen behind the aorta in the long- or short-axis view of the fetal thorax as demonstrated in Figures 3.6, 3.7a and 3.7b. If there are associated complex cardiac abnormalities such as atrioventricular septal defects, the orientation of the fetal heart may be abnormal, with the apex often lying more centrally in the chest (see Chapter 4). In some cases, there may be bilateral superior vena cavae (see Chapters 2 and 4) and anomalies of pulmonary venous drainage can also occur (see Chapter 4). There may be a partial or

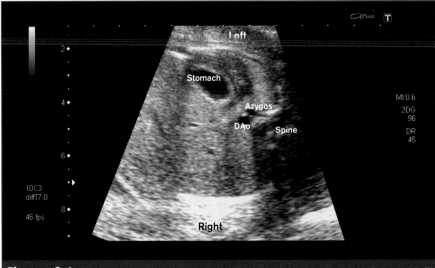

Figure 3.6. The abdominal situs view is abnormal in this example of left atrial isomerism. No inferior vena cava is seen. There is an azygos continuation seen to the left of and behind the descending aorta.

complete atrioventricular septal defect which can be visualised in the four-chamber view (see Chapter 4). The great arteries are usually normally related in left atrial isomerism, but coarctation of the aorta can occasionally be associated (see Chapter 9).

There is a high incidence of cardiac conduction abnormalities, particularly complete heart block. Sometimes there may be sinus node dysfunction producing a bradycardia, but not complete heart block. In cases of complete heart block, cardiomegaly and biventricular hypertrophy are often seen and these cases are frequently associated with an atrioventricular septal defect (see Chapter 4). The diagnosis of complete heart block is made when there is complete dissociation between atrial and ventricular contractions (see Chapter 13).

Occasionally, cases of interrupted inferior vena cava can be seen without any associated cardiac abnormality.

Extracardiac associations
Fetal hydrops can occur particularly in cases with associated complete heart block. Polysplenia is a typical but not consistent finding in left atrial isomerism. The stomach can be left- or right-sided, with malrotation and a risk of bowel obstruction being associated. There may be duodenal or jejunal atresia and rarely, cases of left atrial isomerism can be associated with biliary atresia.

Karyotype abnormalities are very rare, though there has been a report of left atrial isomerism occurring with a microdeletion of chromosome 22.

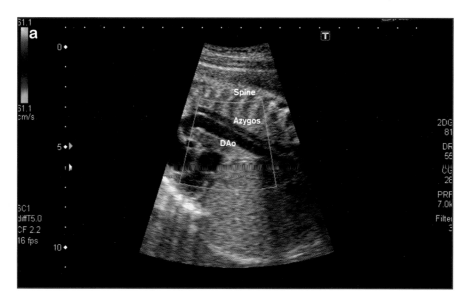

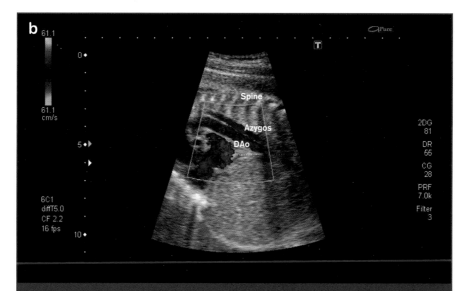

Figure 3.7. a) In a longitudinal view a venous channel (azygos continuation) is seen behind the descending aorta. b) Colour flow shows flow in the venous channel going towards the heart (seen in red). The flow in the descending aorta is seen in blue.

Management and outcome

The management and outcome in all cases of left atrial isomerism will be influenced by the extent of associated lesions, both cardiac and extracardiac (see relevant chapters for specific lesions).

Outcome in a large single-centre fetal series

Of 173 cases of left atrial isomerism diagnosed prenatally, 53% of pregnancies resulted in a termination of pregnancy. If the terminations are excluded then the outcome of the continuing pregnancies was: 16% resulting in spontaneous intrauterine death, 21% died in the neonatal period, 11% died in infancy and 52% were alive at last update.

Of cases seen in the last 10 years, a termination of pregnancy took place in 38% of cases and 57% of the continuing pregnancies were alive at last follow-up.

Summary of fetal echocardiographic features associated with LAI.

- **Abnormal cardiac position**
- **Heart and stomach may be on opposite sides**
- **Interrupted inferior vena cava (IVC is not seen in the normal position in the upper abdomen)**
- **Vascular channel behind the descending aorta (azygos continuation)**
- **Atrioventricular septal defect (common)**
- **Bradycardia (often complete heart block)**
- **Cardiomegaly and cardiac hypertrophy if complete heart block**
- **Anomalies of pulmonary venous drainage**

Right atrial isomerism (RAI)

Definition

Right atrial isomerism is situs ambiguous with bilateral right-handedness. Thus, bilateral structures show features of the normal right-sided structure and the left-sided structure is likely to be absent. The cardiac atrial appendages will both be of right-type morphology, both lungs will be right type (tri-lobed) and the distance from the carina to the first bronchial division will be short in both lungs, as in a normal right lung. Right atrial isomerism is also known as asplenia syndrome or visceral heterotaxy.

Spectrum

There is often complex heart disease associated with this syndrome. Usually there is anomalous pulmonary venous connection (as there is no normal left atrium). Other cardiac abnormalities include an atrioventricular septal defect, double-outlet right ventricle, pulmonary stenosis or atresia.

Fetal echocardiographic features

In the upper abdomen, the relationship of the inferior vena cava to the aorta is abnormal, with both vessels lying on the same side of the body and the inferior vena cava lying directly

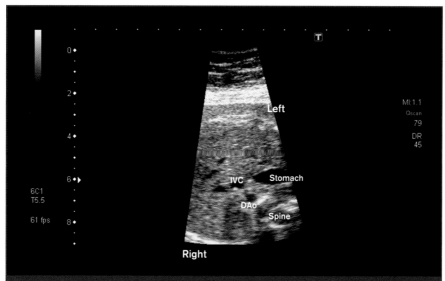

Figure 3.8. The abdominal situs view is abnormal in this example of right atrial isomerism. The inferior vena cava and aorta both lie to the right of the spine and the inferior vena cava is lying directly anterior to the aorta.

anterior to the aorta (Figure 3.8). The cardiac position is often abnormal, with the axis towards the right or midline, though it can also be to the left. There may be bilateral superior vena cavae (see Chapters 2 and 4). The pulmonary venous connection is always anomalous by definition. The pulmonary venous drainage commonly is to a confluence that can drain directly to the atrial mass or to other sites such as the superior or inferior vena cava or to an infra-diaphragmatic site (see Chapter 4). The four-chamber view is often abnormal due to an associated atrioventricular septal defect, which may be of an unbalanced type, with one ventricular chamber being significantly larger than the other (see Chapter 4). The connections of the great arteries are frequently abnormal, usually with both vessels arising from the right ventricle in conjunction with pulmonary obstruction, as in either pulmonary stenosis or pulmonary atresia (see Chapters 6, 7 and 8).

Extracardiac associations

Right atrial isomerism is associated with asplenia, though this is not found in all cases. The liver can be central or to the right and the stomach can be left- or right-sided. Malrotation of the intestines is also associated, with risk of bowel obstruction. Karyotype abnormalities are very rare.

Management and outcome

As with left atrial isomerism, the management and outcome in all cases of right atrial isomerism will be influenced by the extent of associated lesions, both cardiac and extracardiac.

Outcome in a large single-centre fetal series

Of 111 cases of right atrial isomerism diagnosed prenatally, 51% of pregnancies resulted in a termination of pregnancy. If the terminations are excluded then the outcome of the continuing pregnancies was: 11% resulting in spontaneous intrauterine death, 24% died in the neonatal period, 26% died in infancy and 39% were alive at last update.

Of cases seen in the last 10 years, a termination of pregnancy took place in 46% of cases and 39% of the continuing pregnancies were alive at last follow-up.

Summary of fetal echocardiographic features associated with RAI.
• Abnormal cardiac position
• Heart and stomach may be on opposite sides
• Inferior vena cava and descending aorta lie on the same side of the spine
• Inferior vena cava lies directly anterior to the aorta in the abdomen
• Usually associated with complex cardiac malformations
• Anomalous pulmonary venous drainage

Chapter 4

Abnormalities of the four-chamber view (I)
Abnormalities of veno-atrial and atrioventricular connection

Summary

- **Abnormalities of the veno-atrial junction**
  - Variations or abnormalities of systemic venous connection
  - Anomalous pulmonary venous drainage
- **Abnormalities of atrioventricular connection**
  - Mitral atresia
    - hypoplastic left heart syndrome
    - with double-outlet right ventricle
  - Tricuspid atresia
    - with concordant arterial connections
    - with discordant arterial connections
  - Atrioventricular septal defect
    - with normal situs
    - with isomerism (see also Chapter 3)
    - with unbalanced ventricles
  - Double-inlet ventricle

Connection abnormalities at the veno-atrial junction

Abnormalities of the venous connections to the heart consist of a wide spectrum of disease and although they can occur in isolation, they are often found within the context of other forms of cardiac malformation.

Abnormalities and variations of systemic venous connection

Superior vena cava (SVC)
A persistent left superior vena cava is one of the most common systemic venous abnormalities. It can occur in association with other major forms of congenital heart disease, or it can occur in isolation when it is considered to be a normal variant. In fetal life a persistent

left superior vena cava or bilateral superior vena cavae are most easily detected in the three-vessel view of the great arteries (Figure 2.10). A persistent left superior vena cava should also be suspected if there is a dilated coronary sinus, as the drainage of the left SVC is often to the coronary sinus. A section of the heart just inferior to the true four-chamber view will demonstrate the coronary sinus, which is found below the left atrium just above the posterior rim of the mitral valve (Figure 2.11a). It is important to note that a large coronary sinus can make it difficult to visualise the crux of the heart, so that a diagnosis of an atrioventricular septal defect could be made in error (Figures 2.11b, 4.1a and 4.1b).

Isolated cases of persistent left superior vena cava do not require follow-up or any intervention.

Inferior vena cava (IVC)
The most common abnormality of the inferior vena cava is an interrupted inferior vena cava. In such cases the venous return from the lower body reaches the heart via the azygos or hemiazygos vein. These veins connect to a right or left superior vena cava, respectively. Although an interrupted inferior vena cava can occur in isolation, most cases are associated with left atrial isomerism (see Chapter 3).

Abnormalities of pulmonary venous connection – anomalous pulmonary venous connection or drainage (TAPVD, PAPVD)

Prevalence
Total anomalous pulmonary venous connection or drainage (TAPVD) accounts for 1.5-2.6% of all congenital cardiac malformations in postnatal series. In the Evelina fetal series, isolated total anomalous pulmonary venous connection accounted for 0.1% of the total, reflecting the difficulty of detecting this anomaly prenatally.

Definition
Anomalous pulmonary venous connection implies that the pulmonary veins do not connect to the morphological left atrium. Instead the veins drain directly or indirectly through abnormal connections to the right atrium. One or more of the pulmonary veins may be affected.

Spectrum
In total anomalous pulmonary venous drainage (TAPVD), all four pulmonary veins drain to a site other than the left atrium. The site of abnormal drainage can be supracardiac, cardiac or infracardiac. Supracardiac drainage can be to the left brachiocephalic (innominate) vein, directly to the right superior vena cava, to the azygos system, or to a persistent left superior vena cava. Commonly, the pulmonary veins join in a confluence behind the left atrium. From here a vertical vein joins to the left brachiocepalic vein which then joins the superior vena cava. Occasionally, the vertical vein can connect directly to the right superior vena cava. In the cardiac form, the veins usually drain to the coronary sinus and then to the right atrium, or directly into the right atrium. The latter is seen most commonly in the setting of right atrial

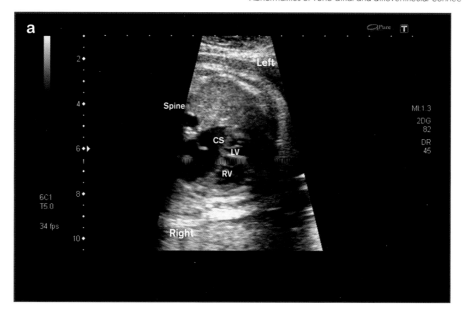

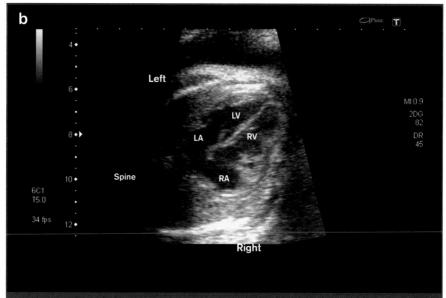

Figure 4.1. a) In this example a large coronary sinus gives the impression of an atrioventricular septal defect (AVSD). b) However, a different view of the same heart shows that the atrioventricular septum is intact.

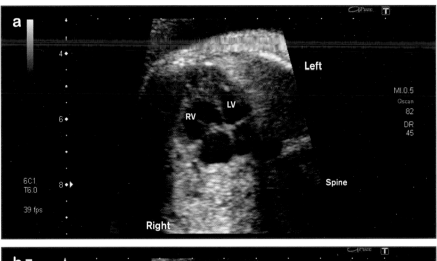

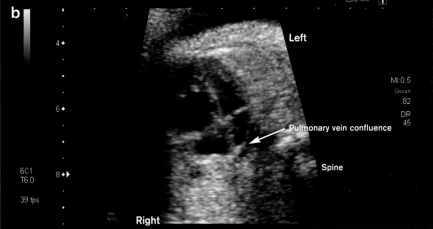

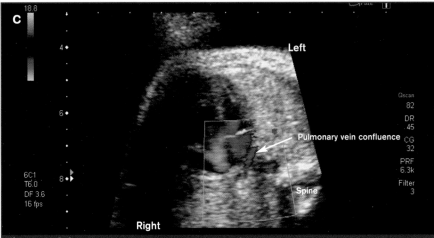

Figure 4.2. An example of isolated TAPVD. a) The four-chamber view showing disproportion with the left-sided structures appearing smaller than right-sided structures. b) A confluence can be seen behind the left atrium (arrow). c) The pulmonary venous confluence is demonstrated with colour-flow mapping (arrow).

isomerism. In the infracardiac (infradiaphragmatic) form, the pulmonary veins enter a descending vertical vein which then drains to the portal venous system. These cases are associated with obstruction following the closure of the venous duct as the blood has to pass through the hepatic veins.

In partial anomalous pulmonary venous connection (PAPVD), up to three of the four pulmonary veins drain into the right atrium, or connect abnormally with a systemic vein. Anomalous venous drainage of the right lower and middle lobe, occurring in association with right lung hypoplasia, is termed the Scimitar syndrome. The right lung hypoplasia typically results in dextroposition of the heart in this condition and there is usually an abnormal arterial supply to the right lung, arising from the descending aorta.

Cardiac associations

This abnormality can be seen as an isolated finding or as part of more complex congenital heart disease, particularly in the setting of isomerism (see Chapter 3).

Fetal echocardiographic features

The diagnosis of anomalous pulmonary venous connection in isolation can be very difficult to make in fetal life and this abnormality is frequently overlooked prenatally, even in experienced centres. The main feature to help make this diagnosis is that the pulmonary veins cannot be seen to be draining into the left atrium in the normal way with colour flow, as described in Chapter 2. The left atrium may appear small with a smooth posterior wall. There may be a gap between the posterior wall of the left atrium and the descending aorta. In some cases where the drainage is supracardiac or cardiac, there may be right atrial and right ventricular dominance, giving an abnormal appearance of the four-chamber view (Figure 4.2a). However, the degree of right ventricular volume overload is influenced by the degree of obstruction and in some cases the four-chamber view may appear normal. A confluence can sometimes be seen behind the left atrium, into which the pulmonary veins drain (Figures 4.2b-c), though this is not always easy to identify. If the veins are draining anomalously to the coronary sinus, this may appear dilated. A dilated coronary sinus can also be associated with a persistent left superior vena cava and with normal pulmonary venous drainage (Figures 2.11a-b). However, it is strongly recommended that in all cases of a dilated coronary sinus the pulmonary venous drainage is carefully checked. It is also important to check that the pulmonary venous drainage is normal in cases with a left-sided superior vena cava or a dilated superior vena cava, as these features can be associated with supracardiac TAPVD. When the drainage is infracardiac there is usually some obstruction and right ventricular volume overload is not a feature. These cases are often associated with complex congenital heart disease and right atrial isomerism (see Chapter 3). A venous channel may be identified in the abdomen and chest with the direction of flow being towards the abdomen as the drainage is infradiaphragmatic. An example of an unbalanced atrioventricular septal defect associated with right atrial isomerism and infracardiac total anomalous pulmonary venous drainage is shown in Figures 4.3a-d.

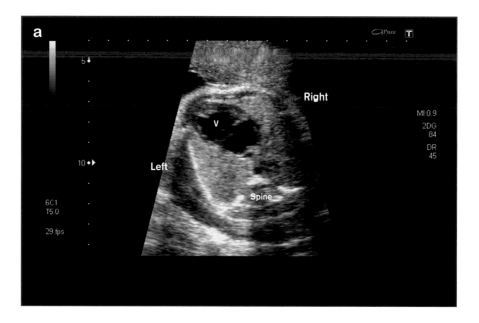

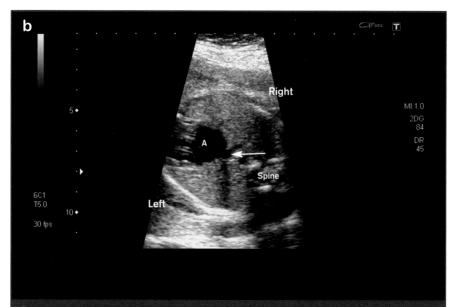

Figure 4.3. An example of a complex AVSD associated with right atrial isomerism and infracardiac TAPVD. a) The four-chamber view shows an AVSD to a large dominant ventricle (V). b) The pulmonary veins do not enter the atrial mass (A) but join in a confluence behind the atrial mass (arrow).
Figure continued overleaf.

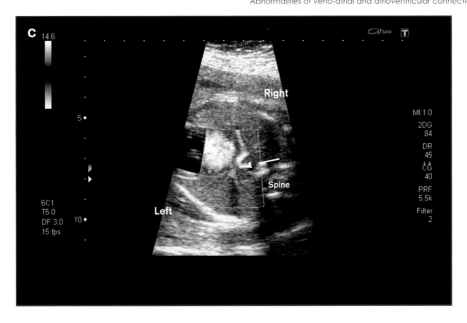

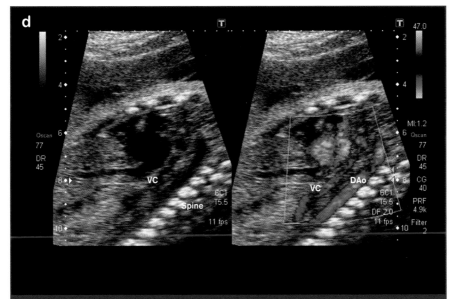

Figure 4.3 *continued.* An example of a complex AVSD associated with right atrial isomerism and infracardiac TAPVD. c) Colour-flow mapping shows that all four pulmonary veins drain to the confluence (arrow). d) The confluence drainage can be seen to be infradiaphragmatic, via a venous channel (VC). In addition to the descending aorta another vessel with flow towards the abdomen can be seen clearly with colour-flow mapping (both vessels seen in blue).

Extracardiac associations

Chromosomal abnormalities are rarely found with anomalous pulmonary venous drainage occurring in isolation. If there is associated isomerism there may be related abnormalities as outlined in Chapter 3.

Management and outcome

Most cases of TAPVD diagnosed prenatally are associated with other cardiac abnormalities and the outcome will be influenced by the extent of associated lesions. By definition all cases of right atrial isomerism will have anomalous pulmonary venous connection. Other forms of cardiac abnormality can also be associated with TAPVD. In the fetal series at Evelina Children's Hospital, in the absence of isomerism, TAPVD has been associated with tetralogy of Fallot, hypoplastic left heart syndrome, atrioventricular septal defect, ventricular septal defect, double-inlet ventricle, double-outlet ventricle, coarctation of the aorta and common arterial trunk.

Isolated cases of TAPVD can usually be repaired surgically with low mortality and a good long-term outcome. However, the long-term outcome will be adversely influenced by development of pulmonary vein stenosis, which is rare but can occur. The overall outcome and success of surgery will be influenced by the site of drainage and whether there is associated obstruction. TAPVD associated with obstructed pulmonary venous drainage is a very severe and critical form of congenital heart disease. Cases of TAPVD seen in association with complex congenital heart disease and isomerism, in particular right atrial isomerism, are associated with a poor outcome.

Outcome in a large single-centre fetal series

In a large single-centre experience there were only four cases of isolated TAPVD. Three were successfully repaired after birth and all the children were well at last review. In one baby there were associated extracardiac abnormalities and the baby died prior to any cardiac surgery.

Summary of fetal echocardiographic features associated with TAPVD.

- Pulmonary veins not seen draining to the left atrium with colour flow
- Left atrium may appear small
- Right heart dominance (sometimes)
- Dilated coronary sinus (possibly)
- Confluence behind the left atrium
- Identification of ascending or descending vein

Summary of possible abnormal drainage sites.

- **Supracardiac**
  - **drainage to the superior vena cava**
  - **drainage to the brachiocephalic vein**
- **Cardiac**
  - **drainage to the coronary sinus**
  - **drainage directly to the right atrium**
- **Infracardiac**
  - **drainage to the portal or hepatic vein**
- **Mixed**

Connection abnormalities at the atrioventricular junction

Mitral atresia (MAT)

Prevalence
The postnatal prevalence of mitral atresia is difficult to ascertain as mitral atresia can occur in different settings (see below). In the Evelina fetal series, mitral atresia accounted for 10.2% of the total. Of these, 6.8% of the total had mitral atresia as part of hypoplastic left heart syndrome and 3.4% of the total had mitral atresia with a double-outlet right ventricle (see below). In the last 10 years of the series, mitral atresia as part of hypoplastic left heart syndrome accounted for 6.4% of the total, and mitral atresia associated with a double-outlet right ventricle accounted for a further 2.2% of the total.

Definition
In mitral atresia there is no connection or flow between the left atrium and the left ventricle. This is usually due to an absent atrioventricular connection.

Spectrum
Mitral atresia comprises a spectrum of abnormality but occurs in three main settings:

- It most commonly occurs in association with aortic atresia in the setting of hypoplastic left heart syndrome (see Chapter 6).
- It can occur with a ventricular septal defect with a normally connected aorta with a patent aortic valve.
- It can occur with a double-outlet right ventricle. In this setting, the aorta is often found arising anterior to the pulmonary artery.

Fetal echocardiographic features
In the four-chamber view, an opening mitral valve is not seen and the left ventricle is hypoplastic (Figure 4.4a). There is no demonstrable flow from the left atrium to the left

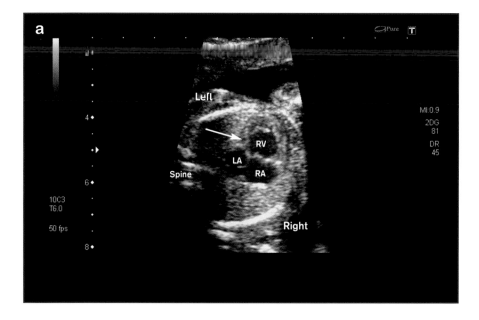

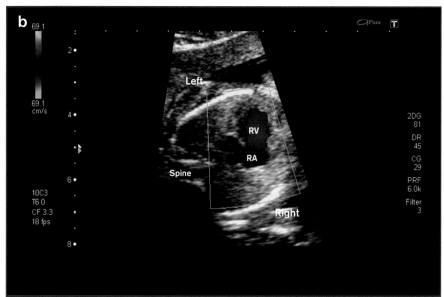

Figure 4.4. a) The four-chamber view of an example of mitral atresia. The left ventricle (arrow) is tiny and no mitral valve can be identified. b) Colour-flow mapping demonstrates the flow across the tricuspid valve from the right atrium to the right ventricle, but no flow is seen on the left side of the heart.

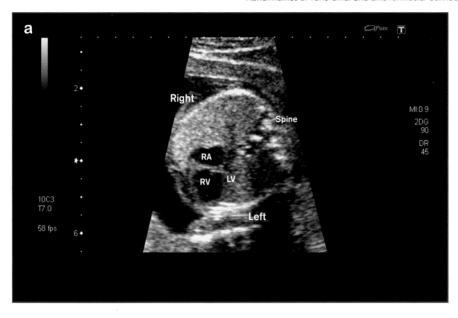

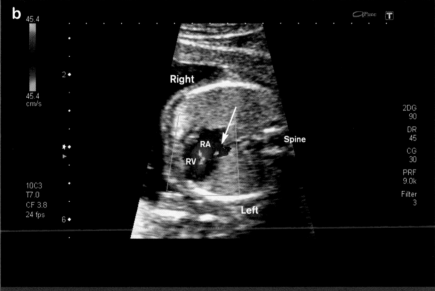

Figure 4.5. a) The four-chamber view of another example of mitral atresia. The left ventricle is tiny and no mitral valve can be identified. b) The flow pattern across the foramen ovale is seen to be left to right (seen in red and arrow).

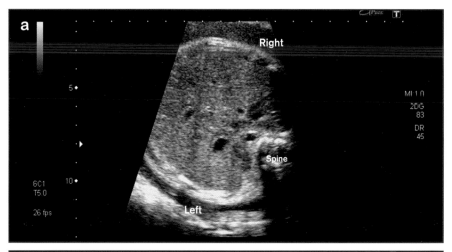

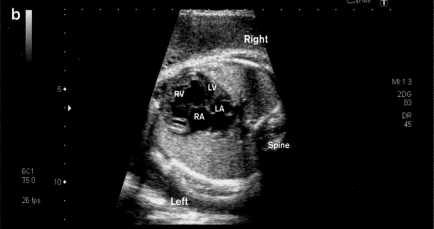

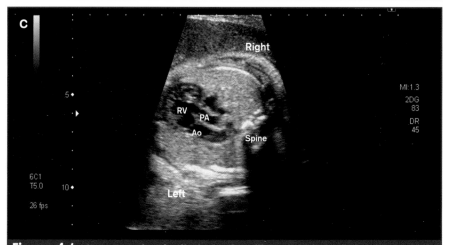

Figure 4.6. An example of mitral atresia with a double-outlet right ventricle associated with dextrocardia. a) The abdominal situs in this example appears normal with the fetal stomach on the left. b) A four-chamber view shows that the apex of the heart is to the right. There is mitral atresia with a very small left ventricle and a large dominant right ventricle. c) Both the great arteries arise in a parallel orientation from the right ventricle.

ventricle on colour flow (Figure 4.4b). The left atrium is small and the flow across the foramen ovale is left to right, which is a reversal of the normal pattern (Figures 4.5a-b). Examination of the great arteries will allow a complete diagnosis, for example, whether there is associated aortic atresia and hypoplastic left heart syndrome (see Chapter 6), or whether there is an associated double-outlet right ventricle (Figures 4.6a-c).

Extracardiac associations

In fetal life, mitral atresia has a significant association with chromosomal anomalies, usually trisomy 18, but trisomy 13 and translocation/deletion syndromes are also possible. In our large fetal series, mitral atresia with a double-outlet right ventricle was associated with chromosomal abnormalities in 17% of cases. Of these, 48% were trisomy 18, 20% were trisomy 13 and the remaining were a variety of chromosomal abnormalities, including unbalanced translocations and deletions. A further 21% of cases, with a normal karyotype, had an extracardiac abnormality, which included cleft lip and palate, diaphragmatic hernia, duodenal atresia, exomphalos, hemivertebrae, hydrocephalus, limb abnormalities, renal abnormalities, talipes and ventriculomegaly. (See Chapter 6 for associations of mitral atresia with aortic atresia and hypoplastic left heart syndrome.)

Management and outcome

This is a severe form of congenital heart disease for which the longer-term management will be a staged surgical palliation aimed towards achieving a single-ventricle circulation (Fontan type circulation). This type of circulation, which is achieved as a staged procedure, leaves the systemic veins (superior vena cava and inferior vena cava) draining directly to the pulmonary arteries (total cavo-pulmonary connection) and the dominant right ventricle pumps systemic arterial blood. The way in which the final circulation is achieved will be influenced by whether there is associated obstruction to either great artery, for example, coarctation of the aorta or pulmonary stenosis.

The longer-term prognosis is uncertain as management is palliative rather than corrective. In this setting the systemic ventricle will be the right ventricle. Longer-term complications include exercise limitation, arrhythmias, heart failure and the potential need for a heart or heart/lung transplantation later.

Outcome for mitral atresia with a double-outlet right ventricle in a large single-centre fetal series (for outcome of hypoplastic left heart syndrome, see Chapter 6)

Of 144 cases of mitral atresia with a double-outlet right ventricle diagnosed prenatally, 60% of pregnancies resulted in a termination of pregnancy. If the terminations are excluded then the outcome of the continuing pregnancies was: 14% resulting in spontaneous intrauterine death, 41% died in the neonatal period, 10% died in infancy and 35% were alive at last update.

Of cases seen in the last 10 years, a termination of pregnancy took place in 42% of cases and 46% of the continuing pregnancies were alive at last follow-up.

Summary of fetal echocardiographic features associated with MAT.

- No opening mitral valve
- Small left ventricle
- Small left atrium
- No flow from the left atrium to the left ventricle
- Left to right flow at atrial level
- +/- ventricular septal defect
- With aortic atresia forms hypoplastic left heart syndrome (see Chapter 6)

Summary of extracardiac associations in fetal MAT.

- Chromosomal
  - 17%
- Extracardiac abnormality (normal chromosomes)
  - 21%

Tricuspid atresia (TAT)

Prevalence

The prevalence of tricuspid atresia in postnatal series is between 0.7-2.5%. In the Evelina fetal series, tricuspid atresia accounted for 3.4% of the total series and 3% of all cases of fetal congenital heart disease seen in the last 10 years.

Definition

In tricuspid atresia there is no direct connection between the right atrium and right ventricle. Usually this is due to complete absence of the right atrioventricular junction and valve, though more rarely this may be due to an imperforate valve. In all cases there must be an inter-atrial communication to allow the blood coming back from the systemic veins to the right atrium out of the heart, via the left atrium and left ventricle.

Spectrum

Virtually all cases of tricuspid atresia will have an associated ventricular septal defect, which can be of variable size and this will influence the size of the right ventricular cavity. The ventriculo-arterial connections are concordant (normally related) in the majority of cases but may be discordant (transposed) in about 20-25% of cases. There may be obstruction to either great artery and this is more likely if the ventricular septal defect is restrictive. In cases with concordant arterial connections, this is likely to be pulmonary obstruction, whereas in cases with discordant connections this is likely to be aortic obstruction, which is usually coarctation of the aorta, though more rarely arch interruption can also occur.

Cardiac associations

As described above, tricuspid atresia can be associated with pulmonary stenosis and more rarely pulmonary atresia, transposed great arteries and coarctation of the aorta. Much more rarely it can occur with atrioventricular discordance (see Chapter 7), common arterial trunk (see Chapter 8), or aortic atresia. A persistent left superior vena cava can also be associated.

Fetal echocardiographic features

In the four-chamber view a patent tricuspid valve is not identified and the right ventricle is hypoplastic, though the size of the right ventricle is variable (Figures 4.7a, 4.8a and 4.9a). There is an associated ventricular septal defect, which can be of varying size. The mitral valve can be seen to open with normal flow across it, but no flow will be detected across the tricuspid valve on pulsed Doppler or colour flow (Figures 4.7b-c and 4.9b). In cases with concordant arterial connections, the pulmonary trunk can vary in size from being near normal to being severely hypoplastic. This is often related to the size of the ventricular septal defect. An example of tricuspid atresia with a good sized pulmonary artery is shown in Figures 4.7a-d and one associated with a small pulmonary artery is shown in Figures 4.8a-b. A small pulmonary artery in this setting is an indicator of pulmonary obstruction and even in cases with significant pulmonary stenosis, it is common for the pulmonary artery Doppler to fall within the normal range. Assessment of the direction of flow in the arterial duct can be very helpful, as reverse flow in the duct indicates that there is likely to be severe pulmonary stenosis or pulmonary atresia.

In cases with discordant arterial connections, there may be different degrees of aortic obstruction, though some cases will have no aortic obstruction, particularly if the ventricular septal defect is unrestrictive. However, in cases where the ventricular septal defect is small and restrictive, the aorta may be smaller than the pulmonary artery due to associated aortic coarctation (Figures 4.9a-d), aortic arch interruption (Figures 4.10a-b) or even aortic atresia in very rare cases.

Extracardiac associations

Tricuspid atresia is rarely associated with chromosomal abnormalities, but can sometimes be associated with extracardiac abnormalities. In our large fetal serieis, tricuspid atresia was associated with chromosomal abnormalities in 0.7% of cases, which was a single case of 47XXY. A further 8% of cases, with a normal karyotype, had an extracardiac abnormality, which included cleft lip and palate, diaphragmatic hernia, ectopia, hydrocephalus and renal abnormalities.

Management and outcome

This is a major form of congenital heart disease for which the surgical approach after birth is staged palliation rather than surgical repair. Initial management will be dictated by the amount of pulmonary blood flow, or in cases with transposed great arteries, whether there is

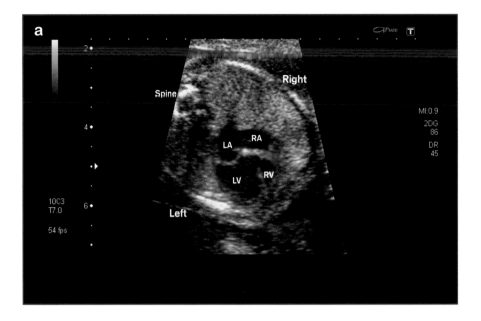

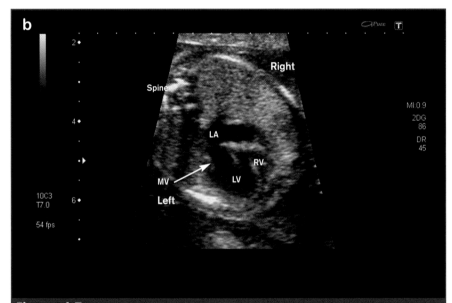

Figure 4.7. An example of tricuspid atresia with a good sized pulmonary artery. a) The four-chamber view in tricuspid atresia. A patent tricuspid valve is not identified and the right ventricle is hypoplastic. b) The mitral valve is seen to open but there is no opening tricuspid valve.

Figure continued overleaf.

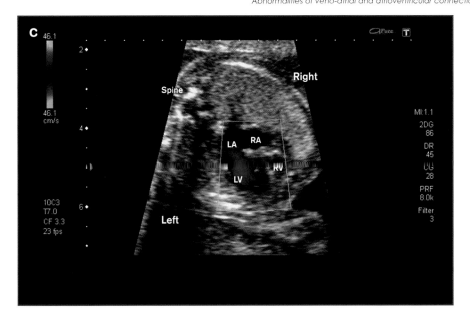

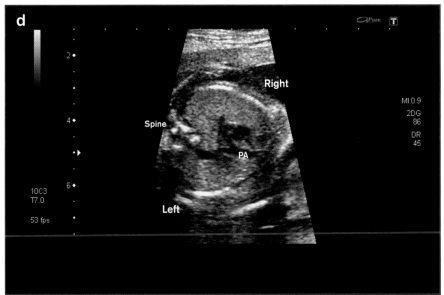

Figure 4.7 *continued.* An example of tricuspid atresia with a good sized pulmonary artery. c) Colour-flow mapping demonstrates flow across the mitral valve (seen in blue) but there is no flow from the right atrium to the right ventricle. d) A good sized pulmonary artery with confluent branches arises from the small right ventricle.

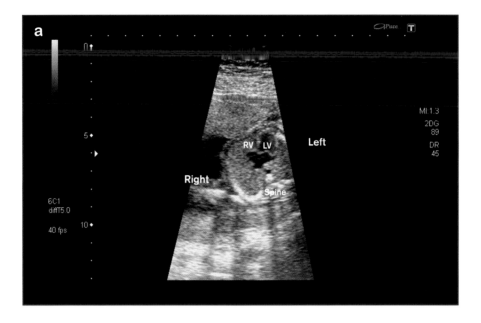

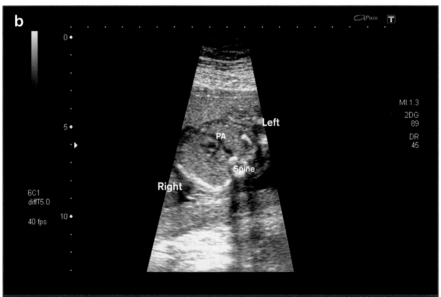

Figure 4.8. An example of tricuspid atresia with a small pulmonary artery. a) The four-chamber view showing a very hypoplastic right ventricle. In this case, the ventricular septal defect is very small. b) A hypoplastic pulmonary artery with confluent branches arises from the small right ventricle.

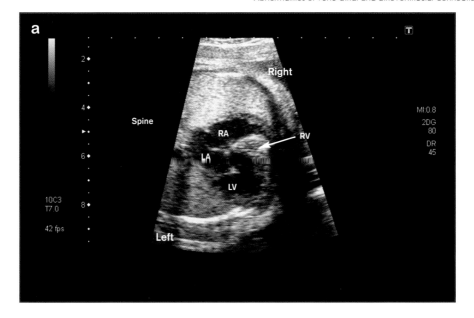

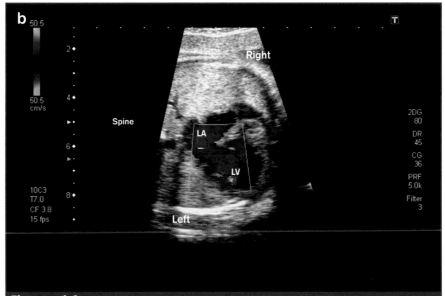

Figure 4.9. An example of tricuspid atresia with discordant ventriculo-arterial connections (transposition) and coarctation. a) The four-chamber view showing tricuspid atresia with a hypoplastic right ventricle. b) Colour flow mapping demonstrates flow across the mitral valve (seen in blue) but there is no flow from the right atrium to the right ventricle.

Figure continued overleaf.

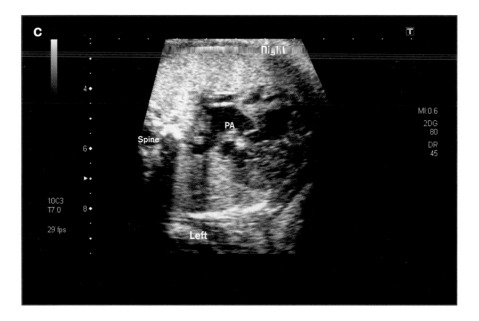

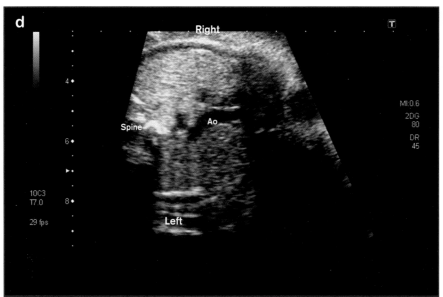

Figure 4.9 *continued.* An example of tricuspid atresia with discordant ventriculo-arterial connections (transposition) and coarctation. c) A large pulmonary artery arises from the left ventricle. d) A smaller aorta arises from the hypoplastic right ventricle.

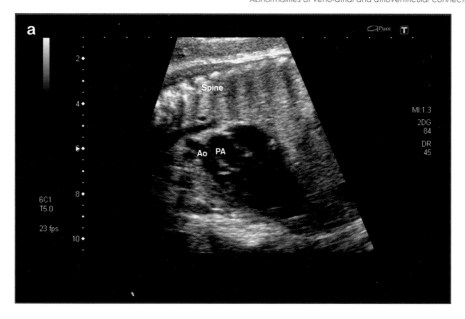

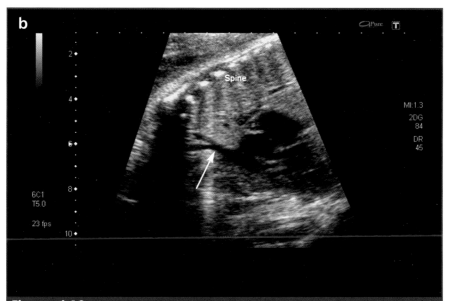

Figure 4.10. An example of tricuspid atresia with associated transposition and with an interrupted aortic arch. a) The two great arteries in this example arise in a parallel orientation with the aorta appearing significantly smaller than the pulmonary artery. b) A 'pronged fork' appearance of the arch is seen which is characteristic of an interrupted aortic arch (arrow) (see Chapter 9).

arch obstruction. If the pulmonary blood flow is satisfactory, then early intervention may not be indicated, though a systemic arterial shunt may be required to augment pulmonary blood flow, in cases with reduced pulmonary blood flow. If there is an associated coarctation of the aorta, or more rarely an interrupted aortic arch, repair of the arch will be required in the early neonatal period. In the longer term, management is towards achieving a single-ventricle circulation (Fontan type circulation). This type of circulation, which is achieved as a staged procedure, leaves the systemic veins (superior vena cava and inferior vena cava) draining directly to the pulmonary arteries and the dominant left ventricle pumps systemic arterial blood. The combined surgical mortality is in the region of 10-15%. However, in later life there may be further complications including functional limitation, arrhythmias, cardiac failure and the need to consider cardiac transplantation.

Outcome in a large single-centre fetal series

Of 144 cases of tricuspid atresia diagnosed prenatally, 59% of pregnancies resulted in a termination of pregnancy. If the terminations are excluded then the outcome of the continuing pregnancies was: 10% resulting in spontaneous intrauterine death, 10% died in the neonatal period, 10% died in infancy and 70% were alive at last update.

Of cases seen in the last 10 years, a termination of pregnancy took place in 48% of cases and 70% of the continuing pregnancies were alive at last follow-up.

Summary of fetal echocardiographic features associated with TAT.

- Hypoplastic right ventricle
- No opening tricuspid valve
- No flow from the right atrium to the right ventricle
- Ventricular septal defect
- May be obstruction to either great artery
- Concordant great arteries in 75-80%
  - more likely to have pulmonary obstruction
- Discordant great arteries (transposition) in 20-25%
  - more likely to have arch obstruction such as coarctation of the aorta

---

Summary of extracardiac associations in fetal TAT.

- Chromosomal
  - 0.7%
- Extracardiac abnormality (normal chromosomes)
  - 8%

Atrioventricular septal defect (AVSD)

Prevalence
Atrioventricular septal defects account for 3-7% of congenital heart disease in various postnatal series. In contrast, atrioventricular septal defects are one of the commonest forms of heart disease diagnosed prenatally. In the Evelina fetal series, atrioventricular septal defects accounted for 16% of the total series and 13.2% of all cases of fetal congenital heart disease seen in the last 10 years.

Definition
Atrioventricular septal defects form a group of abnormalities where there is a common atrioventricular junction, associated with abnormal atrioventricular septation and abnormal atrioventricular valve formation.

Spectrum
The defect can be partial or complete. In the complete form, which is the more common form, there are both atrial and ventricular components to the defect, so that there is an atrial septal defect and a ventricular septal defect at the atrioventricular junction, in association with a common atrioventricular valve. The size of the atrial and ventricular components can be variable. In the partial form, there is a primum atrial septal defect with a common atrioventricular valve, but no ventricular component to the defect. Very rarely, there may be an inlet ventricular septal defect with a common atrioventricular junction.

Cardiac associations
Atrioventricular septal defects can occur as an isolated cardiac abnormality or in conjunction with more complex forms of congenital heart disease. They are associated with isomerism in 20-25% of cases (see Chapter 3). In the Evelina fetal series, 24% of atrioventricular septal defects were associated with isomerism, of which 66% had left atrial isomerism and 34% had right atrial isomerism.

Atrioventricular septal defects can occur with balanced ventricles (both ventricular chambers of equal size) or unbalanced ventricles (one ventricular chamber smaller than the other). Other cardiac lesions that may be associated include coarctation of the aorta, tetralogy of Fallot, double-outlet right ventricle and more rarely a common arterial trunk.

Fetal echocardiographic features
In the four-chamber view there is a defect at the crux of the heart with loss of the normal differential insertion of the atrioventricular valves (Figures 4.11a, 4.12a and 4.13). In the complete form there will be a defect in both the atrial and ventricular septa at the point where the two atrioventricular valves normally insert. The two valves do not form in the normal way and instead, there is a common valve that bridges the defect, resulting in loss of the normal differential insertion. Thus, the echocardiographic appearance is of a single valve opening into both ventricular chambers. Examples of a complete defect, in both systole and diastole, is shown in Figures 4.11a-b and 4.12a-b. In cases with a partial defect, there will be no ventricular component to the defect. In a partial defect, there is a defect in the lower portion

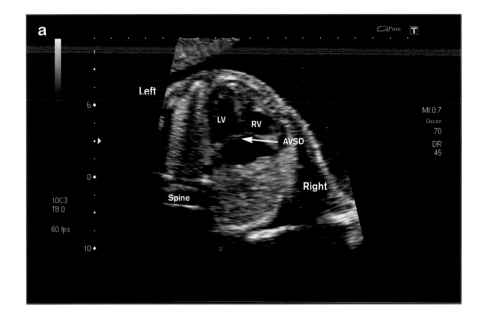

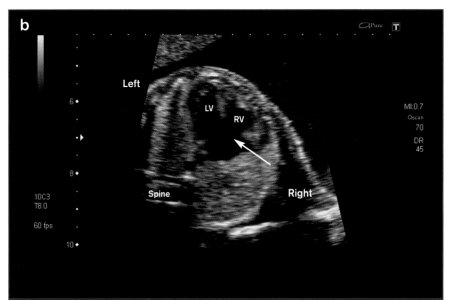

Figure 4.11. An example of an atrioventricular septal defect with balanced ventricles seen in systole and diastole. a) The defect is seen is systole with the atrioventricular valve closed. There is loss of differential insertion. b) The defect is seen in diastole with the atrioventricular valve open. The defect in the atrial and ventricular septum at the crux of the heart is seen (arrow).

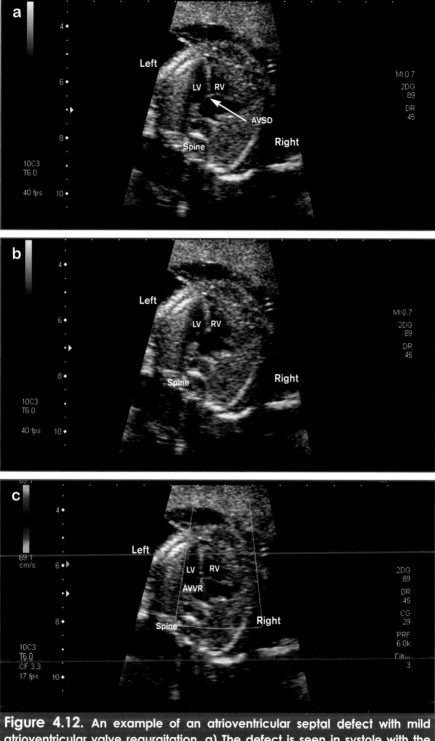

Figure 4.12. An example of an atrioventricular septal defect with mild atrioventricular valve regurgitation. a) The defect is seen in systole with the atrioventricular valve closed. b) The defect is seen is diastole with the atrioventricular valve open. c) There is mild atrioventricular valve regurgitation seen with colour flow.

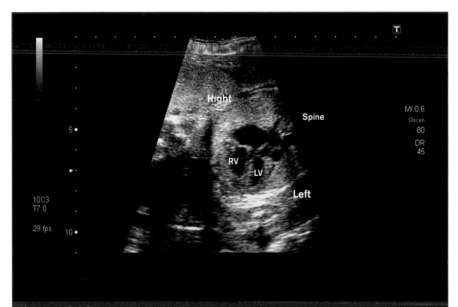

Figure 4.13. An example of an atrioventricular septal defect where the defect is not so obvious but there is loss of differential insertion.

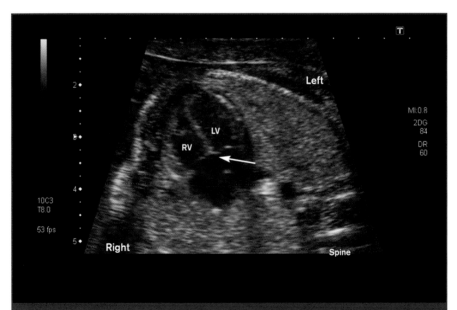

Figure 4.14. A four-chamber view showing a partial atrioventricular septal defect. A defect is seen in the lower portion of the atrial septum, the primum septum and there is loss of the normal differential insertion of the two atrioventricular valves (arrow). No defect in the ventricular septum is seen in this case.

of the atrial septum, the primum septum, associated with loss of the normal differential insertion of the two atrioventricular valves. There is no ventricular component, that is, no defect in the ventricular septum in these cases. Examples of a partial defect are shown in Figures 4.14 and 4.15a.

In some cases there may be unbalanced ventricles, with one ventricle appearing smaller than the other (Figures 4.3a and 4.15a). Unbalanced atrioventricular septal defects are frequently associated with very complex forms of congenital heart disease, which often includes isomerism. Examples of complex forms of an atrioventricular septal defect are shown in Figures 4.3a-d, 4.16a-d, 4.17a-e, 4.18a-b and 4.19a-e. Cases that have a smaller left ventricle may have an associated coarctation of the aorta and this should be excluded as a possibility (Figures 4.15a-c). Occasionally coarctation of the aorta may be associated with atrioventricular septal defects with balanced ventricles (Figures 4.20a-b and see Chapter 9). In cases associated with left atrial isomerism and heart block, the ventricular chambers often appear hypertrophied (Figures 4.16a-d). Atrioventricular valve regurgitation is an adverse associated feature and its presence should be sought in all cases, though mild regurgitation is sometimes not clinically significant (Figures 4.12c, 4.16c and 4.18b).

Extracardiac associations

Atrioventricular septal defects when combined with normal situs are commonly associated with chromosomal anomalies. Most commonly this is trisomy 21, though other chromosome anomalies, such as trisomies 18 and 13 can also occur. Atrioventricular septal defects can also be found with other genetic syndromes such as Ellis van Creveld, Smith-Lemli-Opitz, Cornelia de Lange, Goldenhar, VACTERL and CHARGE syndromes.

In our large fetal series, 36% of all atrioventricular septal defects were associated with chromosomal abnormalities, of which 84% were trisomy 21, 6% were trisomy 18, 1% were trisomy 13 and 9% were a variety of other forms of chromosomal abnormality. Overall, trisomy 21 occurred in 30% of all cases of atrioventricular septal defects, but if cases with isomerism are excluded then trisomy 21 occurred in 39% of cases. Extracardiac abnormalities, without a chromosomal abnormality, were associated in a further 24% of cases, though many of these also had associated isomerism. If cases of isomerism are excluded as well as chromosomal abnormalities, then extracardiac abnormalities occurred in a further 4%. The types of extracardiac abnormalities included an absence of corpus callosum, congenital cystic adenomatoid malformation of the lung, cystic hygroma, diaphragmatic hernia, duodenal atresia, ectopia exomphalos, hydrocephalus, hypospadias, imperforate anus, micrognathia, polydactyly, radial aplasia, renal abnormalities, scoliosis, talipes, tracheo-oesophageal atresia and ventriculomegaly.

Overall in this series, 24% of cases with an atrioventricular septal defect were associated with isomerism (16% were left atrial isomerism and 8% were right atrial isomerism) and these cases usually have a normal karyotype, but other extracardiac abnormalities can occur (see Chapter 3). Although atrioventricular septal defects are often associated with either chromosomal anomalies or with isomerism, they can occur with normal situs, normal chromosomes and no extracardiac abnormality.

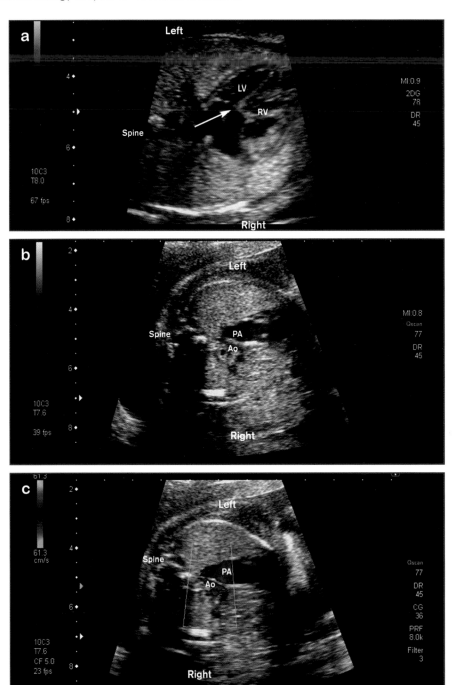

Figure 4.15. An example of a partial atrioventricular septal defect with unbalanced ventricles. a) A four-chamber view showing loss of differential insertion and a partial atrioventricular septal defect (arrow), with no ventricular component. The left ventricle appears smaller than the right ventricle so that there are unbalanced ventricles. b) A three-vessel view in the same example shows that the aorta is significantly smaller than the pulmonary artery suggesting that there is associated coarctation of the aorta. c) Colour shows flow in both great vessels in the same direction towards the spine and confirms there is forward flow in the hypoplastic aortic arch.

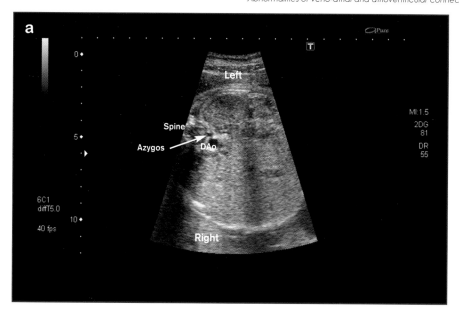

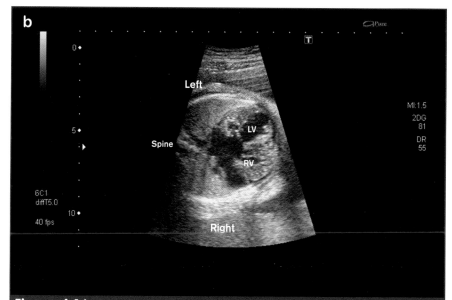

Figure 4.16. A complex atrioventricular septal defect associated with left atrial isomerism and complete heart block. a) The abdominal situs shows features of left atrial isomerism. There is an azygos continuation seen behind the descending aorta. b) The four-chamber view shows an unbalanced atrioventricular septal defect with hypertrophied ventricles. This was in association with complete heart block and left atrial isomerism.

Figure continued overleaf.

95

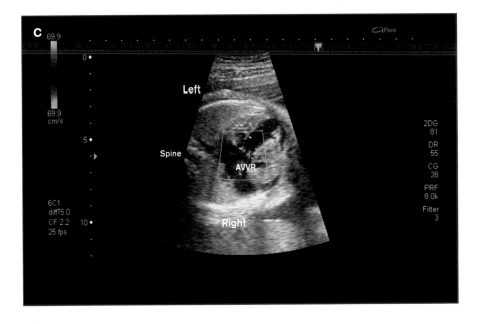

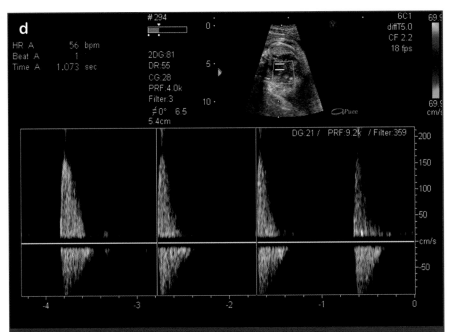

Figure 4.16 *continued.* A complex atrioventricular septal defect associated with left atrial isomerism and complete heart block. c) Moderate to severe atrioventricular valve regurgitation is seen with colour flow. d) The heart rate shown on a Doppler trace was 56 beats per minute.

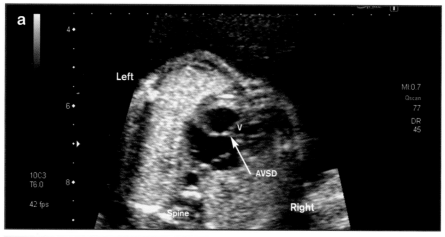

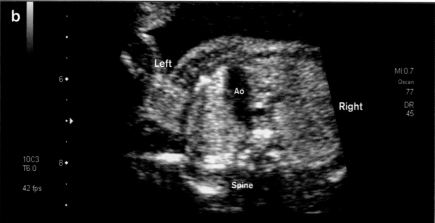

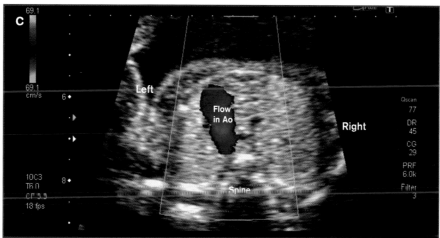

Figure 4.17. A complex atrioventricular septal defect with a dominant ventricle and pulmonary atresia. a) The four-chamber view shows one large ventricular chamber (V). This has a muscle band in it, giving the false impression of two equal ventricles. The second hypoplastic chamber is not seen in this view. b) A large aorta is seen arising from the dominant chamber. c) Forward flow in the aorta is seen with colour flow.

Figure continued overleaf.

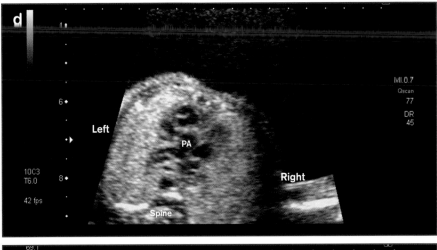

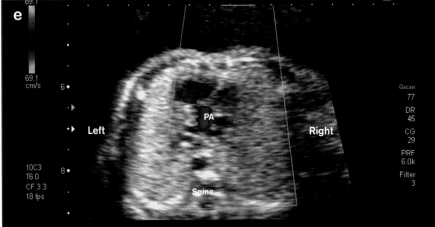

Figure 4.17 *continued.* A complex atrioventricular septal defect with a dominant ventricle and pulmonary atresia. d) A small pulmonary artery is seen with confluent branches. e) Colour flow shows reverse flow in the small pulmonary artery (seen in red) confirming pulmonary atresia.

Management and outcome

The management and outcome of atrioventricular septal defects will be influenced by the extent of associated anomalies, both cardiac and extracardiac.

Isolated cases with balanced ventricles and equal sized great arteries do not typically cause any immediate postnatal problems. However, when the pulmonary vascular resistance falls after birth there may be an increasing left to right shunt, both at atrial level and at ventricular level, depending on the size of the atrial and ventricular components. The size of the ventricular component of the defect is important in terms of the timing of surgery. If the ventricular component is significant, then surgery is usually undertaken at 3-6 months of age. This carries a mortality of around 5%. There is a risk of about 10-15% that further surgery

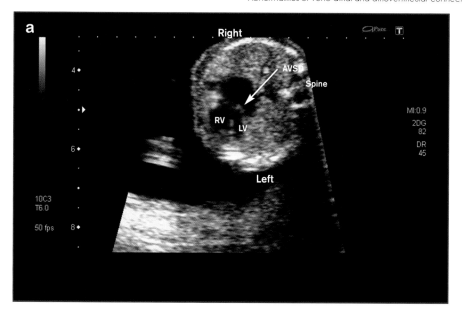

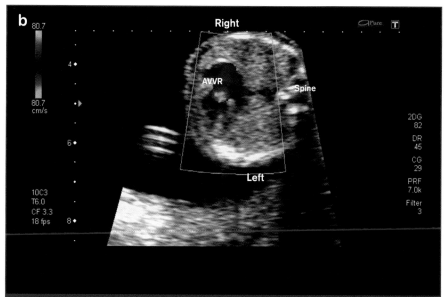

Figure 4.18. A complex atrioventricular septal defect with severe atrioventricular valve regurgitation. a) The four-chamber view showing unbalanced ventricles. b) There is significant atrioventricular valve regurgitation seen with colour flow (shown in red).

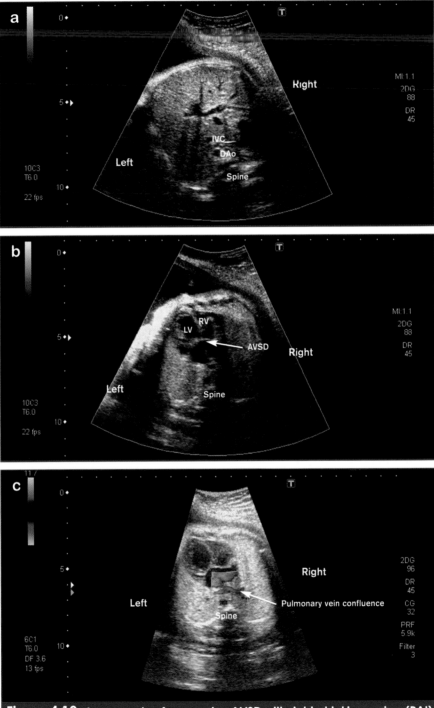

Figure 4.19. An example of a complex AVSD with right atrial isomerism (RAI) and TAPVD. a) The abdominal situs shows features of right atrial isomerism. The stomach is on the right and the descending aorta lies in the midline. The inferior vena cava is lying directly anterior to the aorta. b) The four-chamber view shows that there is a complete AVSD. The heart lies in the midline. c) There is a pulmonary vein confluence behind the left atrium.

Figure continued overleaf.

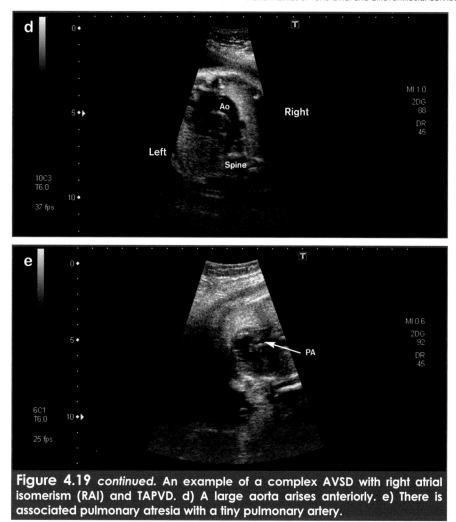

Figure 4.19 *continued.* **An example of a complex AVSD with right atrial isomerism (RAI) and TAPVD. d) A large aorta arises anteriorly. e) There is associated pulmonary atresia with a tiny pulmonary artery.**

on the atrioventricular valve may be required later. If the ventricular component of the defect proves small, or non-existent, then surgery can be safely deferred until later, usually at 2-4 years of age, with a surgical mortality of generally less than 1%.

Adverse factors affecting outcome

The presence of atrioventricular valve regurgitation is an adverse risk factor, which if significant, can lead to the development of fetal hydrops. If there is an imbalance of ventricles, then it may not be possible to achieve a biventricular repair. In these cases, management will be towards surgical palliation. Cases of atrioventricular septal defects associated with other forms of congenital heart disease will generally be associated with a poorer outcome, in particular those cases associated with atrial isomerism.

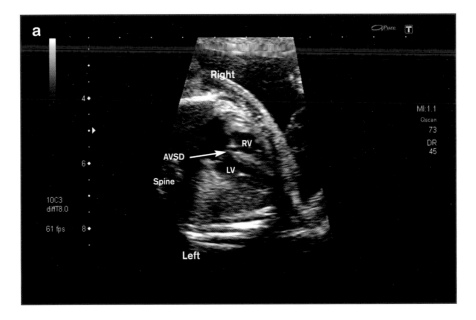

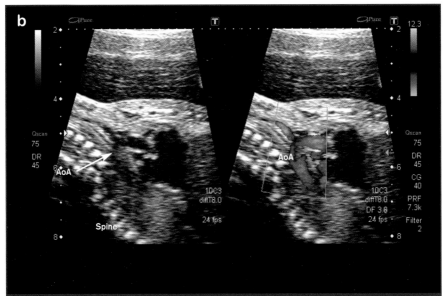

Figure 4.20. An example of an AVSD with coarctation of the aorta. a) The four-chamber view shows an AVSD with balanced ventricular chambers. b) The aortic arch is hypoplastic, though there is forward flow (seen in blue) suggesting coarctation of the aorta.

Outcome in a large single-centre fetal series

Of 687 cases of atrioventricular septal defects diagnosed prenatally, 48% of pregnancies resulted in a termination of pregnancy. Of these cases, 67% had either a chromosomal abnormality (39% of those resulting in termination) or atrial isomerism (28% of those resulting in termination), and further cases had unbalanced ventricles. If the terminations are excluded then the outcome of the continuing pregnancies was: 14% resulting in spontaneous intrauterine death, 21% died in the neonatal period, 11% died in infancy and 53% were alive at last update. Of the continuing pregnancies the outcome is unknown in 1%.

Of cases seen in the last 10 years, a termination of pregnancy took place in 40% of cases and 60% of the continuing pregnancies were alive at last follow-up.

Summary of fetal echocardiographic features associated with AVSD.

- **Common atrioventricular junction**
- **No offset cross at crux due to loss of differential insertion**
- **Atrial and ventricular components of varying sizes**
- **Ventricular imbalance (some cases)**
- **Atrioventricular valve regurgitation (some cases)**

Summary of extracardiac associations in fetal AVSD.

- **Chromosomal**
  - **- 36%**
- **Isomerism**
  - **- 24%**
- **Extracardiac abnormality (normal chromosomes and normal situs)**
  - **- 4%**

Double-inlet ventricle (DIV, DILV)

Prevalence

Double-inlet ventricle accounts for 0.4% of congenital heart disease in postnatal series. In the Evelina fetal series, double-inlet ventricle accounted for 2% of the total. Of these, 93% of cases were a double-inlet left ventricle and 7% were a double-inlet right ventricle.

Definition

In a double-inlet connection, both atria connect predominantly to one ventricular chamber via either two separate atrioventricular valves or a common atrioventricular valve. The ventricle to which both atria drain is usually well formed (dominant ventricle), whereas the other ventricle is usually a rudimentary chamber and communicates with the main chamber via a ventricular septal defect. In most cases the dominant ventricle is a left ventricle (double-inlet left ventricle) with a rudimentary right ventricle. Rarely, the dominant ventricle may be a right ventricle, with a rudimentary left ventricle.

Spectrum

Abnormalities of the atrioventricular valves, such as straddling and leaflet dysplasia may occur. The great arteries can be concordant (normally related) or discordant (transposed). There may be obstruction to the vessel arising from the rudimentary chamber, particularly in cases with a small and restricted ventricular septal defect. In a double-inlet left ventricle with normally related great arteries, there may be some degree of pulmonary stenosis. Aortic arch abnormalities, such as coarctation or an interrupted aortic arch are often associated with cases with transposed great arteries.

Fetal echocardiographic features

In the four-chamber view the ventricular septum cannot be seen to divide the two ventricles equally between the two atrioventricular valves. There is a dominant ventricle and both atrioventricular valves can be seen to open into this dominant ventricle. The flow through both atrioventricular valves demonstrated with colour flow is into the same ventricular chamber (Figures 4.21a-c). Most commonly this chamber is of left ventricular morphology. The great arteries can be concordant or discordant and there may be obstruction to the vessel arising from the rudimentary chamber. In cases with concordant arterial connections, the pulmonary trunk can vary in size from being near normal to being severely hypoplastic. As with tricuspid atresia, this will be dependent on the size of the ventricular septal defect. In cases with discordant arterial connections, the great arteries will arise in parallel orientation. There may be associated aortic obstruction, as in coarctation of the aorta or more rarely an interrupted aortic arch. In such cases the aorta will appear significantly smaller than the pulmonary artery (Figures 4.21d-e).

Extracardiac associations

Double-inlet ventricle is rarely associated with extracardiac or chromosomal abnormalities. However, in our large fetal series, a double-inlet ventricle was associated with chromosomal abnormalities in 2% of cases, which included two cases of trisomy 18. A further 2% had extracardiac abnormalities.

Management and outcome

This is a complex form of congenital heart disease for which management after birth is staged surgical palliation. The initial management will depend on whether there is associated pulmonary obstruction or coarctation of the aorta. Management thereafter is towards achieving a single-ventricle circulation (Fontan type circulation – see section on tricuspid atresia).

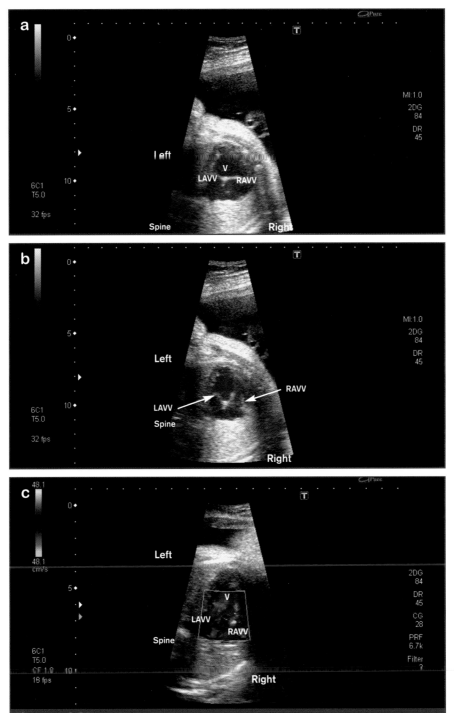

Figure 4.21. An example of a double-inlet ventricle with discordant atrioventricular connections (transposition) and coarctation of the aorta. a) The four-chamber view shows that both atrioventricular valves appear to connect to a dominant ventricle. b) There are two opening atrioventricular valves that appear to drain to the dominant ventricle. c) Colour flow confirms that both atrioventricular valves drain to a dominant ventricle (seen in red). *Figure continued overleaf.*

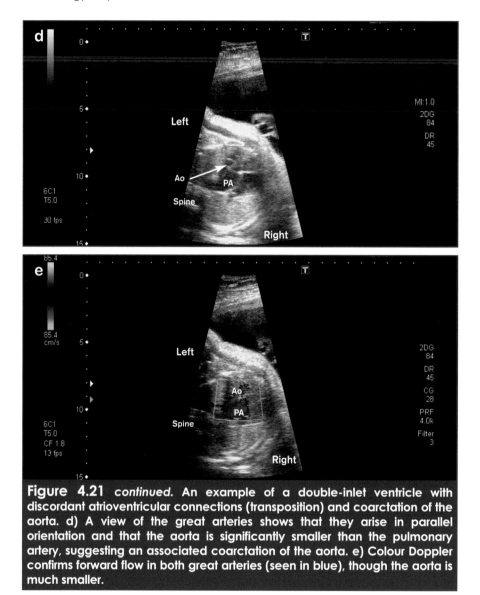

Figure 4.21 *continued.* **An example of a double-inlet ventricle with discordant atrioventricular connections (transposition) and coarctation of the aorta. d) A view of the great arteries shows that they arise in parallel orientation and that the aorta is significantly smaller than the pulmonary artery, suggesting an associated coarctation of the aorta. e) Colour Doppler confirms forward flow in both great arteries (seen in blue), though the aorta is much smaller.**

Outcome in a large single-centre fetal series

Of 89 cases of double-inlet ventricle diagnosed prenatally, the majority of which were a double-inlet left ventricle, 55% of pregnancies resulted in a termination of pregnancy. If the terminations are excluded then the outcome of the continuing pregnancies was: 10% resulting in spontaneous intrauterine death, 10% died in the neonatal period, 5% died in infancy and 75% were alive at last update.

Of cases seen in the last 10 years, a termination of pregnancy took place in 51% of cases and 84% of the continuing pregnancies were alive at last follow-up.

Summary of fetal echocardiographic features associated with DIV.

- Both atrioventricular valves drain predominantly into one dominant ventricle
- Other ventricle usually very hypoplastic
- Great arteries frequently transposed (discordant arterial connection)
- Ventricular septal defect
- May have associated coarctation
    - more frequent with discordant arterial connections
- May have associated pulmonary stenosis
    - more frequent with concordant arterial connections

Summary of extracardiac associations in fetal DIV.

- Chromosomal
    - 2%
- Extracardiac abnormality (normal chromosomes)
    - 2%

Chapter 5

Abnormalities of the four-chamber view (II)
Abnormalities of atrioventricular valves and the ventricular septum with normal connections

Summary

- **Tricuspid valve abnormalities**
  - Ebstein's anomaly of tricuspid valve
  - Tricuspid valve dysplasia
- **Ventricular septal defects**

Tricuspid valve abnormalities

Ebstein's malformation

Prevalence
This is a rare abnormality accounting for approximately 0.3-1.0% of congenital heart disease in postnatal series. In the Evelina fetal series, Ebstein's anomaly accounted for 1.9% of the total series and 1.2% of all cases of fetal congenital heart disease seen in the last 10 years.

Definition
In Ebstein's malformation, the attachments of the septal and mural leaflets of the tricuspid valve are displaced downward into the right ventricle and the anterior leaflet is elongated.

Spectrum
The degree of displacement of the tricuspid valve is variable and there is usually some tricuspid regurgitation (incompetence), though the severity of this can vary. Ebstein's malformation can be associated with other cardiac abnormalities, such as ventricular septal defect, pulmonary stenosis and coarctation of the aorta. More rarely, Ebstein's anomaly can occur in the setting of atrioventricular and ventriculo-arterial discordance (corrected transposition of the great vessels – see Chapter 7). There is also an increased risk of arrhythmias developing.

Fetal echocardiographic features

In the four-chamber view the tricuspid valve will be seen to be displaced apically, with an exaggerated differential insertion. The degree of displacement of the valve is variable and in some cases the tricuspid valve leaflet may appear tethered to the ventricular septum (Figures 5.1, 5.2a, 5.3a and 5.4a-b). The anterior leaflet will appear elongated (Figure 5.4a). There will often be tricuspid regurgitation, the severity of which varies from case to case (Figures 5.2b, 5.3b and 5.4c). Severe tricuspid regurgitation can cause right atrial enlargement, which results in cardiomegaly and an increased cardiothoracic ratio (Figures 5.2a, 5.3a-b and 5.4a-c). However, in some cases there may be little tricuspid regurgitation and minimal or no cardiomegaly (Figures 5.1 and 5.5). Secondary lung hypoplasia as a result of longstanding compression from severe cardiomegaly can be a life-threatening associated feature. Obstruction to the right ventricular outflow tract is common, so that there may be associated pulmonary stenosis or atresia (Figure 5.3c-d). In some cases there may be reduced forward flow into the pulmonary artery as a result of gross tricuspid regurgitation. This may produce functional pulmonary atresia which may be difficult to distinguish from anatomical atresia.

Extracardiac associations

This type of malformation can occasionally be associated with extracardiac anomalies. In our large fetal series, Ebstein's anomaly was associated with chromosomal abnormalities in 1.2% of cases (one case of trisomy 21) and a further 6% had an extracardiac anomaly. The latter included cleft lip and palate, diaphragmatic hernia, duodenal atresia and sacrococcygeal teratoma. Fetal hydrops was associated in 7% of cases, being seen particularly in cases with severe tricuspid regurgitation.

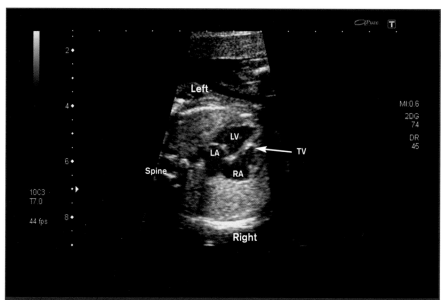

Figure 5.1. An example of Ebstein's anomaly with mild displacement of the tricuspid valve. The four-chamber view shows that the tricuspid valve is displaced apically, with an exaggerated differential insertion. The heart size is within normal limits in this case.

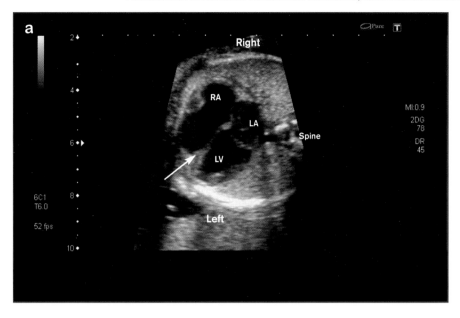

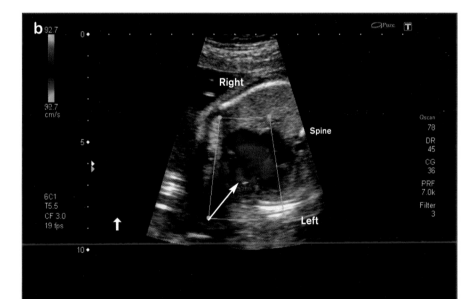

Figure 5.2. An example of Ebstein's anomaly with marked displacement of the tricuspid valve. a) In the four-chamber view the tricuspid valve is not seen in its normal position. The valve is severely displaced towards the apex of the right ventricle (arrow). There is moderate cardiomegaly. b) Colour flow shows tricuspid regurgitation which originates near the apex of the ventricle in the region of the tricuspid valve insertion (arrow).

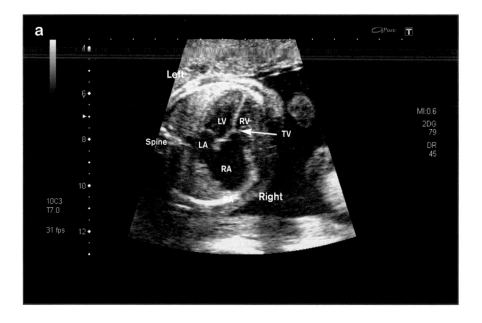

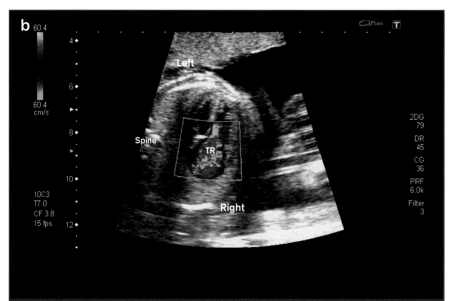

Figure 5.3. An example of Ebstein's anomaly with marked cardiomegaly and associated pulmonary atresia. a) The four-chamber view in this example shows marked cardiomegaly with an increased cardiothoracic ratio. The tricuspid valve is displaced apically. b) There is significant tricuspid regurgitation associated with the displaced tricuspid valve resulting in right atrial enlargement and cardiomegaly.

Figure continued overleaf.

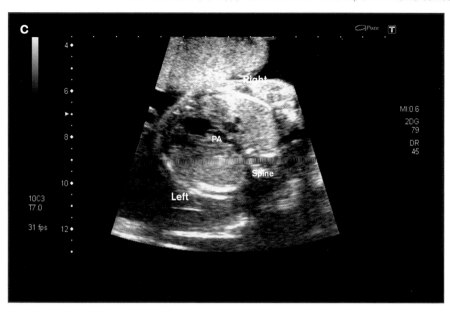

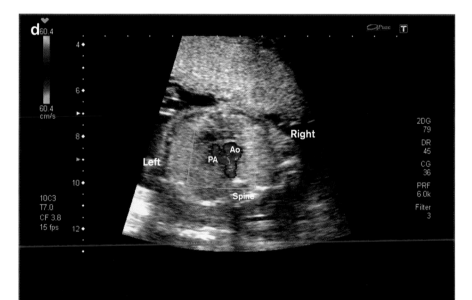

Figure 5.3 *continued.* An example of Ebstein's anomaly with marked cardiomegaly and associated pulmonary atresia. c) A small pulmonary artery can be seen arising from the right ventricle. d) There is reverse flow from the duct in the pulmonary artery (seen in red) confirming severe obstruction to the right ventricular outflow. The forward flow in the aorta is seen in blue.

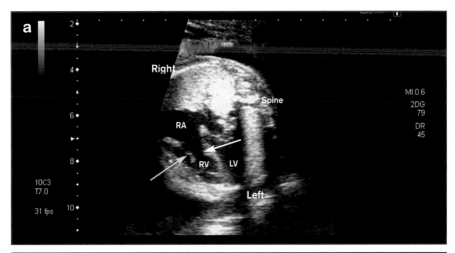

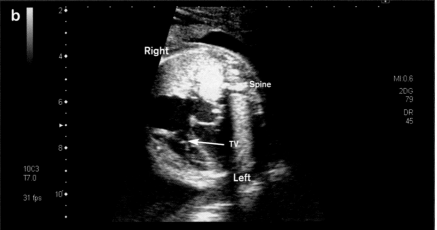

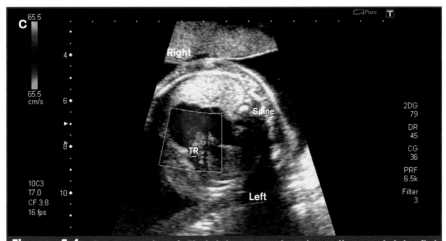

Figure 5.4. An example of Ebstein's anomaly where the septal leaflet appears tethered to the septum. a) There is moderate cardiomegaly. The septal leaflet of the tricuspid valve appears tethered to the ventricular septum (white arrow). The anterior leaflet is elongated (yellow arrow). b) The tricuspid valve leaflets do not meet completely when the valve is closed. c) Colour flow shows significant tricuspid regurgitation (seen In red).

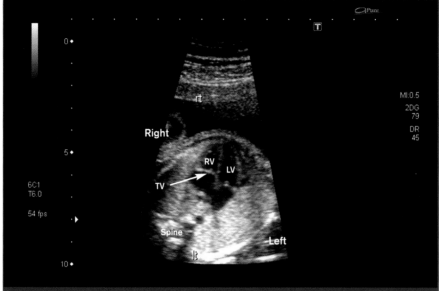

Figure 5.5. An example of mild Ebstein's anomaly associated with dextroposition of the heart. The heart size is within normal limits.

Management and outcome

Ebstein's anomaly is a spectrum disorder with a very wide range of immediate, medium-term and longer-term problems. During fetal life the cardiac findings may remain stable but, in some cases, tricuspid regurgitation can worsen as pregnancy advances, resulting in increasing cardiomegaly and the development of hydrops. This has a major adverse impact on the prognosis.

After birth the immediate concern is adequate ventilation, particularly in cases where there has been marked cardiomegaly compromising lung development. Some babies are duct-dependent and require an urgent systemic to pulmonary artery shunt (Blalock-Taussig shunt) to maintain pulmonary blood flow, whilst others do not need any early surgical intervention or support.

Outcome in a large single-centre fetal series

Of 82 cases of Ebstein's anomaly diagnosed prenatally, 44% of pregnancies resulted in a termination of pregnancy. If the terminations are excluded then the outcome of the continuing pregnancies was: 24% resulting in spontaneous intrauterine death, 22% died in the neonatal period, 4% died in infancy and 50% were alive at last update.

Of cases seen in the last 10 years, a termination of pregnancy took place in 23% of cases and 65% of the continuing pregnancies were alive at last follow-up.

Summary of fetal echocardiographic features associated with Ebstein's anomaly.

- Downward displacement of tricuspid valve leaflets (septal and mural) into the right ventricle
- Long anterior leaflet
- Right atrial enlargement
- Tricuspid regurgitation (incompetence)
- Increased cardiothoracic ratio
- Right ventricular outflow tract obstruction

Summary of extracardiac associations in fetal Ebstein's anomaly.

- Chromosomal
  - 1.2%
- Extracardiac abnormality (normal chromosomes)
  - 6%

Tricuspid valve dysplasia (TVD)

Prevalence
This lesion is not commonly diagnosed as a separate entity in postnatal life. In the Evelina fetal series, tricuspid valve dysplasia accounted for 1.5% of the total series and 0.7% of all cases of fetal congenital heart disease seen in the last 10 years.

Definition
In tricuspid valve dysplasia the attachments of the tricuspid valve leaflets are normal but the leaflets are dysplastic. As a result, the valve is usually incompetent. Tricuspid dysplasia can sometimes be difficult to distinguish from Ebstein's malformation, as the two overlap each other anatomically.

Fetal echocardiographic features
There is usually some degree of cardiomegaly, but as in Ebstein's anomaly the level of this is variable. In the four-chamber view the tricuspid valve appears thick, nodular and dysplastic (Figures 5.6a). There is often associated tricuspid regurgitation which results in right atrial enlargement (Figure 5.6b). The severity of this is variable, but in severe cases this can result in secondary pulmonary hypoplasia, as in similar cases with Ebstein's anomaly. Obstruction to the right ventricular outflow tract is common so there may be associated pulmonary stenosis or atresia, which in some cases may be functional.

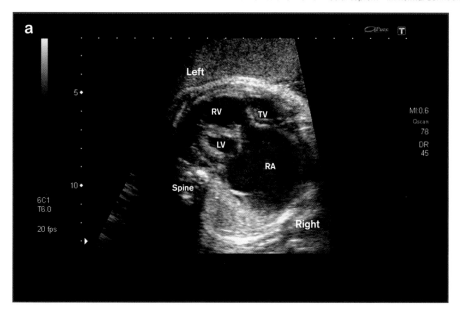

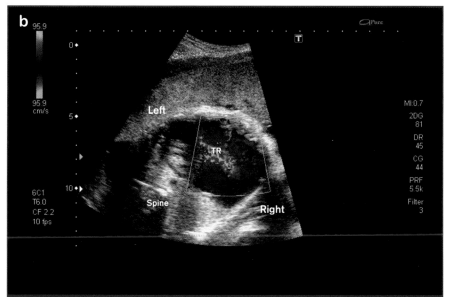

Figure 5.6. An example of tricuspid valve dysplasia at the severe end of the spectrum. a) In the four-chamber view there is marked cardiomegaly with a 'wall to wall' heart. The right atrium in particular is grossly dilated. The tricuspid valve leaflets are dysplastic and do not co-apt (do not meet). b) Colour flow demonstrates severe tricuspid regurgitation.

Extracardiac associations

Tricuspid valve dysplasia can be associated with extracardiac abnormalities. In our large fetal series, tricuspid valve dysplasia was associated with chromosomal abnormalities in 8% of cases, which included trisomy 21, trisomy 13 and trisomy 18. A further 11% had other extracardiac abnormalities and 13% had associated fetal hydrops.

Management and outcome

As with Ebstein's anomaly, tricuspid valve dysplasia has a wide spectrum from mild to severe forms. The management and outcome when diagnosed in fetal life is similar to that for Ebstein's anomaly described above.

Outcome in a large single-centre fetal series

Of 64 cases of tricuspid valve dysplasia diagnosed prenatally, 44% of pregnancies resulted in a termination of pregnancy. If the terminations are excluded then the outcome of the continuing pregnancies was: 32% resulting in spontaneous intrauterine death, 30% died in the neonatal period, 2% died in infancy and 36% were alive at last update.

Of cases seen in the last 10 years, a termination of pregnancy took place in 46% of cases and 71% of the continuing pregnancies were alive at last follow-up. The higher percentage of survivors is a reflection of improved obstetric screening so that cases at the less severe end of the spectrum of abnormality are increasingly being detected.

Summary of fetal echocardiographic features associated with TVD.

- Dysplastic but normally positioned tricuspid valve leaflets
- Right atrial enlargement
- Right ventricular enlargement
- Tricuspid regurgitation (incompetence)
- Increased cardiothoracic ratio
- Right ventricular outflow tract obstruction

Summary of extracardiac associations in fetal TVD.

- Chromosomal
  - 8%
- Extracardiac abnormality (normal chromosomes)
  - 11%

Ventricular septal defect (VSD)

Prevalence

Ventricular septal defects are the commonest type of congenital heart disease in infancy, accounting for up to 25-30% of all cases of congenital heart disease in postnatal series. In the Evelina fetal series, isolated ventricular septal defects accounted for 11.3% of the total series and 14.2% of all cases of fetal congenital heart disease seen in the last 10 years.

Definition

A ventricular septal defect is a hole in the septum between the two ventricular chambers. The ventricular septum is a curvilinear structure and can be divided into four areas by anatomic landmarks in the right ventricle. The four areas are the membranous septum, the muscular septum, the inlet septum and the outlet septum. Thus, ventricular septal defects can be classified depending on their site and can be:

- Perimembranous (also have been described as membranous or infracristal). These are the most common types of ventricular septal defects and occur in the membranous septum (small fibrous area in continuity with the tricuspid valve and the aortic valve) with extension to the adjacent muscular portion of the septum. These can be further classified as perimembranous inlet, perimembranous outlet, or perimembranous muscular.
- Muscular (also known as trabecular). These defects are entirely surrounded by the muscular septum. They may be single or multiple and can be further subdivided depending on their location, for example, they may be mid-muscular or apical.
- Inlet (also called posterior or inferior). The location of these defects is between the two atrioventricular valves (mitral and tricuspid) and similar to that seen in atrioventricular septal defects, but these are not usually associated with abnormalities of the atrioventricular valves.
- Outlet (also have been described as supracristal, infundibular, conal, subpulmonary or doubly committed subarterial). These defects are located below the arterial valves and involve the infundibular or conal septum.

Spectrum

Ventricular septal defects can occur in any part of the ventricular septum, as described above, and may be single or multiple. A ventricular septal defect can occur in isolation or may be a component of many complex forms of congenital heart disease.

Fetal echocardiographic features

The ventricular septum can be visualised in the four-chamber view and in views imaging the outflow tracts, where the septum should normally appear intact. A defect may be seen in any part of the septum, though some defects may be difficult to visualise because of their size or position. Care should be taken when imaging the four-chamber view with the ultrasound beam parallel to the ventricular septum, as drop out is often seen at the crux of the heart where the septum is thin (Figure 5.7). A real defect may have bright edges at its border helping to distinguish a true defect from a false positive. It is also helpful in this situation to

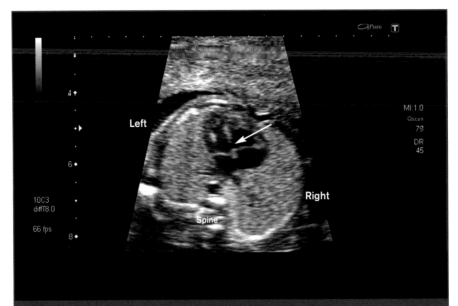

Figure 5.7. In this four-chamber view drop-out is seen in the region of the crux (arrow). This appearance was not seen in any other views and this heart was confirmed to be normal after birth.

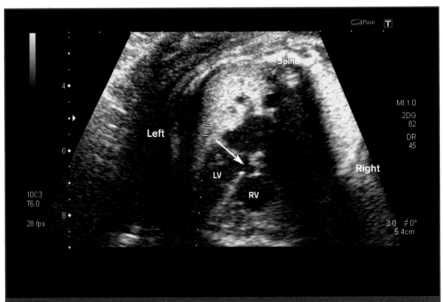

Figure 5.8. An example of a perimembranous ventricular septal defect (arrow) seen in a four-chamber view.

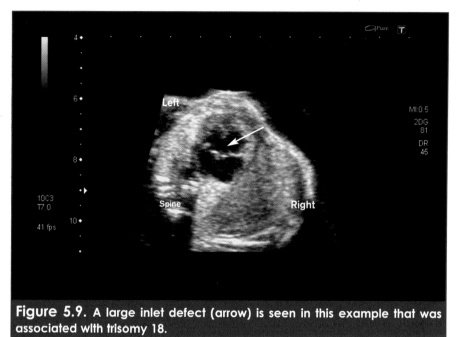

Figure 5.9. A large inlet defect (arrow) is seen in this example that was associated with trisomy 18.

obtain a four-chamber view in a different orientation with the ultrasound beam perpendicular to the ventricular septum. An example of a perimembranous defect is shown in Figure 5.8. A large inlet defect is shown in Figure 5.9. An example of a large muscular defect is shown in Figures 5.10a-c. Colour flow can help to confirm cases, if flow can be clearly demonstrated crossing the septum. The shunting is usually bidirectional in fetal life (Figure 5.10b-c). Small muscular defects may not always be visible without the use of colour flow but are detected when the colour map is turned on (Figures 5.11a-c). However, care is required in interpretation, as colour is sometimes seen smearing across the septum in the absence of a ventricular septal defect, particularly if the colour flow map is not adequately set. Multiple defects can occur and may be in any part of the ventricular septum (Figure 5.12). An example of a malalignment type of defect, where there is associated great artery override, is shown in Figure 5.13. This can be associated with other great artery abnormalities which are discussed in Chapter 8. An example of a large ventricular septal defect that was associated with a double-outlet right ventricle is shown in Figure 5.14 (see also Chapter 7).

Extracardiac associations

Ventricular septal defects can be associated with chromosomal abnormalities as well as extracardiac structural abnormalities, though the risk of this is dependent on the type of defect. Large perimembranous or inlet defects may be associated with trisomies and other chromosomal abnormalities. Malalignment type of defects, where there is aortic override, are strongly associated with extracardiac abnormalities and chromosomal anomalies, in particular trisomy 18. In contrast, small muscular defects often occur in isolation and are rarely associated with other abnormalities.

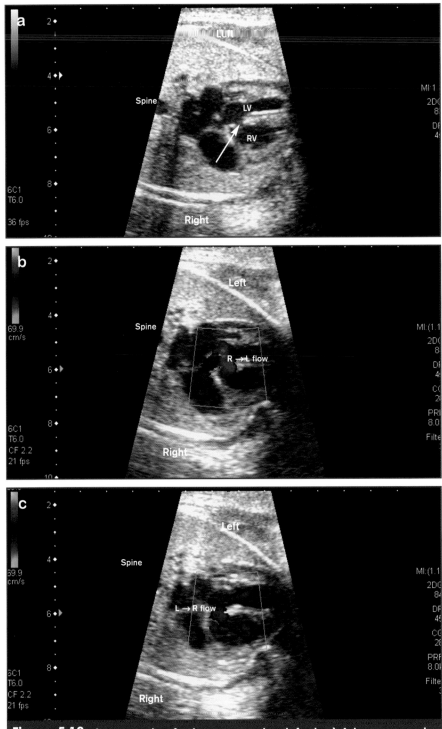

Figure 5.10. An example of a large muscular defect. a) A large muscular defect is seen near the crux of the heart (arrow). b-c) Colour flow demonstrates bidirectional flow across the defect, with right to left flow (red) seen in b and left to right flow (blue) seen in c.

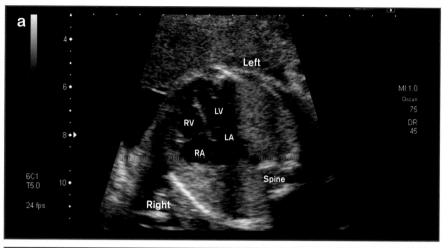

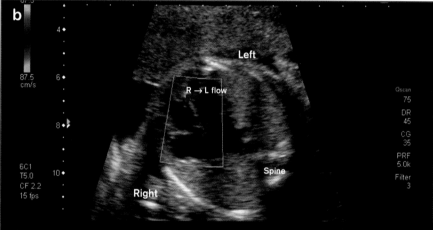

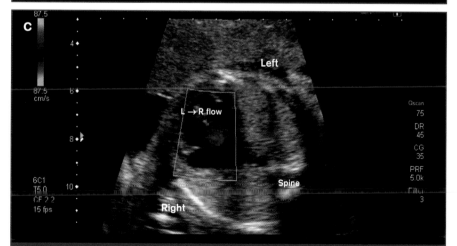

Figure 5.11. A small muscular defect detected with colour Doppler. a) In the four-chamber view no definite defect is seen in the ventricular septum. b-c) Colour flow demonstrates bidirectional shunting across a small muscular defect with right to left flow (red) seen in b and left to right flow (blue) seen in c.

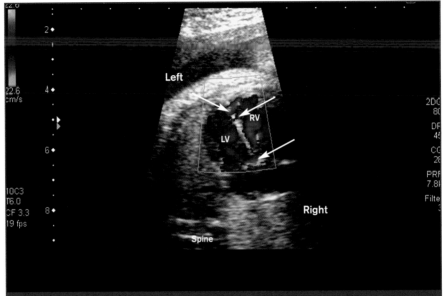

Figure 5.12. An example of multiple ventricular septal defects demonstrated with colour flow (arrows).

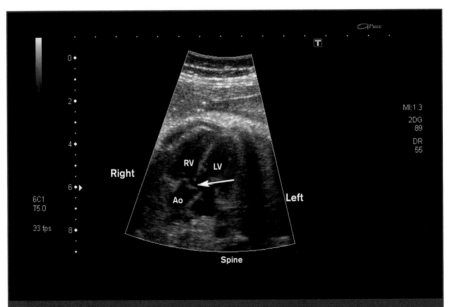

Figure 5.13. A malalignment type of ventricular septal defect with great artery override is seen in this example. The arrow indicates the aortic valve overriding the crest of the ventricular septum.

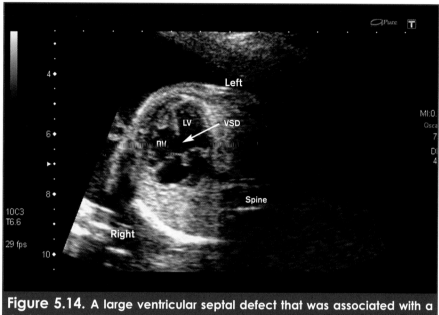

Figure 5.14. A large ventricular septal defect that was associated with a double-outlet right ventricle (see Chapter 7).

In our large fetal series, 23% of all cases of ventricular septal defect (with no other cardiac lesion) had a chromosomal abnormality. Of those with an abnormal karyotype, 47% had trisomy 18, 31% had trisomy 21 and 10% had trisomy 13. The remaining cases included triploidy, Turner's syndrome, trisomy 22, 22q11 deletion and other translocations and deletions.

A further 17% had extracardiac abnormalities, which included anal atresia, anterior chest wall defects, cleft lip and palate, cystic hygroma, diaphragmatic hernia, duodenal atresia, encephalocoele, exomphalos, holoprosencephaly, hydrocephalus, hypospadias, microcephaly, oesophageal atresia, polydactyly, radial aplasia, renal abnormalities, talipes, scoliosis and ventriculomegaly. In addition, a few cases were associated with genetic syndromes with normal chromosomes, such as VACTERL and CHARGE associations.

Management and outcome

The management and outcome of ventricular septal defects will depend on the size, number and position of the defect. Isolated ventricular septal defects do not usually cause cardiac compromise before birth. After birth, once the pulmonary vascular resistance falls, there will be an increasing left to right shunt of blood through the ventricular septal defect and if the defect is of significant size, this will lead to symptoms. In these cases, the definitive treatment is with surgical closure of the ventricular septal defect, which is usually undertaken at 3-4 months of age. The surgical mortality is less than 2%. The long-term prognosis following effective closure of the ventricular septal defect is very good. In some cases with multiple defects or defects in inaccessible regions such as the apex, surgical closure may not be possible. In these cases, if there is a significant shunt across the ventricular septum, then the surgical management is with a pulmonary artery band. Small ventricular septal defects may not be of any haemodynamic significance and thus require no treatment and some of these may close spontaneously.

The overall prognosis for babies with isolated ventricular septal defects will be influenced by associated abnormalities, which can include structural extracardiac abnormalities, chromosomal abnormalities or other genetic syndromes.

Outcome in a large single-centre fetal series

Of 482 cases of isolated ventricular septal defect diagnosed prenatally, 16% of pregnancies resulted in a termination of pregnancy. Of these cases, 67% had a chromosomal abnormality and a further 30% had an extracardiac abnormality. If the terminations are excluded then the outcome of the continuing pregnancies was: 7% resulting in spontaneous intrauterine death, 8% died in the neonatal period, 2% died in infancy and 78% were alive at last update. Of the continuing pregnancies the outcome is unknown in 5%.

Summary of fetal echocardiographic features associated with a VSD.

- **Discontinuity in ventricular septum suggesting defect**
- **Bright edges to defect**
- **Colour flow demonstrated across defect**

Summary of extracardiac associations in fetal VSD.

- **Chromosomal**
  - 23%
- **Extracardiac abnormality (normal chromosomes)**
  - 17%

Chapter 6

Abnormalities of the four-chamber view (III)

Obstructive lesions at the ventriculo-arterial junction that may be associated with an abnormal four-chamber view

Summary

- **Aortic valve**
  - **Aortic atresia**
    - hypoplastic left heart syndrome
    - aortic atresia with ventricular septal defect (see Chapter 8)
    - aortic atresia with other congenital heart disease
  - **Aortic stenosis**
    - critical aortic stenosis
    - non-critical forms of aortic stenosis
- **Pulmonary valve**
  - **Pulmonary atresia with an intact interventricular septum**
  - **Pulmonary stenosis**
    - critical pulmonary stenosis
    - non-critical forms of pulmonary stenosis

Obstructive lesions of both the arterial valves and the aortic arch can produce an abnormal four-chamber view. Although it is the severe end of the spectrum that will be associated with an abnormal four-chamber view, these lesions are discussed in their entirety in this section, apart from coarctation of the aorta which is discussed in Chapter 9.

Obstructive lesions of the aortic valve associated with an abnormal four-chamber view

Aortic atresia and hypoplastic left heart syndrome (HLH)

Prevalence

The prevalence of hypoplastic left heart syndrome (HLH) varies from 3.8-9% in different postnatal series of congenital heart disease. Hypoplastic left heart syndrome is one of the commonest types of cardiac abnormality in fetal series. In the Evelina fetal series, hypoplastic left heart syndrome accounted for 15.5% of the total, with cases with aortic atresia accounting for 12.3% of the total. Thus, although aortic atresia is not associated in all cases of hypoplastic left heart syndrome, it is present in the majority (see below). Hypoplastic left heart syndrome accounted for 12.4% of all cases of fetal congenital heart disease seen in the last 10 years.

Definition

Aortic atresia implies a complete obstruction at the level of the aortic valve. This is usually associated with a very hypoplastic ascending aorta and arch.

Spectrum of aortic atresia

Aortic atresia is most commonly seen in the context of hypoplastic left heart syndrome where it is associated with an underdeveloped left ventricle. There may be associated mitral atresia (see Chapter 4), or the mitral valve may be very small but still patent. All these cases are associated with an abnormal four-chamber view.

Rare forms of aortic atresia exist, which can be associated with a normally developed left ventricle. These cases are associated with a ventricular septal defect, but the diagnosis of aortic atresia may be overlooked unless the arterial connections are carefully examined (see Chapter 8). In addition, aortic atresia can also very rarely be associated with atrioventricular septal defects, corrected transposition (atrioventricular and ventriculo-arterial discordance), Ebstein's anomaly of the tricuspid valve and tricuspid atresia (see Chapters 4, 5 and 7).

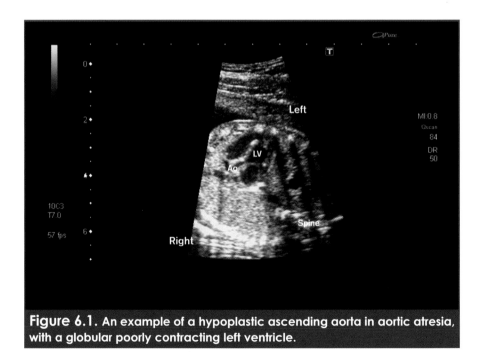

Figure 6.1. An example of a hypoplastic ascending aorta in aortic atresia, with a globular poorly contracting left ventricle.

Spectrum of hypoplastic left heart syndrome

The majority of cases of hypoplastic left heart syndrome will have either mitral and aortic atresia or aortic atresia with a small but patent mitral valve. Around 5-6% may be cases at the severe end of the spectrum of critical aortic stenosis with a hypoplastic poorly functioning left ventricle, and 6-7% may be at the severe end of the spectrum of coarctation of the aorta with a very small left ventricle and aorta, but with both mitral and aortic valves being patent.

Fetal echocardiographic findings

In all cases of aortic atresia, the aortic valve is atretic and the ascending aorta and aortic arch are hypoplastic (Figures 6.1, 6.2a and 6.3a). No forward flow is detected in the ascending aorta and there is retrograde flow in the aortic arch from the arterial duct, which may be easily detected in the three-vessel view (Figure 6.2b), but may also be detected in the longitudinal view of the arch (Figure 6.3b).

Hypoplastic left heart syndrome

In cases of mitral and aortic atresia, the left ventricle is tiny and often not discernable (Figures 4.4a and 4.5a – see Chapter 4). In cases where the mitral valve is still patent, the left ventricle is globular, echogenic and poorly contracting (Figure 6.4a and 6.5a). The left ventricle in these latter cases is usually hypoplastic, but its size can be variable. Even though the mitral valve may be patent, little inflow is detectable into the left ventricle (Figures 6.4b and 6.5b) and occasionally there may be mitral regurgitation (Figure 6.5c). In hypoplastic left heart syndrome, there will be a left to right shunt at atrial level (Figure 6.6). In a small number of cases the foramen ovale may be restrictive or intact (Figures 6.7 and 6.8). In these cases, the pulmonary veins may appear dilated (Figure 6.9a) and the pulmonary venous Doppler may be helpful in predicting a severely restricted or intact atrial septum (Figures 6.9b-c), as there will be an increase in the velocity of the reversal wave and loss of normal diastolic flow.

Aortic atresia with other forms of congenital heart disease
(For aortic atresia with ventricular septal defect see Chapter 8)

When aortic atresia is associated with other forms of congenital heart disease such as atrioventricular septal defects, corrected transposition (atrioventricular and ventriculo-arterial discordance), Ebstein's anomaly of the tricuspid valve or tricuspid atresia, the echocardiographic features of the associated lesions (see Chapters 4, 5 and 7) will be seen in addition to the features of aortic atresia.

Extracardiac associations

It is very unusual for cases of aortic atresia with a patent mitral valve to be associated with extracardiac abnormalities. However, hypoplastic left heart syndrome with aortic and mitral atresia can occasionally be associated with chromosomal anomalies, including Turner's syndrome, trisomy 18, trisomy 13, and various translocations or deletions. In our large fetal series, hypoplastic left heart syndrome was associated with chromosomal abnormalities in 4% of cases (none of which had aortic atresia with a patent mitral valve). Of these, 36% had trisomy 18, 14% had trisomy 13, 11% had 45XO Turner's karyotype and the remaining had various chromosomal abnormalities including unbalanced translocations and deletions. A further 4% of cases had an extracardiac abnormality, which included cases with cystic

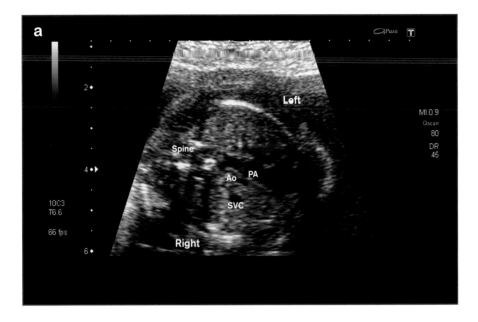

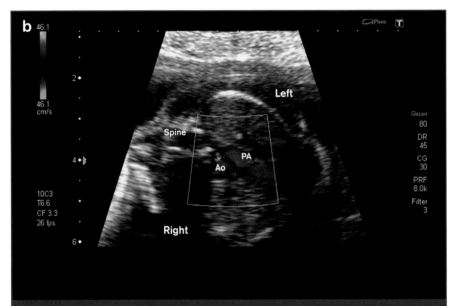

Figure 6.2. a) In the three-vessel view the aortic arch is very hypoplastic. b) No forward flow is detected in the ascending aorta and there is retrograde flow in the aortic arch from the arterial duct (seen in blue).

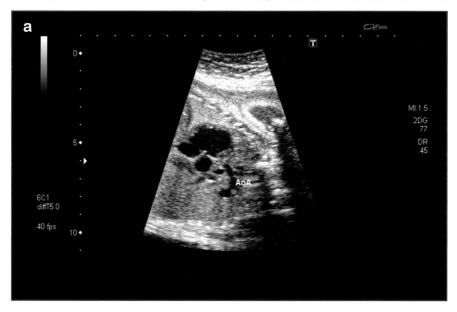

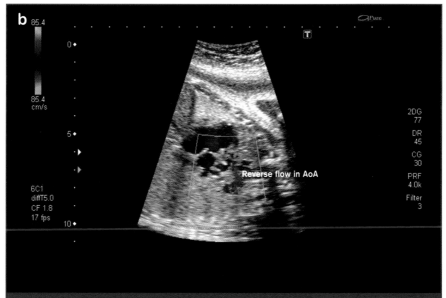

Figure 6.3. a) A longitudinal view of the aortic arch showing it is very hypoplastic. b) No forward flow is detected in the aortic arch and there is retrograde filling from the arterial duct (seen in red).

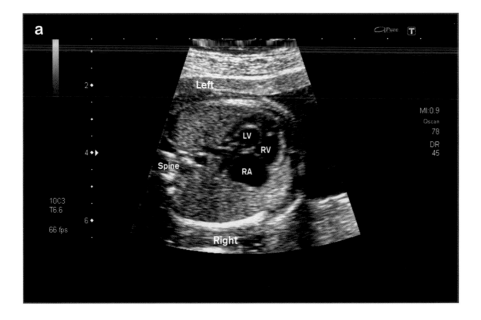

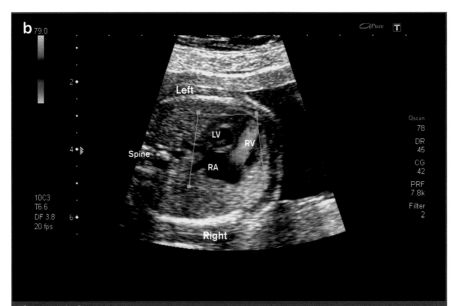

Figure 6.4. The four-chamber view in aortic atresia. a) The left ventricle is hypoplastic, globular and echogenic. b) Colour flow shows the flow across the tricuspid valve (seen in red) but there is little forward flow seen into the left ventricle.

Obstructive lesions at the ventriculo-arterial junction that may be associated with an abnormal four-chamber view

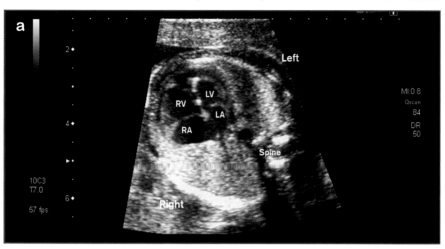

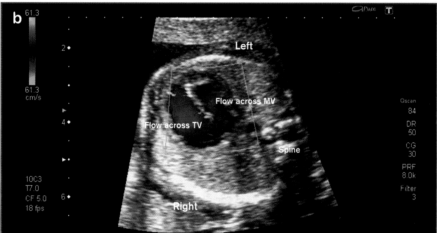

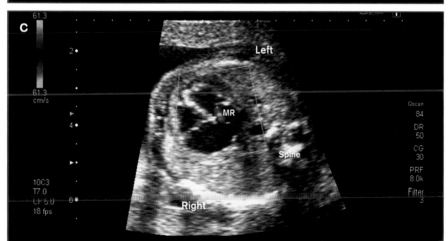

Figure 6.5. The four-chamber view in aortic atresia showing a reasonable sized left ventricle. a) The left ventricle in this example is only slightly small, though it is globular, echogenic and was contracting poorly. b) Colour Doppler shows the normal flow across the tricuspid valve and a reduced amount of flow across the mitral valve (both seen in red). c) There is a small amount of mitral regurgitation detected in this example (seen in blue).

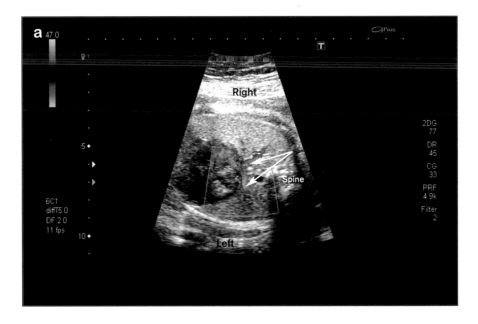

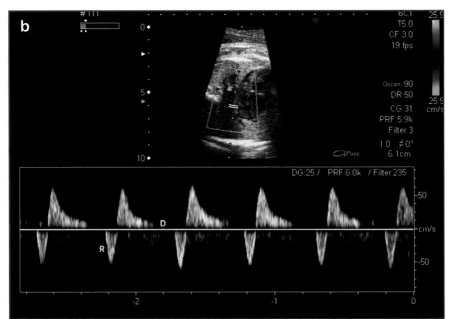

Figure 6.9. a) The four-chamber view of an example of aortic atresia with a very restricted atrial septum showing dilated pulmonary veins (arrows). b) The pulmonary venous pattern indicative of a restricted atrial septum. There is an increase in the velocity of the reversal wave (R) and loss of diastolic flow (D). This can be compared to the normal pattern in Figure 2.24 or a common pattern for hypoplastic left heart syndrome as shown in c) where there is some reversal of flow during atrial systole (R) but diastolic flow is present.

Figure continued overleaf.

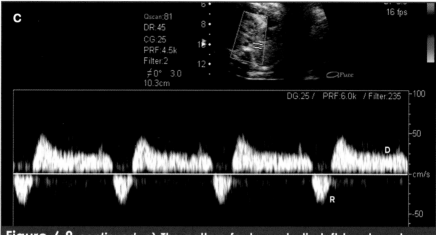

Figure 6.9 *continued.* **c) The pattern for hypoplastic left heart syndrome where there is some reversal of flow during atrial systole (R) but diastolic flow is present.**

Outcome of hypoplastic left heart syndrome in a large single-centre fetal series
Of 663 cases of hypoplastic left heart syndrome diagnosed prenatally, 62% of pregnancies resulted in a termination of pregnancy. If the terminations are excluded then the outcome of the continuing pregnancies was: 8% resulting in spontaneous intrauterine death, 45% died in the neonatal period, 8% died in infancy and 37% were alive at last update. Of the continuing pregnancies the outcome is unknown in 2%.

Of cases seen in the last 10 years, a termination of pregnancy took place in 45% of cases and 49% of the continuing pregnancies were alive at last follow-up. Not all cases proceeded to surgery, so that the survival here does not represent the survival from surgery alone.

Summary of fetal echocardiographic features of aortic atresia when associated with HLH.

- **Hypoplastic left ventricle**
- **Echogenic left ventricle (if mitral valve patent)**
- **Hypoplastic aorta**
- **No forward flow across the aortic valve**
- **Retrograde flow in the aortic arch**
- **Left to right shunt at atrial level**

Summary of fetal echocardiographic features of aortic atresia when associated with other CHD.

- Features of other congenital heart disease
- Hypoplastic aorta and aortic arch
- No forward flow across aortic valve
- Retrograde flow in aortic arch

Summary of extracardiac associations in fetal HLH.

- Chromosomal
  - 4%
- Extracardiac abnormality (normal chromosomes)
  - 4%

Aortic stenosis (AS)

Prevalence
Aortic stenosis accounts for approximately 2.9% of congenital heart disease in postnatal series. In the Evelina fetal series, aortic stenosis accounted for 2% of the total, with 91% of cases having critical aortic stenosis.

Definition
Aortic stenosis means that there is an obstruction to blood flow in the left ventricular outflow tract from the left ventricle into the aorta. The site of obstruction may be subvalvar, valvar or supravalvar, though in fetal life the aortic stenosis is predominantly valvar.

Spectrum
Aortic stenosis often occurs in isolation but can also commonly occur with other left heart obstructive lesions, such as coarctation of the aorta and mitral valve abnormalities. Shone syndrome is a complex of left heart disease which includes mitral stenosis, aortic stenosis and coarctation of the aorta. Less commonly, aortic stenosis can occur in association with other forms of congenital heart disease.

The stenotic aortic valve can be bicuspid or even unicuspid, instead of having three leaflets as in the normal aortic valve. The severity of obstruction can vary from mild to severe or critical.

Fetal echocardiographic features

The appearance of the fetal heart will vary depending on the degree of obstruction to the aortic valve.

Mild to moderate cases

The four-chamber view will usually appear normal if the obstruction is at the milder end of the spectrum. In particular, the left ventricle will appear to be of normal size with normal function (Figures 6.10a-b). The aortic root and ascending aorta size will be normal. The aortic valve may appear bright or dysplastic (Figure 6.10c). There will be turbulent flow across the aortic valve, with the Doppler velocity across the valve being elevated (Figures 6.10d-e).

Moderate to severe cases

In moderate to severe cases, the left ventricle may appear normal or sometimes hypertrophied (Figure 6.11a). The left ventricular function may be preserved. Mitral regurgitation, which can be detected using colour flow, can be associated in some cases. The aortic root and ascending aorta size are usually within the normal range in the mid-trimester, but can become small for the gestational age as pregnancy advances. The aortic valve will appear dysplastic, thickened and doming (Figures 6.10c and 6.11b). Colour flow will demonstrate turbulent flow across the valve and the aortic arch in some cases (Figures 6.10d and 6.11c). Pulsed Doppler will show an increased aortic Doppler velocity above the normal range and will confirm that the valve is stenotic. In cases where left ventricular function is preserved, high velocities ranging from 2-4m/second may be documented (Figures 6.10e and 6.11d).

Critical cases

In critical aortic stenosis, the left ventricle is typically dilated with very poor function. Often there is increased echogenicity of the left ventricular walls and papillary muscles of the mitral valve (Figures 6.12a and 6.13a). This appearance correlates well with the finding of endocardial fibroelastosis at post mortem examination and implies damage to the ventricular wall. The mitral valve often appears abnormal and is usually very restricted in opening. There is reduced flow demonstrated across the mitral valve (Figure 6.12b) and mitral regurgitation may often be detected in these cases (Figures 6.13b and 6.14b). This will usually be at a high velocity and can help to predict left ventricular pressure. The aortic valve may appear thick and dysplastic with restricted movement (Figure 6.12c). The aortic root and ascending aorta are commonly small for gestational age in critical cases, though their sizes can be variable (Figures 6.12c-d). Forward flow can occasionally be detected across the aortic valve, but often it can be difficult to demonstrate. If forward flow is detected in cases with significant left ventricular compromise, the aortic Doppler velocities may be within the normal range for gestation or only mildly elevated, thus not reflecting the severity of the obstruction. There may be reversed flow in the transverse aortic arch from the arterial duct (Figure 6.12e), which is an important discriminating feature for those cases with a poor prognosis for postnatal treatment. As seen with other forms of severe left heart obstruction, the direction of flow across the atrial communication will be left to right, the reverse of normal (Figure 6.12f). The interatrial communication may be restrictive, or in some cases the atrial septum may be intact. In these cases, there will be left atrial enlargement with an increased cardiothoracic ratio (Figures 6.14a-b).

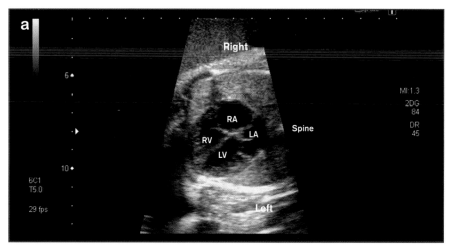

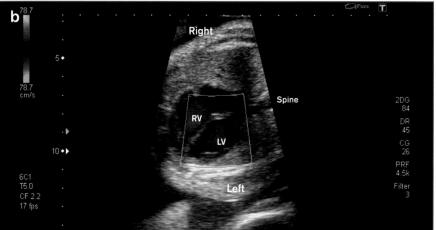

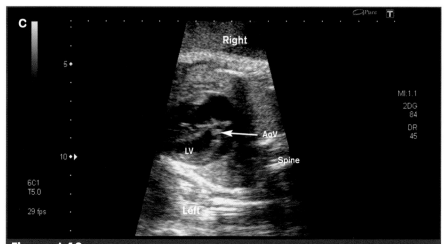

Figure 6.10. An example of moderate aortic stenosis. a) The four-chamber view appears normal. The left ventricle is a normal size and was contracting well. There is no left ventricular hypertrophy. b) There is equal inflow into both ventricular chambers seen with colour flow (seen in blue). c) The aortic valve appears dysplastic.

Figure continued overleaf.

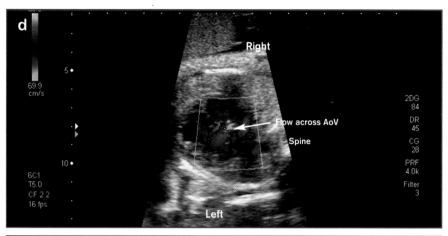

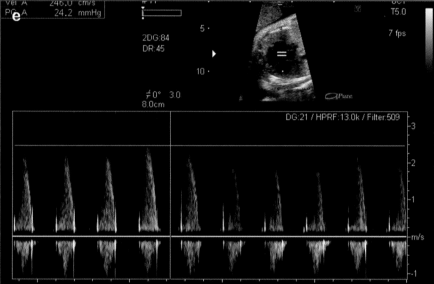

Figure 6.10 *continued.* **An example of moderate aortic stenosis. d) There is turbulent flow across the aortic valve with an elevated Doppler velocity. e) Pulsed Doppler shows an increased velocity of 2.46m/second across the aortic valve.**

Extracardiac associations

Isolated valvar aortic stenosis is rarely associated with extracardiac malformations, though occasionally aortic stenosis is seen in Turner's syndrome. Fetal hydrops can be associated in cases with critical aortic stenosis. In our large fetal series, 6% of cases with critical aortic stenosis had fetal hydrops.

Management and outcome

Non-critical cases (not duct-dependent)

Early postnatal echocardiographic assessment is recommended to evaluate the Doppler gradient across the aortic valve in the postnatal circulation. If the gradient is significant then

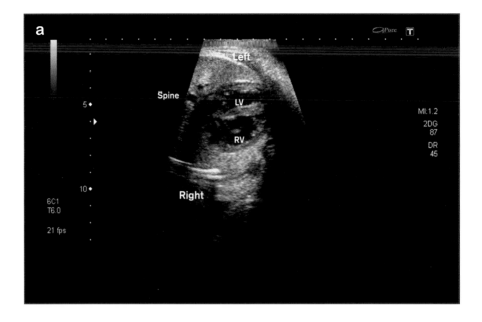

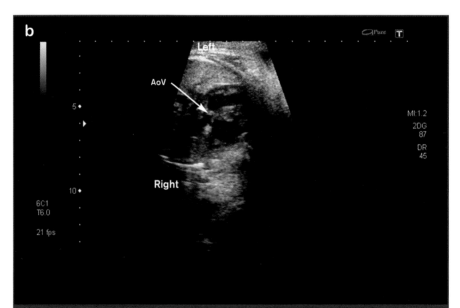

Figure 6.11. An example of moderate to severe aortic stenosis. a) The four-chamber view shows a good sized left ventricle that was contracting well, though there is some left ventricular hypertrophy. b) The aortic valve appears dysplastic.

Figure continued overleaf.

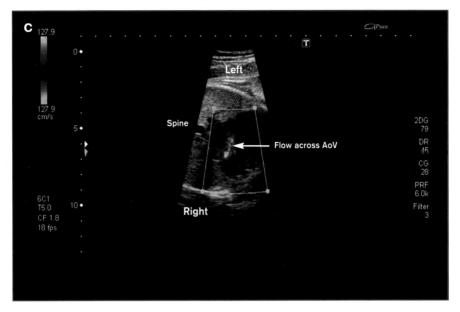

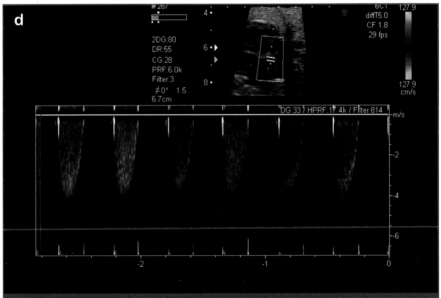

Figure 6.11 *continued.* **An example of moderate to severe aortic stenosis. c) Colour flow shows turbulent flow across the aortic valve. d) Pulsed Doppler shows an increased velocity of 4m/second across the aortic valve.**

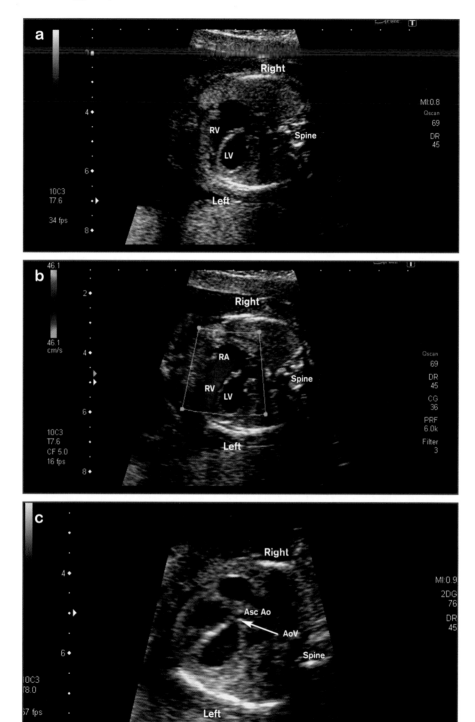

Figure 6.12. An example of critical aortic stenosis. a) The four-chamber view shows a dilated echogenic left ventricle which was poorly contracting. b) Colour flow shows the flow from the right atrium to the right ventricle (seen in blue) but there is little flow from the left atrium to the left ventricle. c) The ascending aorta is slightly small and the aortic valve is dysplastic.

Figure continued overleaf.

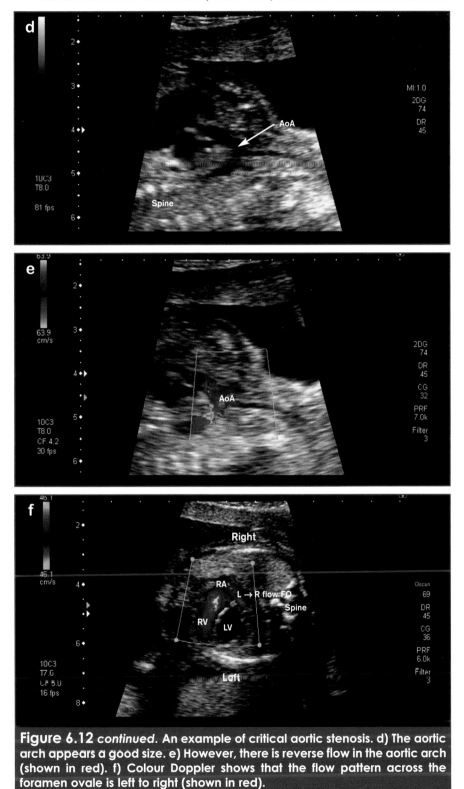

Figure 6.12 *continued*. **An example of critical aortic stenosis. d) The aortic arch appears a good size. e) However, there is reverse flow in the aortic arch (shown in red). f) Colour Doppler shows that the flow pattern across the foramen ovale is left to right (shown in red).**

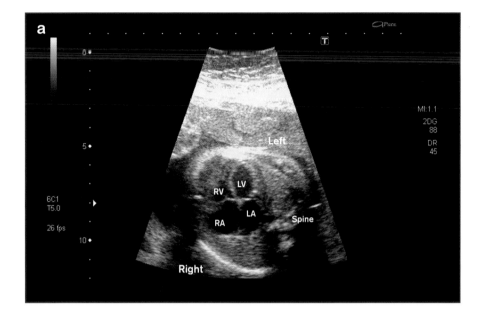

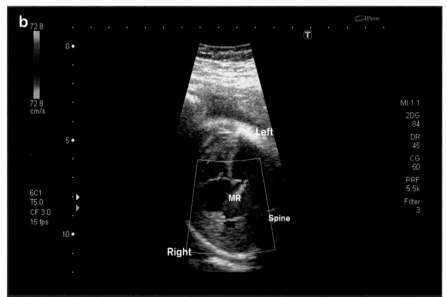

Figure 6.13. Another example of critical aortic stenosis. a) The four-chamber view shows a dilated echogenic left ventricle which was poorly contracting. b) Colour flow shows moderate mitral regurgitation in this example (shown in blue).

Obstructive lesions at the ventriculo-arterial junction that may be associated with an abnormal four-chamber view

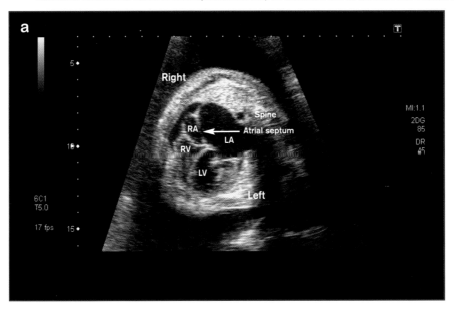

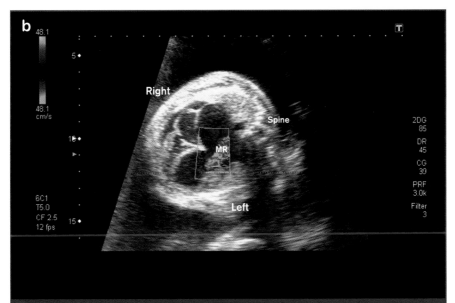

Figure 6.14. An example of critical aortic stenosis with a very restricted atrial septum. a) The four-chamber view shows left atrial enlargement with an increased cardiothoracic ratio. The atrial septum appears intact. The left ventricle is dilated and was poorly contracting. b) There is significant associated mitral regurgitation (shown in red).

early intervention may be required. This is most likely with balloon dilation of the aortic valve. Many children who have had early ballooning of the aortic valve will require intervention at some stage later in life on the aortic valve.

Critical cases (duct-dependent)

The major decision after birth is whether the baby is suitable for a biventricular repair or not. There is a tendency for critical aortic stenosis to progress, so that by term the appearances are likely to be more similar to hypoplastic left heart syndrome. In such cases a biventricular repair is not feasible and management is towards single-ventricle circulation, as for hypoplastic left heart syndrome (see above). In cases where a biventricular repair seems feasible, the initial postnatal management will most likely be balloon dilation of the aortic valve to relieve obstruction at this level. However, the success of this will be dependent on whether the mitral valve and left ventricle prove adequate to maintain the systemic circulation in the longer term. In borderline cases the option of a 'hybrid' procedure may be considered. This is a part-surgical, part-interventional procedure which has been recently developed and involves placing a stent in the arterial duct and banding of the branch pulmonary arteries. This allows deferment of the decision making with regard to the eventual type of repair, as assessment can be made of the ability of the left ventricle to support the systemic circulation with time.

Outcome in a large single-centre fetal series

Of 77 cases of critical aortic stenosis diagnosed prenatally, 44% of pregnancies resulted in a termination of pregnancy. If the terminations are excluded then the outcome of the continuing pregnancies was: 2% resulting in spontaneous intrauterine death, 60% died in the neonatal period, 5% died in infancy and 33% were alive at last update.

Of cases seen in the last 10 years, a termination of pregnancy took place in 42% of cases and 50% of the continuing pregnancies were alive at last follow-up.

In addition to the above cases, there were eight cases of aortic stenosis that were not critical. Of these, there are seven survivors and one pregnancy resulted in a termination.

Progression

Occasionally, the echocardiographic findings can be normal in early pregnancy but aortic stenosis may develop in later gestation. In cases where the diagnosis has been made in the mid-trimester, there is potential for progression in severity as pregnancy advances. This may be seen as an increase in the Doppler velocity, or in cases of severe left ventricular outflow tract obstruction, there may be a reduced rate of growth of left heart structures with advancing gestation. In some fetuses with aortic stenosis, the apex of the heart may be gradually taken over by the right ventricle with advancing pregnancy, as the right ventricle grows normally and the left ventricle does not. In such cases at term, the left ventricle may not be of adequate size for a biventricular repair, even though there is still forward flow through the left heart. Thus, critical aortic stenosis can progress to fall in the spectrum of hypoplastic left heart syndrome by term, due to failure of growth of the left ventricle (Figures 6.15a-c).

Obstructive lesions at the ventriculo-arterial junction that may be associated with an abnormal four-chamber view

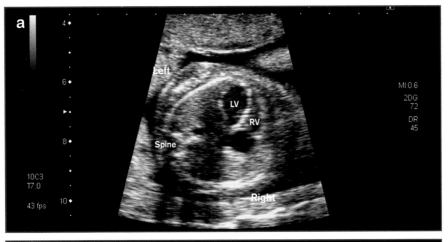

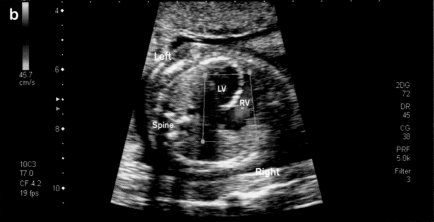

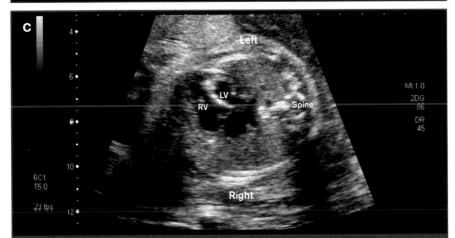

Figure 6.15. Progression of critical aortic stenosis to hypoplastic left heart syndrome. a) The four-chamber views shows a dilated echogenic left ventricle which was poorly contracting. The left ventricle reaches the apex. b) Colour flow shows the flow from the right atrium to the right ventricle (seen in red) but there is little flow from the left atrium to the left ventricle. c) The four-chamber view of the same example seen in later pregnancy. At this stage the left ventricle appears hypoplastic and no longer reaches the apex.

Fetal intervention

In order to prevent the progression of critical aortic stenosis during fetal life, prenatal catheter intervention has been advocated and undertaken in some cases. However, although technical success has been reported, from current published series a biventricular circulation is achieved in around 20-25% of fetuses following prenatal intervention. Many babies will therefore still be managed in a manner similar to hypoplastic left heart syndrome.

Summary of fetal echocardiographic features associated with AS.

Mild to moderate
- Normal four-chamber view
- Aortic root normal size
- Mild dysplasia of the aortic valve
- Mildly elevated Doppler velocity across the aortic valve

Moderate to severe
- Four-chamber view may be normal
- May be some left ventricular hypertrophy or some impairment of left ventricular function
- Aortic valve dysplastic with restriction in its opening
- Turbulent flow across the aortic valve usually with increased Doppler velocity

Critical
- Dilated, poorly contracting, hypertrophied left ventricle
- Increased echogenicity of the left ventricular walls
- Restricted mitral valve motion
- Mitral regurgitation
- Reversal of interatrial shunt
- Small aortic root and ascending aorta
- Thickened restricted aortic valve
- Difficult to detect forward flow across the aortic valve
- Velocity of forward flow across the aortic valve may be low or in the normal range
- Reverse flow from the arterial duct in the aortic arch

Obstructive lesions of the pulmonary valve associated with an abnormal four-chamber view

Pulmonary atresia with an intact ventricular septum (PAT IVS)

Prevalence
Pulmonary atresia with an intact ventricular septum accounts for approximately 2.5-4% of congenital heart disease in postnatal series. In the Evelina fetal series, pulmonary atresia with an intact ventricular septum accounted for 3.2% of the total series and 2.5% of all cases of fetal congenital heart disease seen in the last 10 years.

Definition
In pulmonary atresia with an intact ventricular septum there is complete obstruction to blood flow from the right ventricle to the pulmonary artery in association with an intact ventricular septum.

Pulmonary atresia can occur in association with a ventricular septal defect, but this is a different type of lesion and is discussed in Chapter 8. Pulmonary atresia can also occur with complex cardiac malformations such as those associated with atrial isomerism. This section is confined to cases of pulmonary atresia with an intact ventricular septum only.

Spectrum
In fetal life, two forms of pulmonary atresia with an intact interventricular septum are encountered. The majority are those associated with a hypoplastic right ventricle and in these cases the cardiothoracic ratio is normal. However, the size of the right ventricle can vary from being very hypoplastic to near normal in size. This relates to whether there is valvar atresia only, or whether the infundibulum below the pulmonary valve is also atretic. The latter group is usually associated with very hypoplastic right ventricles.

In a smaller number of cases, the heart may be dilated in association with either Ebstein's malformation or with tricuspid valve dysplasia (see Chapter 5).

Fetal echocardiographic findings
The four-chamber view will be abnormal whether the right ventricle is hypoplastic or the heart is dilated.

Normal sized heart
In the majority of cases, the right ventricle is hypoplastic, hypertrophied and poorly contracting, though occasionally the right ventricle may be of near normal size (Figures 6.16a, 6.17, 6.18a and 6.19a). The tricuspid valve is often small with restricted movement and there will be reduced flow from the right atrium to the right ventricle (Figure 6.18b). There may be a narrow jet of tricuspid regurgitation detected with colour flow (Figures 6.18c and 6.19b) and this is usually at a high velocity (Figure 6.18d). The size of the pulmonary artery is variable

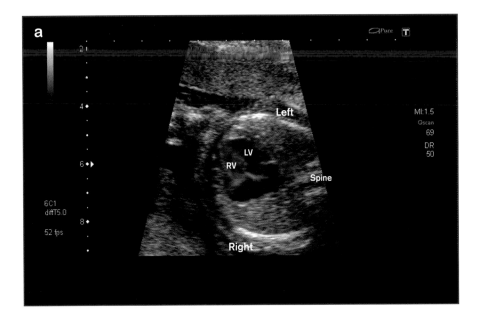

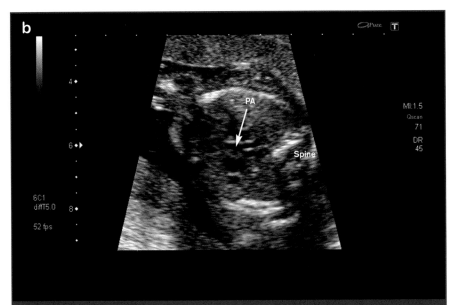

Figure 6.16. An example of pulmonary atresia with an intact septum with a very hypoplastic right ventricle and a small pulmonary artery. a) The four-chamber view shows a very hypoplastic right ventricle with no discernible right ventricular cavity. b) The pulmonary artery in this example was very small.

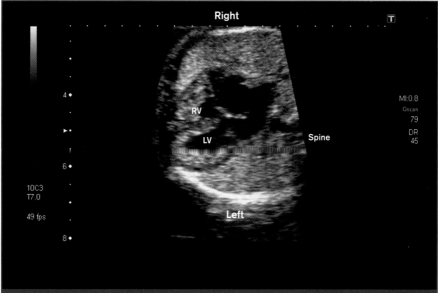

Figure 6.17. The four-chamber view of an example of pulmonary atresia with an intact septum with a hypertrophied right ventricle.

and though it is usually small, it can sometimes be a normal size (Figures 6.16b, 6.18e and 6.19c). In cases where the valve leaflets can be visualised, they appear thick with no opening movement. There is no forward flow detectable into the pulmonary artery, but reverse flow from the arterial duct is frequently seen (Figure 6.18f and 6.19d). The branch pulmonary arteries fill retrogradely from the duct. The arterial duct is often said to be a 'curly' shape . Whilst this is seen in some cases, it is not always seen in this setting. A curly or tortuous duct can also sometimes be seen with a normal heart before birth (Figures 6.20a-b). An example of the diagnosis of pulmonary atresia made at 15 weeks is shown in Figures 6.21a-d.

Connections between the coronary arteries and the right ventricle, or sinusoids, are frequently encountered in cases with a hypoplastic right ventricle.

In some cases with a very hypoplastic tricuspid valve, the distinction from tricuspid atresia can be difficult, though the jet of tricuspid regurgitation will confirm patency of the tricuspid valve and differentiate this condition from tricuspid atresia.

Enlarged heart

Less frequently, pulmonary atresia with an intact interventricular septum can be seen with a dilated right atrium and dilated right ventricle. This form is usually associated with either tricuspid valve dysplasia or Ebstein's malformation (see Chapter 5). There is usually marked tricuspid regurgitation associated with the tricuspid valve abnormality. The pulmonary artery is often small. No forward flow is detected across the pulmonary valve or in the main

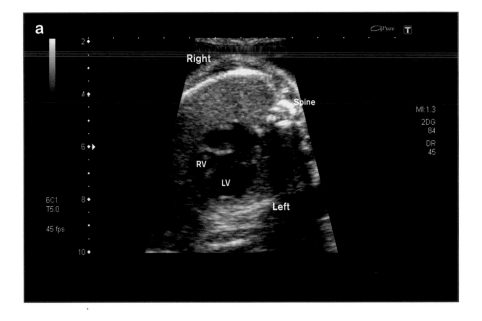

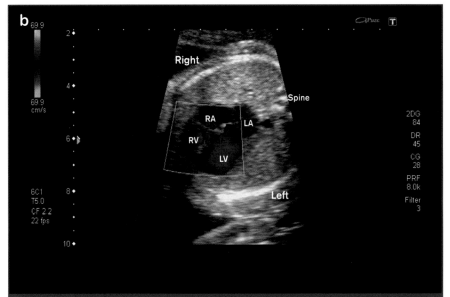

Figure 6.18. An example of pulmonary atresia with an intact septum with a hypoplastic right ventricle and a moderate sized pulmonary artery. a) The four-chamber view shows a hypoplastic right ventricle. b) Colour flow shows the flow from the left atrium to the left ventricle (seen in blue) but there is little flow from the right atrium into the right ventricle.

Figure continued overleaf.

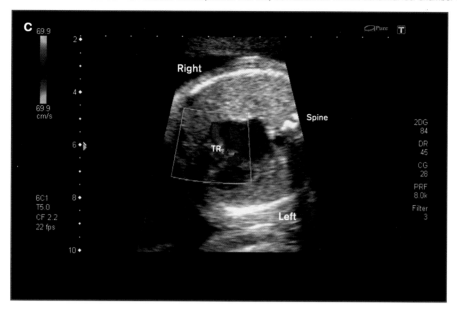

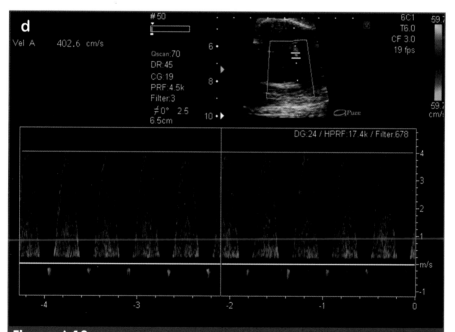

Figure 6.18 *continued.* **An example of pulmonary atresia with an intact septum with a hypoplastic right ventricle and a moderate sized pulmonary artery. c) Colour Doppler shows a narrow jet of tricuspid regurgitation (shown in red). d) Pulsed Doppler shows the tricuspid regurgitation jet has a high velocity of 4m/second.**

Figure continued overleaf.

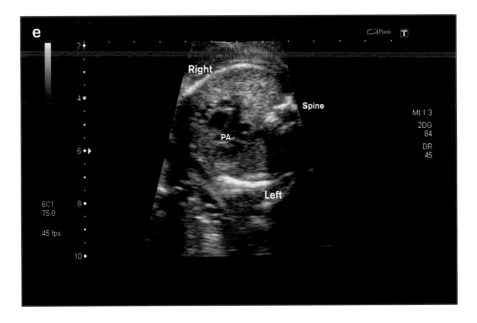

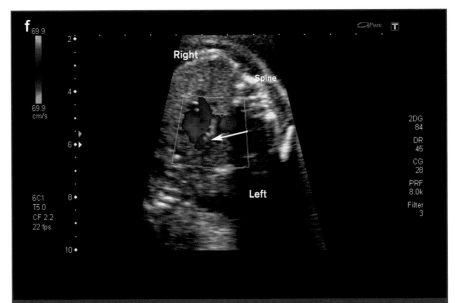

Figure 6.18 *continued.* **An example of pulmonary atresia with an intact septum with a hypoplastic right ventricle and a moderate sized pulmonary artery. e) The pulmonary artery in this example is smaller than normal but is of a moderate size with confluent branch pulmonary arteries. f) There is reverse flow in the pulmonary artery from the arterial duct (shown in blue).**

Obstructive lesions at the ventriculo-arterial junction that may be associated with an abnormal four-chamber view

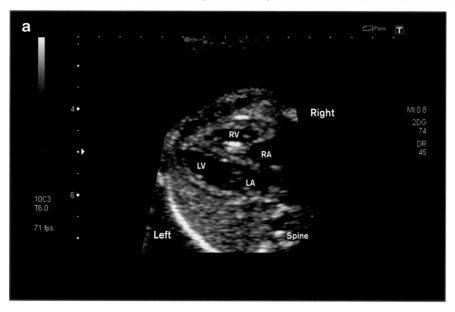

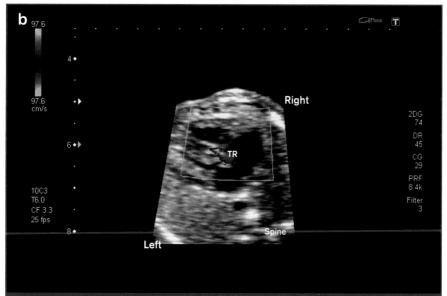

Figure 6.19. An example of pulmonary atresia with an intact septum with a good sized right ventricle and a normal sized pulmonary artery. a) The four-chamber view shows a near normal sized right ventricle, though there is an echogenic focus present. b) Colour flow shows a narrow jet of tricuspid regurgitation (shown in blue).

Figure continued overleaf.

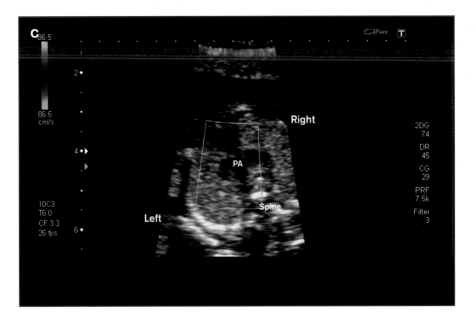

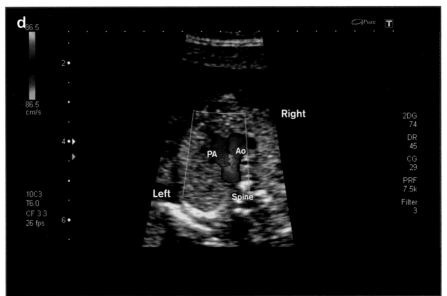

Figure 6.19 *continued*. An example of pulmonary atresia with an intact septum with a good sized right ventricle and a normal sized pulmonary artery. c) The pulmonary artery in this example is of normal size. d) There is reverse flow in the pulmonary artery from the arterial duct (shown in red). The normal forward flow in the aorta is seen in blue.

Obstructive lesions at the ventriculo-arterial junction that may be associated with an abnormal four-chamber view

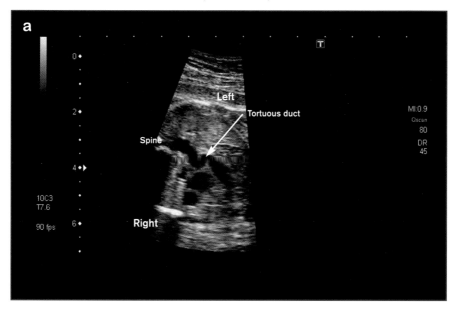

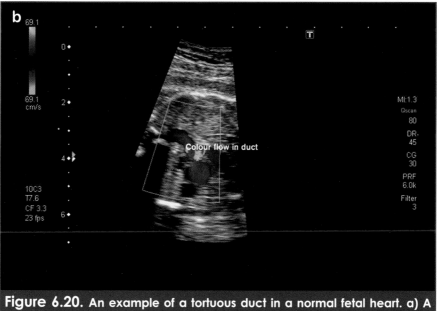

Figure 6.20. An example of a tortuous duct in a normal fetal heart. a) A view of the tortuous duct. b) The tortuous duct is seen with colour flow.

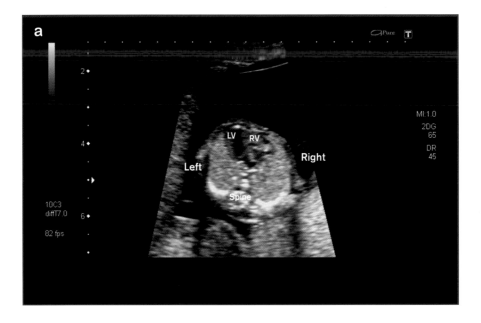

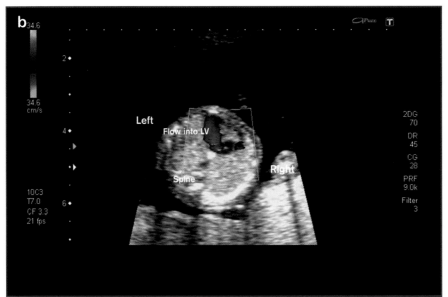

Figure 6.21. An example of pulmonary atresia with an intact ventricular septum at 15 weeks. a) The four-chamber view shows a very hypoplastic right ventricle. b) Colour flow shows the flow from the left atrium to the left ventricle (seen in red) but no flow is seen from the right atrium into the right ventricle.

Figure continued overleaf.

Obstructive lesions at the ventriculo-arterial junction that may be associated with an abnormal four-chamber view

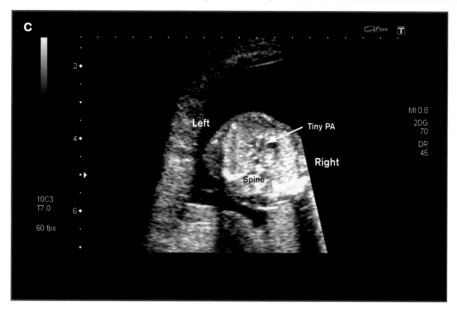

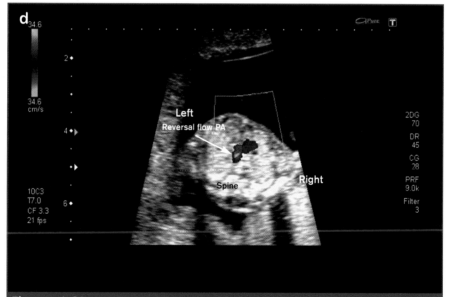

Figure 6.21 *continued.* An example of pulmonary atresia with an intact ventricular septum at 15 weeks. c) The pulmonary artery is very small. d) There is reverse flow in the pulmonary artery from the arterial duct (seen in red).

pulmonary artery. In this setting where there is severe tricuspid regurgitation, there may be little or no forward flow out of the right ventricle into the pulmonary artery, as most of the blood is going backwards into the right atrium. Thus, in this situation the pulmonary atresia can sometimes be functional, rather than anatomical and it can be difficult to distinguish between the two.

Extracardiac associations

Pulmonary atresia with an intact ventricular septum is not commonly associated with extracardiac malformations. In our large fetal series, pulmonary atresia with an intact ventricular septum was associated with chromosomal abnormalities in 1.5% of cases, which were two cases of trisomy 18. A further 3% had an extracardiac anomaly, which included anal atresia, oesophageal atresia, renal abnormalities and tracheo-oesophageal fistula. Fetal hydrops was associated in 1% of cases.

Management and outcome

This is a major form of congenital cardiac abnormality which will be duct-dependent after birth. Usually the first cardiac intervention would be either a systemic to pulmonary artery shunt (Blalock-Taussig shunt), or an interventional cardiac catheterisation to perforate the pulmonary valve, and re-establish continuity between the right ventricle and the pulmonary artery. This may need to be supplemented by placing a stent in the arterial duct or by a shunt. Further management will depend on the size and function of the right ventricle. In many of the cases detected prenatally, a biventricular circulation is not possible and management is towards staged surgical palliation (Fontan type circulation). This type of circulation, which is achieved as a staged procedure, leaves the systemic veins (superior vena cava and inferior vena cava) draining directly to the pulmonary arteries and the dominant left ventricle supports the systemic arterial circulation. There is a guarded long-term prognosis with a risk of heart failure, arrhythmias and a potential need for heart transplantation later in life.

Outcome in a large single-centre fetal series

Of 135 cases of pulmonary atresia with an intact interventricular septum diagnosed prenatally, 56% of pregnancies resulted in a termination of pregnancy. If the terminations are excluded then the outcome of the continuing pregnancies was: 10% resulting in spontaneous intrauterine death, 27% died in the neonatal period, 8% died in infancy and 53% were alive at last update. Of the continuing pregnancies the outcome is unknown in 2%.

Of cases seen in the last 10 years, a termination of pregnancy took place in 46% of cases and 64% of the continuing pregnancies were alive at last follow-up.

Summary of fetal echocardiographic features associated with PAT IVS with a normal sized heart.

- Hypoplastic right ventricle (usually)
- Hypertrophied right ventricle
- Poorly contracting right ventricle
- Small and restricted tricuspid valve
- Tricuspid regurgitation jet (high velocity)
- Small pulmonary artery (occasionally may be normal size)
- No forward flow in pulmonary artery
- Reverse flow in arterial duct

Summary of fetal echocardiographic features associated with PAT IVS in cases with a large heart.

- Dilated right atrium
- Dilated right ventricle (sometimes)
- Abnormal tricuspid valve
  - Ebstein's anomaly
  - tricuspid valve dysplasia
- Tricuspid regurgitation
- Small pulmonary artery
- No forward flow in pulmonary artery
- Reverse flow in arterial duct

Summary of extracardiac associations in fetal PAT IVS.

- Chromosomal
  - 1.5%
- Extracardiac abnormality (normal chromosomes)
  - 3%

Pulmonary stenosis (PS)

Prevalence

Isolated pulmonary stenosis accounts for approximately 9% of congenital heart disease in postnatal series. In the Evelina fetal series, isolated pulmonary stenosis accounted for 1.4% of the total.

Definition

Pulmonary stenosis implies an obstruction to blood flow into the pulmonary circulation. This occurs most commonly at the level of the pulmonary valve, but can also occur in the subvalvar or infundibular region of the right ventricle, or in the branch pulmonary arteries.

Spectrum and other cardiac associations

Pulmonary stenosis can occur as an isolated finding or as part of more complex heart lesions, such as tetralogy of Fallot, a double-outlet right ventricle, transposition of the great arteries, Ebstein's malformation and atrial isomerism (see Chapters 3, 5, 7 and 8). This section will deal with pulmonary stenosis as an isolated finding. The severity of obstruction can vary from mild to severe or critical.

Fetal echocardiographic features

The echocardiographic findings are variable depending on the severity of pulmonary obstruction. The right ventricle can be hypoplastic, dilated, or of normal size and may be hypertrophied (Figures 6.22a, 6.23a, 6.24 and 6.25a). The size of the pulmonary artery can also be variable, from normal to hypoplastic or, in some cases, dilated. The pulmonary valve usually appears dysplastic (Figures 6.22b, 6.23b and 6.25b) and there is an increased Doppler velocity across the valve, with turbulent flow seen on colour flow (Figures 6.22c-d and 6.23c-d). However, in cases with marked pulmonary artery hypoplasia, although there may be forward flow into the pulmonary artery across the pulmonary valve, the Doppler velocity may not be increased. In these cases, the diagnosis of pulmonary obstruction in fetal life is made because of the small size of the pulmonary artery. This is often the case where pulmonary stenosis occurs with more complex forms of congenital heart disease, but rarely this is also noted in isolated cases. In cases with severe obstruction, reverse flow from the arterial duct may be detected in addition to forward flow across the pulmonary valve (Figures 6.23c and 6.25c). Occasionally, pulmonary stenosis can be associated with a dilated pulmonary artery. These cases often have associated pulmonary regurgitation with a very dysplastic pulmonary valve (Figures 6.26a-d) and there is overlap with absent pulmonary valve syndrome (see Chapter 8).

Mild pulmonary stenosis

Mild forms of pulmonary stenosis are often not detected before birth. The four-chamber view will appear normal and the Doppler velocities may also be normal during fetal life. The pulmonary valve may appear slightly thickened or bright and the Doppler velocity across the valve may be at the upper end of the normal range or mildly elevated.

Moderate to severe pulmonary stenosis

The right ventricle may appear normal or may be hypertrophied (Figures 6.22a and 6.23). The pulmonary artery may appear a normal size or may appear small in some cases. The pulmonary valve will usually appear thickened and restricted in motion (Figure 6.22b) and colour flow will demonstrate turbulent flow across the pulmonary valve (Figure 6.22c). The pulsed Doppler velocity across the pulmonary valve will be increased above the normal range (Figure 6.22d).

Critical pulmonary stenosis

In these cases, the right ventricle will have impaired function and may be hypoplastic and hypertrophied or, in some cases, may be dilated (Figures 6.25a-c). The tricuspid valve will be restricted in opening. The size of the pulmonary artery can vary and may be small or normal. In critical pulmonary stenosis, it can sometimes be difficult to demonstrate forward flow across the pulmonary valve, due to poor ventricular function. If forward flow can be detected, the Doppler velocity in the pulmonary artery may be within the normal range for gestation, though there is likely to also be some reversed flow from the arterial duct, indicating severe obstruction (Figure 6.25c).

Progression

Sequential studies have shown that right heart obstructive lesions can be progressive in nature. In some cases, the initial fetal heart study may be normal, with obstruction developing later in gestation, or even after birth. When pulmonary stenosis is diagnosed during fetal life, the severity can increase with advancing gestational age. In a few instances, pulmonary stenosis has been documented to progress to pulmonary atresia.

Extracardiac associations

Pulmonary stenosis can occur as part of Noonan's, Alagille's or Williams syndromes. It is very rare for isolated pulmonary stenosis to be associated with chromosomal anomalies.

Management and outcome

The management of pulmonary stenosis will depend on the severity of the lesion.

Mild cases

In cases with mild pulmonary valve stenosis, conservative management is usually indicated unless obstruction becomes more significant.

Moderate to severe cases

In moderate or severe cases of pulmonary valve stenosis that are not duct-dependent, treatment is usually required but not urgently. This is usually balloon dilation of the pulmonary valve via catheter intervention.

Critical cases

In cases of duct-dependent pulmonary valve stenosis, or critical stenosis, urgent treatment is needed after birth. In these cases, the first cardiac intervention may be either a systemic to pulmonary artery shunt (Blalock-Taussig shunt), or an interventional cardiac catheterisation to dilate the pulmonary valve, in order to improve pulmonary blood flow. The latter procedure may need to be supplemented by placing a stent in the arterial duct or a systemic to pulmonary shunt. Further management depends on the growth and development of the right ventricle. If the right ventricle is adequate to support the pulmonary blood flow, then a

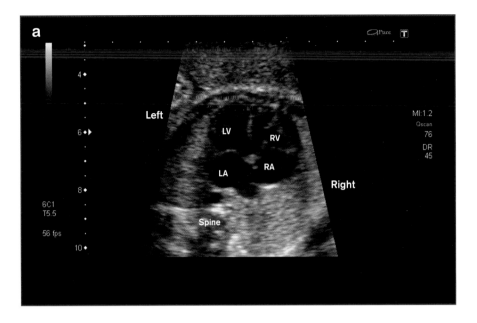

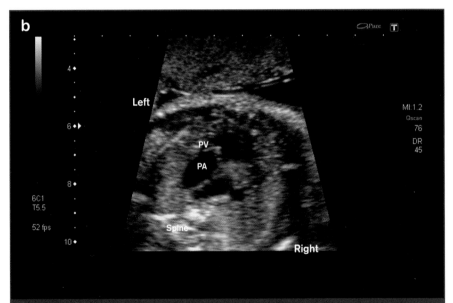

Figure 6.22. An example of pulmonary stenosis with a normal sized right ventricle that showed reasonable contraction. a) The four-chamber view appears normal. b) The pulmonary valve is very dysplastic and thickened. The main pulmonary artery appears slightly dilated.

Figure continued overleaf.

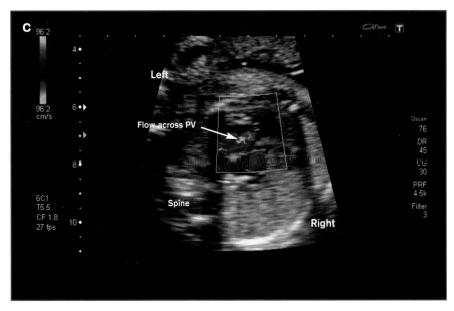

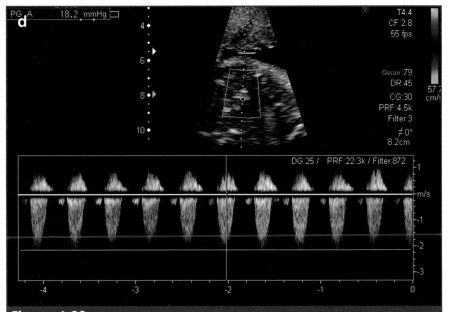

Figure 6.22 *continued.* **An example of pulmonary stenosis with a normal sized right ventricle that showed reasonable contraction. c) Colour flow shows turbulent flow across the pulmonary valve. d) Pulsed Doppler shows an increased velocity of 2m/second across the pulmonary valve.**

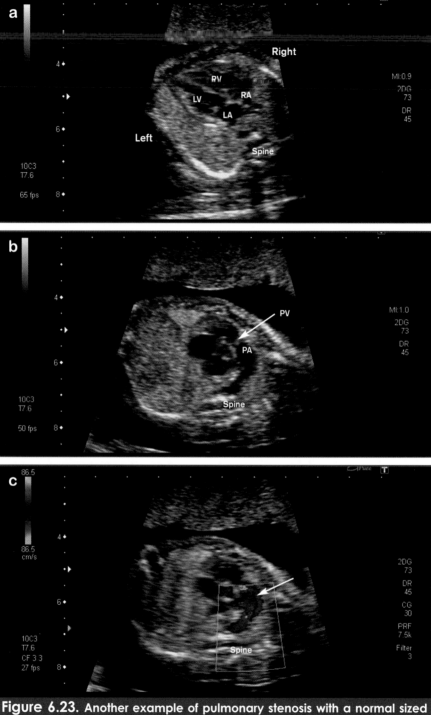

Figure 6.23. Another example of pulmonary stenosis with a normal sized right ventricle. a) The four-chamber view appears normal. b) The pulmonary valve is dysplastic. c) Colour flow shows that there is forward flow across the pulmonary valve (arrow and seen in blue), but there is also reverse flow (seen in red) indicating significant right ventricular outflow tract obstruction. *Figure continued overleaf.*

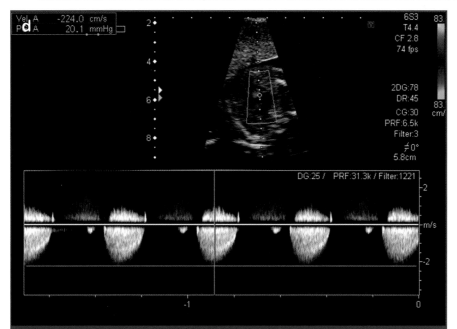

Figure 6.23 *continued.* **Another example of pulmonary stenosis with a normal sized right ventricle. d) Pulsed Doppler shows an increased velocity of 2m/second across the pulmonary valve.**

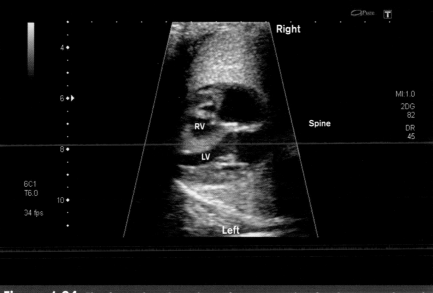

Figure 6.24. The four-chamber view of an example of pulmonary stenosis showing right ventricular hypertrophy.

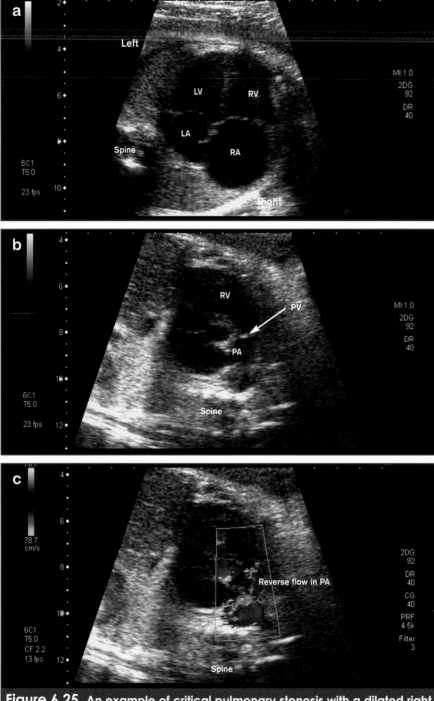

Figure 6.25. An example of critical pulmonary stenosis with a dilated right atrium and right ventricle. a) The four-chamber view shows cardiomegaly with the right atrium and right ventricle both appearing dilated. b) The pulmonary valve appears dysplastic with restricted opening. c) Reverse flow in the main pulmonary artery can be seen (shown in red) indicating severe obstruction, though some forward flow was detected across the pulmonary valve.

Obstructive lesions at the ventriculo-arterial junction that may be associated with an abnormal four-chamber view

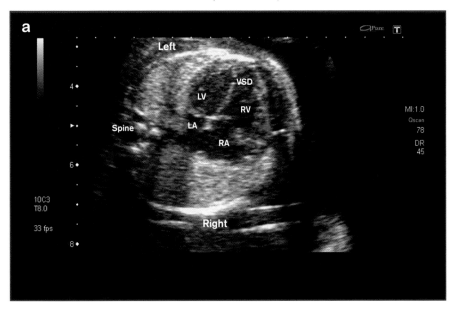

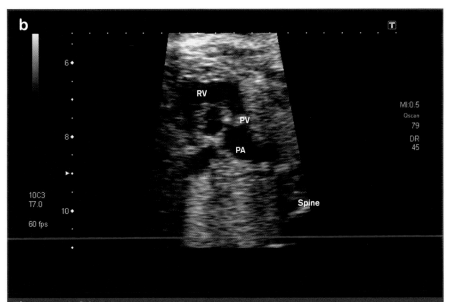

Figure 6.26. An example of pulmonary stenosis with a dysplastic pulmonary valve that was stenotic and regurgitant. a) The four-chamber view shows a dilated and hypertrophied right ventricle. There is also a small muscular ventricular septal defect. b) The pulmonary valve appears very dysplastic.

Figure continued overleaf.

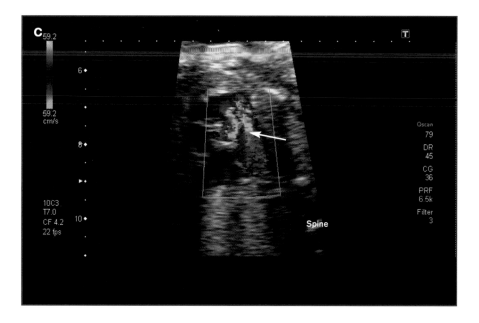

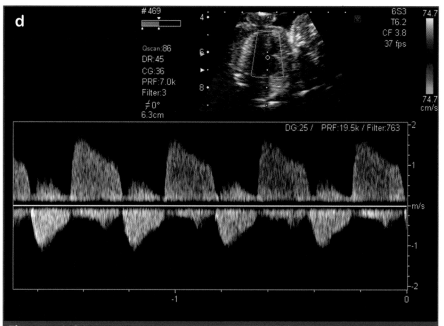

Figure 6.26 *continued.* An example of pulmonary stenosis with a dysplastic pulmonary valve that was stenotic and regurgitant. c) Colour flow shows turbulent and regurgitant flow across the pulmonary valve (arrow). d) Pulsed Doppler shows to and fro flow across the pulmonary valve.

biventricular circulation can be attained with a positive longer-term prognosis. However, if the right ventricle is not adequate then the management would be towards single-ventricle circulation (see under pulmonary atresia).

Outcome in a large single-centre fetal series

Of 60 cases of isolated pulmonary stenosis diagnosed prenatally, 22% of pregnancies resulted in a termination of pregnancy, most of which were cases of critical pulmonary stenosis. If the terminations are excluded then the outcome of the continuing pregnancies was: 6% resulting in spontaneous intrauterine death, 17% died in the neonatal period, and 77% were alive at last update.

Summary of fetal echocardiographic features associated with PS.

Mild to moderate
- Normal four-chamber view
- Pulmonary artery of normal size
- Mild dysplasia of the pulmonary valve
- Mildly elevated Doppler velocity across the pulmonary valve

Moderate to severe
- Four-chamber view may be normal
- May be some right ventricular hypertrophy or some impairment of right ventricular function
- Small or normal sized pulmonary artery
- Pulmonary artery may be dilated (occasionally)
- Thickened restricted pulmonary valve leaflets
- Turbulent flow across the pulmonary valve
- Pulmonary artery Doppler flow velocity increased above normal

Critical cases
- Poorly contracting right ventricle
- Hypertrophied right ventricle
- Occasionally dilated poorly functioning right ventricle
- Restricted tricuspid valve motion
- Pulmonary artery may be small for the gestational age
- Pulmonary artery may be dilated (occasionally)
- Thickened restricted pulmonary valve
- Difficult to detect forward flow across the pulmonary valve
- Velocity of forward flow across the pulmonary valve may be low or within the normal range
- Reverse flow from the arterial duct in the main pulmonary artery

Chapter 7

Great artery abnormalities (I)
Abnormalities of ventriculo-arterial connection

Summary

- **Ventriculo-arterial discordance**
  - Simple transposition of the great arteries
  - Transposition with ventricular septal defect
- **Atrioventricular and ventriculo-arterial discordance**
  - Corrected transposition of the great arteries
- **Double-outlet right ventricle**
  - With normally related great arteries
  - With transposed great arteries

Ventriculo-arterial discordance

Transposition of the great arteries (discordant ventriculo-arterial connection, TGA)

Prevalence
Transposition of the great arteries accounts for about 5-7% of congenital heart disease in postnatal series. In the Evelina fetal series, transposition of the great arteries (either simple transposition or transposition with a ventricular septal defect) accounted for 3.7% of the total series and 5.3% of all cases of fetal congenital heart disease seen in the last 10 years. (Simple transposition accounted for 2% of the total series and 2.9% of all cases of fetal congenital heart disease seen in the last 10 years.)

Definition
In transposition of the great arteries the aorta arises from the right ventricle, instead of the left, and the pulmonary artery arises from the left ventricle, instead of the right.

Spectrum
The majority of cases will have simple transposition, where there are no associated cardiac lesions, or just a small ventricular septal defect. However, in some cases, there may be a significant ventricular septal defect, and obstruction in either great artery, pulmonary stenosis or

coarctation of the aorta, may occur as associated lesions. Fetal series are generally biased towards cases with associated abnormality, where the four-chamber view may be abnormal. More rarely, transposition can also occur in the context of other, often complex, forms of congenital heart disease, for example, tricuspid atresia and double-inlet ventricle (see Chapter 4).

Fetal echocardiographic features

Simple transposition (TGA)

In most cases of simple transposition of the great arteries, the four-chamber view will appear normal (Figures 7.1a, 7.2a, 7.3a and 7.4a) and the diagnosis can only be made if views of the great arteries are examined. Moving cranially from the four-chamber view, the first vessel seen in transposition will be the branching pulmonary artery (Figure 7.1b and 7.4b). In the normal heart the first vessel seen moving cranially from the four-chamber view is the aorta (Figure 2.13a in Chapter 2). In transposition the aorta will be identified arising more cranially and anterior to the pulmonary artery (Figures 7.1c and 7.4c). The two great arteries arise from the heart in a parallel orientation and there will be loss of the normal cross-over of the great arteries (Figures 7.2b and 7.3b). Colour flow will demonstrate flow into both great arteries in a parallel orientation (Figure 7.2c) A normal three-vessel view will usually not be identified and often a 'two-vessel' view will be seen (Figure 7.4c). In this view, the aorta and superior vena cava can be seen, but the pulmonary artery is not visualised. Since the aorta arises more anteriorly from the right ventricle, the aortic arch will appear to be more wide-sweeping (Figure 7.5) compared to the normal, tight-hooked arch (Figures 2.19 and 2.20 in Chapter 2).

In simple transposition, the interventricular septum is usually intact, though some cases with a very small muscular ventricular septal defect may be classified as simple transposition.

Transposition with a ventricular septal defect (TGA VSD)

The aorta arises from the right ventricle and the pulmonary artery arises from the left ventricle, as above, but there is an associated ventricular septal defect, which can be of variable size. This condition can be associated with either pulmonary stenosis or coarctation of the aorta. In the former, the pulmonary valve may be thickened or the pulmonary artery may be smaller in size than the aorta (Figures 7.6a-e). Turbulent flow across the pulmonary valve may be demonstrated in some cases. This condition overlaps with a double-outlet right ventricle with a subpulmonary ventricular septal defect. In cases with a coarctation (Figures 7.7a-f), the aorta is smaller than the pulmonary artery, the arch appears hypoplastic and there may be associated sub-aortic narrowing.

Transposition with other congenital heart disease (complex TGA)

The features of the associated congenital heart disease will be present. As with all cases of transposition, the aorta arises from the right ventricle and the pulmonary artery arises from the left ventricle. In the context of complex congenital heart disease, either ventricular chamber may be rudimentary or small; for example, in cases of a double-inlet left ventricle or tricuspid atresia, the aorta will arise from a rudimentary or small right ventricular chamber. With complex forms of transposition, obstruction to either great artery can occur and is quite common in this setting. Thus, there may be pulmonary stenosis or coarctation of the aorta as described above.

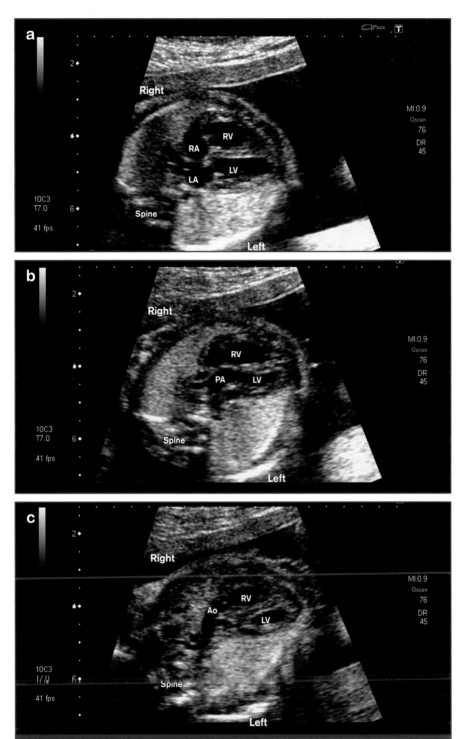

Figure 7.1. An example of simple transposition of the great arteries. a) The four-chamber view appears normal. b) Moving cranially from the four-chamber view, the first vessel seen in transposition is the branching pulmonary artery. c) The aorta arises more cranially to the pulmonary artery.

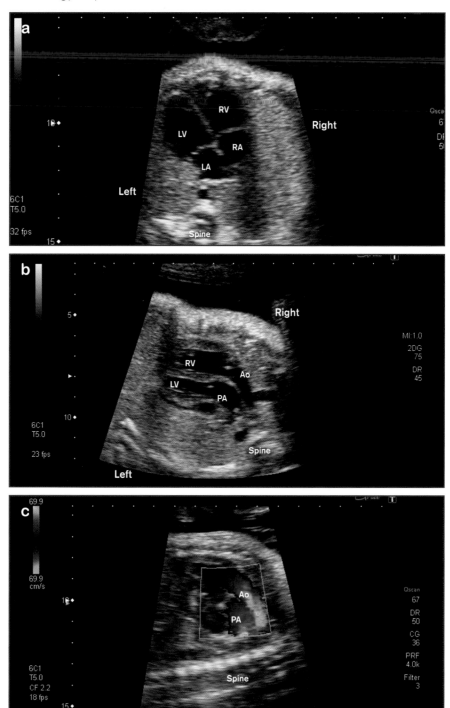

Figure 7.2. Another example of simple transposition. a) The four-chamber view appears normal. b) The two great arteries arise from the heart in a parallel orientation and there is loss of the normal cross-over of the great arteries. c) Colour flow shows forward flow in both the great arteries (shown in blue), which are arising in parallel orientation.

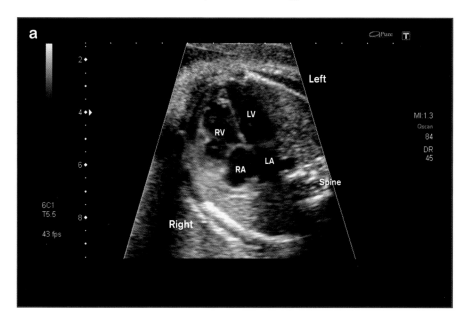

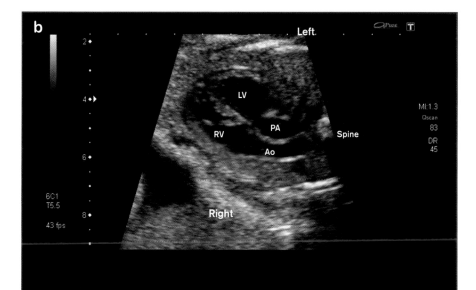

Figure 7.3. Another example of simple transposition. a) In the four-chamber view the heart appears slightly prominent but otherwise the view is normal. b) The two great arteries arise from the heart in a parallel orientation and there is loss of the normal cross-over of the great arteries. Branching of the pulmonary artery is clearly seen and this vessel is arising from the left ventricle.

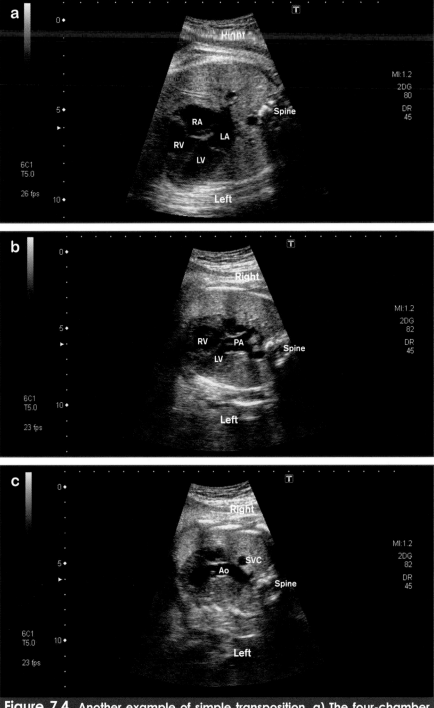

Figure 7.4. Another example of simple transposition. a) The four-chamber view appears normal. b) Moving cranially from the four-chamber view, the first vessel seen in transposition is the branching pulmonary artery. c) The aorta arises more cranially to the pulmonary artery. A normal three-vessel view is usually not identified and a 'two-vessel' view is seen. In this view, the aorta and superior vena cava can be seen, but the pulmonary artery is not visualised.

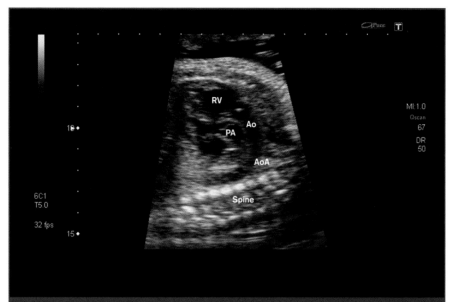

Figure 7.5. The aortic arch is more wide-sweeping compared to the normal tight-hooked arch as the aorta arises more anteriorly from the right ventricle.

Extracardiac associations

Transposition of the great arteries usually occurs in isolation and is rarely associated with chromosomal abnormalities, though extracardiac abnormalities can sometimes be associated. In our large fetal series, none of the cases of simple transposition had a chromosomal abnormality, but 5% had an extracardiac abnormality. These included dextrocardia, hemivertebrae, a lemon- shaped head and stomach on the right side. Of the cases with transposition of the great arteries with a ventricular septal defect, 2% had a chromosomal abnormality, which were two cases of 47XXX. A further 4% had extracardiac abnormalities which included duodenal atresia and renal abnormalities.

Management and outcome

Simple transposition is a major but repairable form of congenital heart disease. The baby will be duct-dependent after birth and a balloon atrial septostomy is sometimes required initially. The definitive surgical management is the arterial switch operation, which is usually undertaken in the first week or two of life. This consists of switching the great arteries back to their normal positions, with transfer of the coronary arteries. The surgical mortality is less than 5%, with good long-term results. Abnormal coronary artery patterns can increase the surgical risk.

More complex forms of transposition, for example, those associated with a ventricular septal defect and pulmonary stenosis may not be suitable for an arterial switch procedure. In these cases, more complex surgery, such as the Rastelli procedure, may be required. This involves closure of the ventricular septal defect with a patch in a way to direct the blood flow from the left ventricle to the aorta. The right ventricle is connected to the pulmonary artery via a conduit.

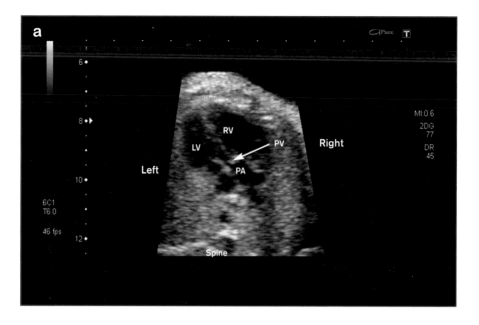

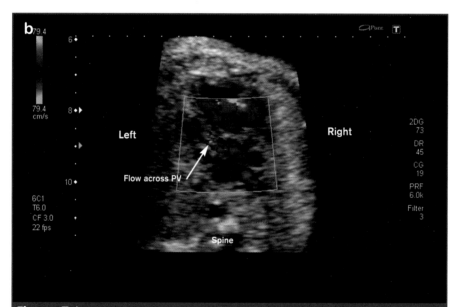

Figure 7.6. An example of transposition associated with a ventricular septal defect and pulmonary stenosis. a) The pulmonary artery arises from the left ventricle. The pulmonary valve is dysplastic. b) Colour flow shows turbulent flow across the pulmonary valve.

Figure continued overleaf.

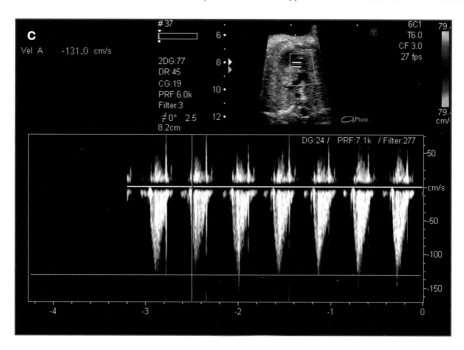

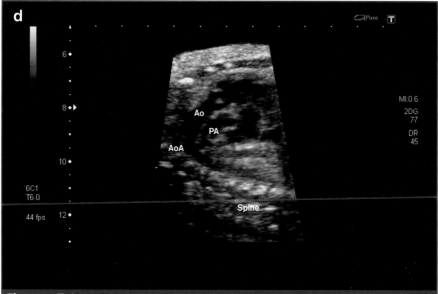

Figure 7.6 *continued.* An example of transposition associated with a ventricular septal defect and pulmonary stenosis. c) Pulsed Doppler shows a velocity of over 1m/second, which is increased for mid-gestation. d) The parallel great arteries are seen in a longitudinal view of the arches.

Figure continued overleaf.

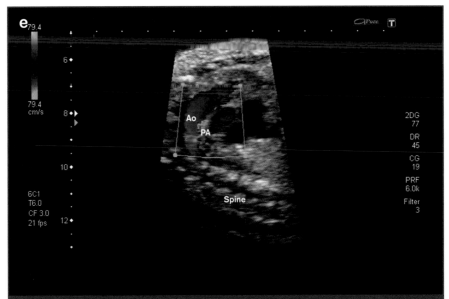

Figure 7.6 *continued.* **An example of transposition associated with a ventricular septal defect and pulmonary stenosis. e) There is reversed flow from the duct in the pulmonary artery (shown in red) suggesting significant pulmonary obstruction.**

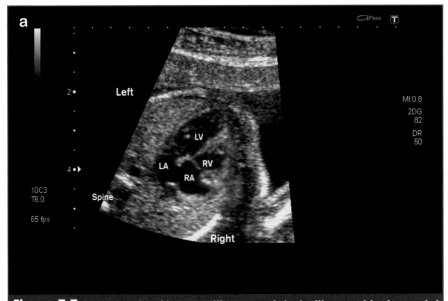

Figure 7.7 An example of transposition associated with a ventricular septal defect and coarctation of the aorta. a) The four-chamber view appears normal.

Figure continued overleaf.

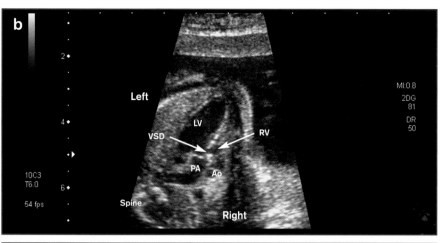

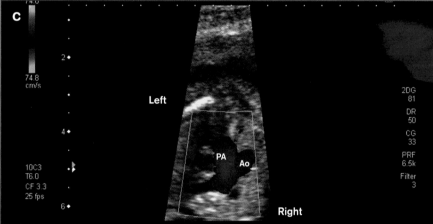

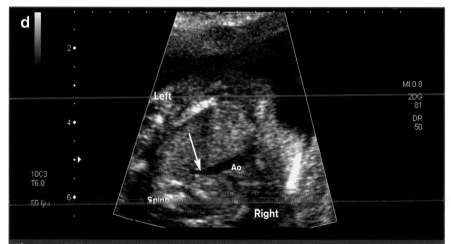

Figure 7.7 *continued.* An example of transposition associated with a ventricular septal defect and coarctation of the aorta. b) The great arteries arise in parallel orientation and there is a ventricular septal defect. The aorta appears smaller than the pulmonary artery. c) Colour flow shows forward flow in both the great arteries (shown in blue). d) A view of the aorta shows it tapering towards the descending aorta (arrow).

Figure continued overleaf.

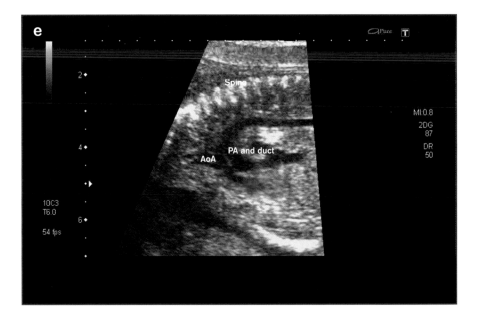

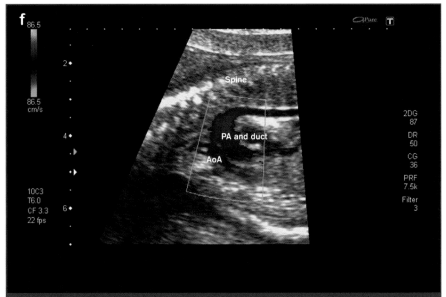

Figure 7.7 *continued.* **An example of transposition associated with a ventricular septal defect and coarctation of the aorta. e) Parallel great arteries are seen in a longitudinal view of the arches. The aortic arch appears smaller than the pulmonary artery and duct. f) Colour flow shows forward flow in both the arches (shown in red), though the aortic arch appears smaller.**

Outcome in a large single-centre fetal series

Simple transposition

Of 84 cases of simple transposition diagnosed prenatally, 8% of pregnancies resulted in a termination of pregnancy. If the terminations are excluded then the outcome of the continuing pregnancies was: 8% died in the neonatal period, and 90% were alive at last update. Of the continuing pregnancies the outcome is unknown in 2%.

Of cases seen in the last 10 years, a termination of pregnancy took place in 5% of cases and 94% of the continuing pregnancies were alive at last follow-up.

Transposition with a ventricular septal defect

Of 71 cases of transposition with a ventricular septal defect diagnosed prenatally, 23% of pregnancies resulted in a termination of pregnancy. If the terminations are excluded then the outcome of the continuing pregnancies was: 2% died in the neonatal period, 7% died in infancy and 87% were alive at last update. Of the continuing pregnancies the outcome is unknown in 4%.

Summary of fetal echocardiographic features associated with TGA.

Simple transposition of the great arteries
- Four-chamber view usually normal
- Pulmonary artery (branching artery) arises from the left ventricle
- Pulmonary artery is the first vessel seen moving cranially from a four-chamber view
- Aorta (gives rise to head and neck vessels and forms most cranial arch) arises from the right ventricle
- Parallel arrangement of the great arteries
- Wide sweeping aortic arch
- Abnormal three-vessel view
  - only two vessels seen

Transposition with VSD or other CHD
- Four-chamber view may be abnormal depending on associated abnormality
- Ventricular septal defect
- Aorta arises from the right ventricle
- Pulmonary artery arises predominantly from the left ventricle
- Pulmonary artery may override a ventricular septal defect
- May be evidence of pulmonary stenosis (pulmonary artery smaller than the aorta or increased Doppler velocity across the pulmonary valve)
- May be evidence of coarctation of the aorta (aorta smaller than the pulmonary artery and hypoplastic aortic arch)

Summary of extracardiac associations in fetal simple TGA.

- **Chromosomal**
  - 0%
- **Extracardiac abnormality (normal chromosomes)**
  - 5%

Summary of extracardiac associations in fetal TGA VSD.

- **Chromosomal**
  - 2%
- **Extracardiac abnormality (normal chromosomes)**
  - 4%

Of cases seen in the last 10 years, a termination of pregnancy took place in 13% of cases and 90% of the continuing pregnancies were alive at last follow-up.

Atrioventricular and ventriculo-arterial discordance

Congenitally corrected transposition of the great arteries (discordant atrioventricular connection with discordant ventriculo-arterial connection, CCTGA)

Prevalence
This is a rare and complex anomaly, accounting for approximately 1% of congenital heart disease in postnatal series. In the Evelina fetal series, corrected transposition accounted for 1.4% of the total series and 1.6% of all cases of fetal congenital heart disease seen in the last 10 years.

Definition
In this malformation, there is an abnormality at two levels, with discordance at both the atrioventricular connection and the ventriculo-arterial connection. Thus, the right atrium is connected to the left ventricle, which gives rise to the pulmonary artery. The left atrium is connected to the right ventricle, which gives rise to the aorta. However, the systemic venous return reaches the pulmonary artery and the pulmonary venous return reaches the aorta, so the circulation is anatomically 'corrected', even though the ventricular anatomy is inverted.

Spectrum
Atrioventricular and ventriculo-arterial discordance can occur as an isolated lesion, but often it will be associated with other cardiac abnormalities. Commonly associated cardiac

lesions are a ventricular septal defect, pulmonary stenosis or atresia, and Ebstein's anomaly. Complete congenital heart block is also a well-recognised association.

More rarely it may be associated with other cardiac anomalies such as an absent left-sided connection (tricuspid atresia in the setting of atrioventricular discordance), aortic stenosis or atresia and arch abnormalities, such as coarctation of the aorta and, very rarely, interrupted aortic arch.

Fetal echocardiographic features

The position of the heart is often abnormal in this condition, though it may be normal in some cases (Figures 7.8 and 7.9a). The heart may lie more centrally in the chest, with the ventricular septum in a more anteroposterior position than normal (Figure 7.9a and 7.10a). In the majority of cases the morphological right ventricle lies to the left of the morphologically left ventricle and the aorta usually arises to the left of the pulmonary artery. Thus, in the four-chamber view, the more apically attached atrioventricular valve and the moderator band, which are both features of the morphological right ventricle, will be in the left-sided ventricle (Figure 7.8). A ventricular septal defect may be evident in the four-chamber view (Figures

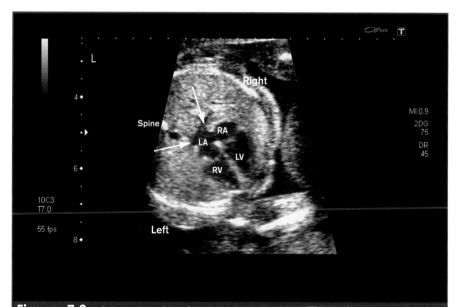

Figure 7.8, An example of corrected transposition with normal heart position. The four-chamber view shows that the posterior left-sided atrioventricular valve is more apically positioned than the anterior right-sided atrioventricular valve. This is the reverse of normal and indicates that the right ventricle is left-sided and the left ventricle is right-sided. The pulmonary veins (arrows) drain to the left atrium which connects to the right ventricle (atrioventricular discordance).

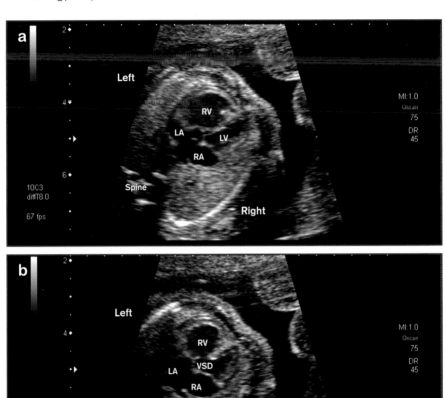

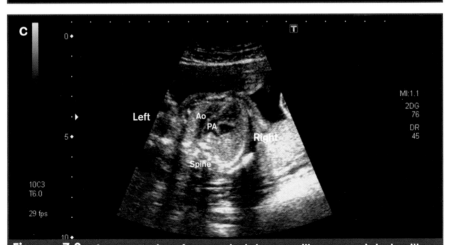

Figure 7.9. An example of corrected transposition associated with a ventricular septal defect. a) The heart lies centrally in the chest. The right ventricle is left-sided and the left ventricle is right-sided. b) An associated ventricular septal defect is seen in this view. c) A view of the great arteries shows that they arise in parallel orientation and the aorta arises to the left of the pulmonary artery.

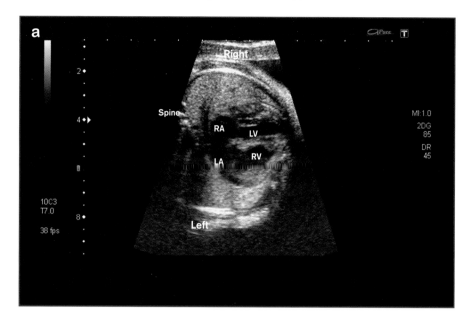

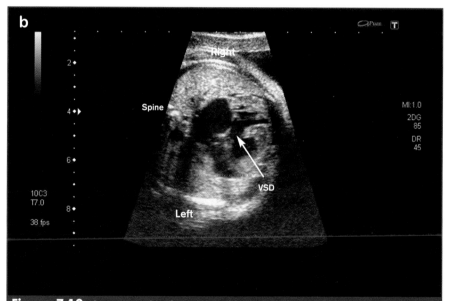

Figure 7.10. An example of corrected transposition with a ventricular septal defect and pulmonary stenosis. a) The four-chamber view shows atrioventricular discordance (left atrium connects to a left-sided morphologically right ventricle, right atrium connects to a right-sided morphologically left ventricle). The heart lies in the midline with the apex towards the right. b) There is a large ventricular septal defect.

Figure continued overleaf.

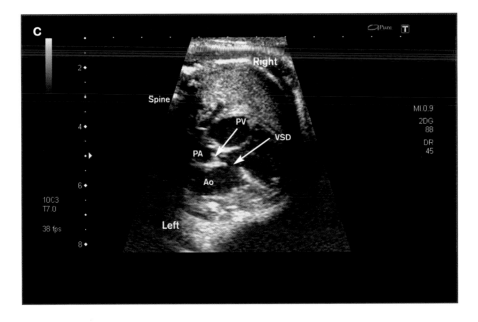

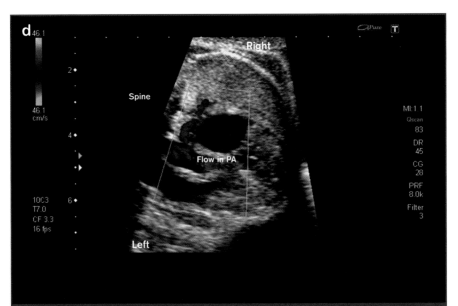

Figure 7.10 *continued.* **An example of corrected transposition with a ventricular septal defect and pulmonary stenosis. c) The great arteries arise in parallel orientation, with the aorta arising from the morphologically right ventricle and the pulmonary artery arising predominantly from the morphologically left ventricle. The pulmonary valve appears dysplastic and the sub-pulmonary area appears narrowed. d) There is some forward flow across the pulmonary valve, but there is also some reversed flow suggesting significant pulmonary stenosis.**

Figure continued overleaf.

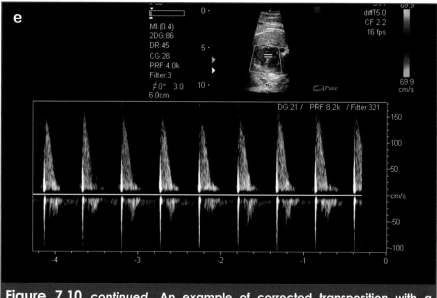

Figure 7.10 *continued.* **An example of corrected transposition with a ventricular septal defect and pulmonary stenosis. e) There is a slightly elevated Doppler velocity (1.5m/second) across the pulmonary valve, confirming pulmonary stenosis.**

7.9b and 7.10b). The great arteries usually arise in a parallel orientation, with the aorta arising from the left-sided morhologically right ventricle and the pulmonary artery more rightwards from the morphologically left ventricle (Figure 7.9c and 7.10c). An example with associated pulmonary stenosis is shown in Figures 7.10a-e and a further example associated with coarctation of the aorta is shown in Figures 7.11a-d.

Extracardiac associations

Extracardiac abnormalities, including chromosomal anomalies are very rare in this condition, though the position or cardiac axis of the heart can often be abnormal.

Management and outcome

In atrioventricular and ventriculo-arterial discordance, with no other cardiac lesions, the circulation is functionally corrected and there may not be any symptoms or problems for many years. However, the pulmonary ventricle is a morphological left ventricle and the systemic ventricle is a morphological right ventricle. This is of significance in the long term if the right ventricle struggles to cope with the systemic circulation. Associated lesions such as ventricular septal defect, Ebstein's anomaly, pulmonary obstruction (stenosis or atresia) or coarctation may require early intervention. Another associated feature of corrected transposition is complete heart block (see Chapter 13), the risk of which increases with age.

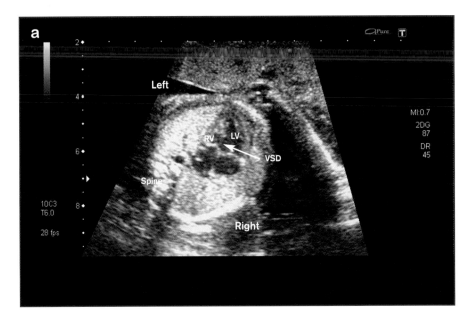

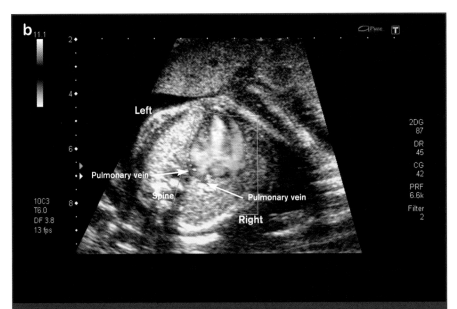

Figure 7.11. An example of complex corrected transposition associated with coarctation of the aorta. a) The four-chamber view shows a hypoplastic left-sided morphologically right ventricle and a large ventricular septal defect. b) The pulmonary veins drain to the left-sided atrium which is connected to the hypoplastic morphologically right ventricle.

Figure continued overleaf.

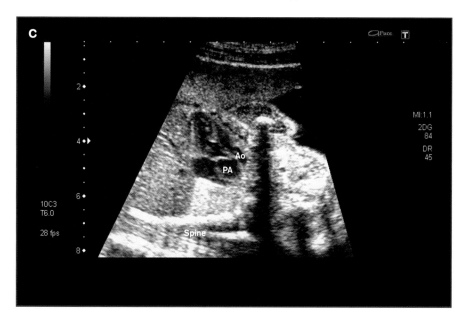

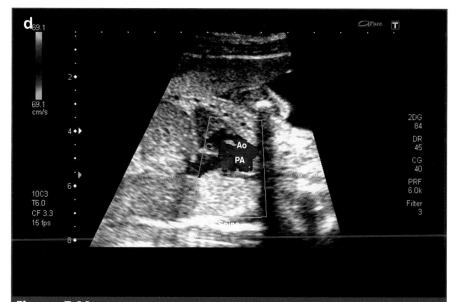

Figure 7.11 *continued.* An example of complex corrected transposition associated with coarctation of the aorta. c) The two great arteries arise in parallel orientation. The aorta arises anterior to and is smaller than the pulmonary artery, suggesting associated coarctation of the aorta. d) Colour flow shows forward flow in both the great arteries (shown in blue).

Outcome in a large single-centre fetal series
Of 60 cases of atrioventricular and ventriculo-arterial discordance diagnosed prenatally, 37% of pregnancies resulted in a termination of pregnancy. If the terminations are excluded then the outcome of the continuing pregnancies was: 8% died in the neonatal period, 13% died in infancy and 76% were alive at last follow-up. Of the continuing pregnancies the outcome is unknown in 3%.

Of cases seen in the last 10 years, a termination of pregnancy took place in 43% of cases and 83% of the continuing pregnancies were alive at last follow-up.

Summary of fetal echocardiographic features associated with CCTGA.

- **Abnormal four-chamber view**
- **Centrally positioned heart**
- **'Reversed' differential insertion of the atrioventricular valves**
- **Moderator band in a left-sided ventricle**
- **Pulmonary veins drain to the atrium (left atrium) that is connected to the right ventricle**
- **Parallel great arteries (aorta arises from the right ventricle, pulmonary artery arises from the left ventricle)**
- **Aorta arises to the left of the pulmonary artery**

Summary of extracardiac associations in fetal CCTGA.

- **Very rare**

Double-outlet right ventricle (DORV)

Prevalence
A double-outlet right ventricle accounts for 1-1.5% of all congenital heart disease in postnatal series. In the Evelina fetal series, a double-outlet right ventricle accounted for 5.2% of the total series and 3.3% of all cases of fetal congenital heart disease seen in the last 10 years.

Definition
In a double-outlet right ventricle both great arteries arise completely or predominantly from the right ventricle. There is always an associated ventricular septal defect (VSD).

Spectrum

The term double-outlet right ventricle covers a heterogeneous group of conditions and the anatomical variations are classified based on the position of the VSD relative to the position of the great arteries. DORV can occur as an isolated cardiac finding or in association with other cardiac malformations.

There are four types of double-outlet right ventricle (DORV):

- DORV with a subaortic VSD. The VSD is located below the aortic valve and is more related to the aortic valve than the pulmonary valve. In this type, blood from the left ventricle flows across the VSD into the aorta.
- DORV with a subpulmonary VSD. The VSD is located below the pulmonary valve. This type is also known as a Taussig-Bing anomaly and the great arteries are transposed. Thus, in this type, blood from the left ventricle flows across the VSD into the pulmonary artery.
- DORV with a doubly committed VSD. The VSD is located below the aortic and pulmonary valves.
- DORV with a non-committed or remote VSD. The VSD is in a position away from both arterial valves, such as the muscular septum or the inlet septum.

Thus, a double-outlet right ventricle covers a spectrum of abnormality, which includes tetralogy of Fallot (see Chapter 8) and transposition of the great arteries (see above). A double-outlet right ventricle can also occur in the setting of more complex heart disease, for example, with an atrioventricular septal defect, mitral atresia or isomerism.

Some cases in the spectrum of double-outlet right ventricle have associated pulmonary atresia. However, strictly speaking these cannot be termed double outlet, as one of the outlets is completely obstructed and the correct terminology would be, for example, VSD (or AVSD or mitral atresia) with the aorta from the right ventricle and pulmonary atresia.

Fetal echocardiographic features

The fetal echocardiographic features will depend on the type of double outlet and the relative positions of the great arteries, as well as associated cardiac lesions. In cases with no associated cardiac lesions, the four-chamber view may appear normal, though the ventricular septal defect may sometimes be seen in this view (Figures 7.12a and 7.13a). There can be imbalance of the ventricular chambers, with one side appearing smaller than the other; this will be detectable in the four-chamber view. If there is an associated cardiac lesion such as an atrioventricular septal defect or mitral atresia, then the four-chamber view will appear abnormal (see Chapter 4).

Views of the great arteries will be abnormal in all cases with both great arteries arising predominantly from the right ventricle (Figures 7.12b and 7.13b). As well as arising in an abnormal position, either great artery can be obstructed. This is often inferred by the obstructed vessel appearing small. Thus, if the pulmonary artery is small there is likely to be

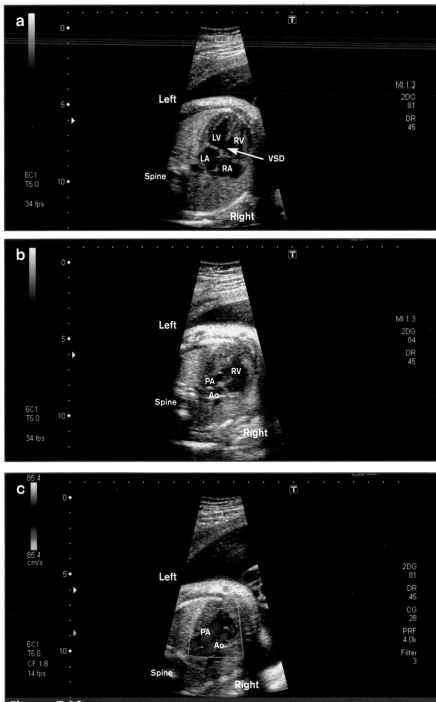

Figure 7.12. An example of a double-outlet right ventricle with the aorta anterior (TGA type). a) The four-chamber view shows equal sized ventricles but there is a large ventricular septal defect. b) Both great arteries arise from the right ventricle in a parallel orientation. The great arteries are of equal size. The aorta in this example is arising anterior to the pulmonary artery. c) There is forward flow in both great arteries (shown in blue).

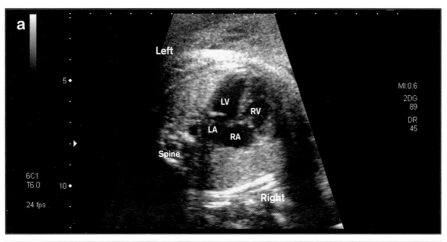

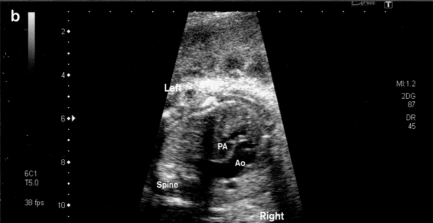

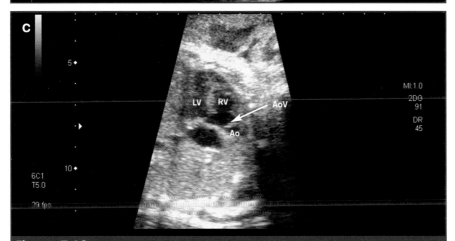

Figure 7.13. An example of a double-outlet right ventricle of tetralogy type. a) In the four-chamber view there are equal sized ventricles. b) Both the great arteries appear to arise from the right ventricle with the aorta being significantly larger than the pulmonary artery. In this particular view the aorta appears to be anterior to the pulmonary artery. c) However, in this long axis view the aorta is clearly seen overriding the crest of the ventricular septum and the ventricular septal defect.

Figure continued overleaf.

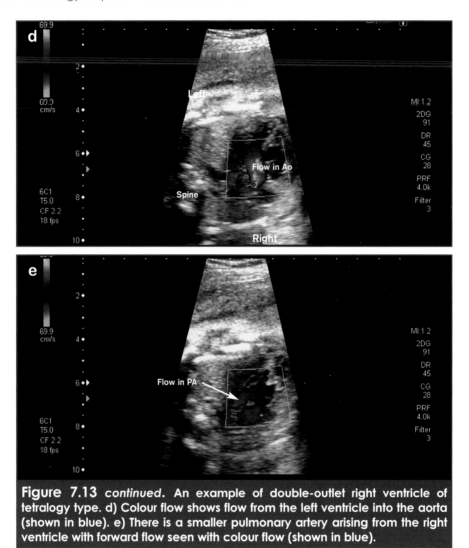

Figure 7.13 *continued*. **An example of double-outlet right ventricle of tetralogy type. d) Colour flow shows flow from the left ventricle into the aorta (shown in blue). e) There is a smaller pulmonary artery arising from the right ventricle with forward flow seen with colour flow (shown in blue).**

pulmonary stenosis and if the aorta and arch appear small there is likely to be associated coarctation of the aorta, or more rarely an interrupted aortic arch (see Chapters 6 and 9).

When the arteries are normally related (Figures 7.13a-e), there will be aortic override, but with more than 50% of the vessel arising from the right ventricle. In these cases, the pulmonary artery arises from the right ventricle and can be a normal size with no obstruction to outflow, or there may be some degree of pulmonary obstruction. In cases of pulmonary stenosis, the pulmonary artery will be small but there will be forward flow across the pulmonary valve, which may be at a normal velocity. This form of double-outlet right ventricle falls in the same spectrum as tetralogy of Fallot, in terms of clinical manifestation and management (see Chapter 8). In cases with pulmonary atresia, the pulmonary artery will be small or tiny with no forward flow and reverse flow from the arterial duct will be detected. In other cases, there may be no obstruction to the pulmonary artery, but there may be obstruction to the aorta, such as coarctation of the aorta. In these the aorta will appear small and the aortic arch will appear hypoplastic. There will, however, be forward flow across the aortic valve. In some cases, there may be no obstruction to either great artery; the clinical manifestation in these will be similar to a large ventricular septal defect.

In cases with a transposed arrangement of the great arteries (Figures 7.12a-c), the pulmonary artery may override the ventricular septal defect, but with more than 50% of the vessel arising from the right ventricle. These cases fall into the spectrum of transposition of the great arteries, in terms of clinical manifestation and management. The great arteries will arise from the heart in a parallel orientation. In this setting it is less common to have pulmonary obstruction and more common to have aortic obstruction, though either can occur.

Extracardiac associations

A double-outlet right ventricle can be associated with chromosomal anomalies such as trisomies 13 and 18 and more rarely trisomy 21. It has also been reported with 22q11 deletion and trisomy 9. Generally, chromosomal abnormalities are more likely in cases with a subaortic VSD and those with other cardiac abnormalities such as an atrioventricular septal defect. Cases with a sub-pulmonary defect are less likely to be associated with a chromosomal defect.

A double-outlet right ventricle can also occur with extracardiac abnormalities including central nervous abnormalities, cleft lip and palate, diaphragmatic hernia, exomphalos, limb and renal abnormalities.

In our large fetal series, a double-outlet right ventricle was associated with chromosomal abnormalities in 14% of cases. Of these, 44% were trisomy 18, 19% were trisomy 13, 6% were trisomy 21, 6% were 22q11 deletion and the remaining were various abnormalities including a case of trisomy 9. A further 17% had an extracardiac anomaly, which included cleft lip and palate, cystic hygroma, dextrocardia, diaphragmatic hernia, duodenal atresia, exomphalos, limb, renal and spinal abnormalities and ventriculomegaly.

Management and outcome

The postnatal management and outcome of infants with a double-outlet right ventricle is dependent upon the variable aspects of the diagnosis which will influence whether the surgical management will be a corrective or a palliative procedure. These include the size of both ventricles and atrioventricular valves, the position and size of the ventricular septal defect, the relationship of the great arteries to each other and to the ventricular septal defect, and the presence of pulmonary or aortic outflow tract obstruction.

Outcome in a large single-centre fetal series

Of 223 cases of a double-outlet right ventricle diagnosed prenatally, 56% of pregnancies resulted in a termination of pregnancy. If the terminations are excluded then the outcome of the continuing pregnancies was: 13% resulting in spontaneous intrauterine death, 24% died in the neonatal period, 12% died in infancy and 51% were alive at last update.

Of cases seen in the last 10 years, a termination of pregnancy took place in 31% of cases and 59% of the continuing pregnancies were alive at last follow-up. It should be noted, however, that this is a heterogeneous group of abnormalities with many associations, both cardiac and non-cardiac.

Summary of fetal echocardiographic features associated with DORV.

- Four-chamber view may be normal in isolated cases
- Ventricular septal defect
- Both great arteries arise predominantly from the right ventricle
- Aortic override if VSD is subaortic
- Pulmonary override and parallel great arteries if VSD is subpulmonary
- Small pulmonary artery if pulmonary stenosis
- Small aorta if aortic obstruction (coarctation or interrupted aortic arch)
- May have associated cardiac lesions such as AVSD, mitral atresia, isomerism

---

Summary of extracardiac associations in fetal DORV.

- Chromosomal
  - 14%
- Extracardiac abnormality (normal chromosomes)
  - 17%

Chapter 8

Great artery abnormalities (II)
Abnormalities of ventriculo-arterial connection

Summary

- **Ventricular septal defect with great artery override**
  - Malalignment ventricular septal defect
  - Tetralogy of Fallot
  - Pulmonary atresia with a ventricular septal defect
  - Common arterial trunk
  - Absent pulmonary valve syndrome
  - Aortic atresia with a sub-pulmonary VSD

Ventricular septal defect with great artery override

In this group of lesions the findings are of a ventricular septal defect with great artery override in the absence of transposed great arteries. It is important to search for the second great artery in order to make a correct diagnosis.

Malalignment ventricular septal defect

In these cases, there is a ventricular septal defect with aortic override. The aorta is of normal size and there is no evidence of aortic obstruction. The pulmonary artery arises normally from the right ventricle, is a normal size and there is no evidence of pulmonary obstruction. Ventricular septal defects are discussed in Chapter 5.

Tetralogy of Fallot (ToF/tetralogy)

Prevalence
Tetralogy of Fallot accounts for up to 10% of all cases of congenital heart disease in postnatal series. In the Evelina fetal series, tetralogy of Fallot accounted for 5.2% of the total series and 7.2% of all cases of fetal congenital heart disease seen in the last 10 years.

Definition

Tetralogy of Fallot is described as an anomaly consisting of four components: a ventricular septal defect, infundibular pulmonary stenosis (the pulmonary valve is also often stenotic and hypoplastic), anterior deviation of the aorta causing the aorta to override the ventricular septal defect, and right ventricular hypertrophy. In practice the significant clinical features are the ventricular septal defect and the pulmonary stenosis.

Spectrum

Tetralogy of Fallot constitutes a spectrum of abnormality. If there is minimal or no obstruction to the right ventricular outflow tract, then it is hard to distinguish from a ventricular septal defect with aortic override. If there is complete obstruction to the right ventricular outflow tract, then the condition overlaps with pulmonary atresia with a ventricular septal defect (see below). There is another variant of tetralogy, which is less common, known as absent pulmonary valve syndrome (see below).

Tetralogy of Fallot can occur with other cardiac lesions, including a right-sided aortic arch, total anomalous pulmonary venous drainage, atrioventricular septal defect, multiple ventricular septal defects and coronary artery fistula.

Fetal echocardiographic features

The axis of the fetal heart may be abnormal in some cases (Figure 8.1a). However, the four-chamber view of the fetal heart is often normal, though a ventricular septal defect may sometimes be seen in this view (Figure 8.2a). Long-axis views of the left ventricle, to image the aorta arising from the left ventricle, will demonstrate the ventricular septal defect and the aorta overriding the crest of the ventricular septum (Figures 8.1b, 8.2b and 8.3a). Colour flow will demonstrate flow into the aorta from both the left and right ventricles (Figures 8.1c and 8.2c). Note that it is the aortic valve that overrides the ventricular septal defect. Occasionally the impression of aortic override can be produced by artefact, but in these cases, the appearance of a defect is above the aortic valve (Figure 8.4) and therefore this cannot be true override. Further examples of the four-chamber view and override are shown in Figures 8.5a-b and 8.6a-b. In cases with tetralogy of Fallot, the aorta may appear dilated. The pulmonary artery arises from the right ventricle and is usually small, though its size can vary from being within the normal range to very hypoplastic (Figures 8.2d-e, 8.3b, 8.5c-d and 8.6c-d). A small pulmonary artery indicates some degree of right ventricular outflow tract obstruction, even though the Doppler velocities may fall in the normal range, with laminar flow across the valve into the small pulmonary artery (Figure 8.2f). In cases with severe pulmonary outflow tract obstruction, the pulmonary artery is likely to be very hypoplastic and reversal of flow in the arterial duct may be detected. Colour flow may be helpful in identifying very small pulmonary arteries which may not be easily visualised and for identifying reverse flow from the arterial duct (Figures 8.7a-d). These cases overlap with pulmonary atresia with a ventricular septal defect (see below).

In some cases of tetralogy, the aortic arch will be right-sided (Figures 8.6a-d). This association can be easily identified in the three-vessel view (Figure 8.6d).

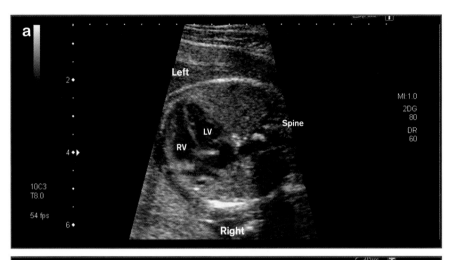

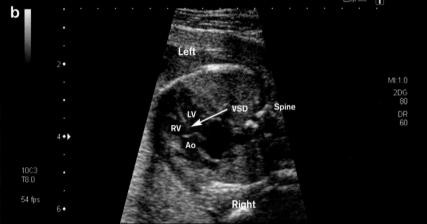

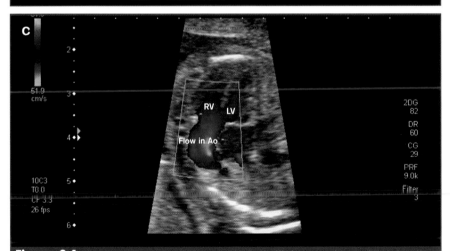

Figure 8.1. An example of tetralogy of Fallot with levoposition of the cardiac axis. a) The four-chamber view shows that the cardiac axis is rotated towards the left axilla. b) The aorta is overriding the crest of the ventricular septum and the ventricular septal defect. c) Colour flow shows flow from both ventricles in the aorta (shown in blue).

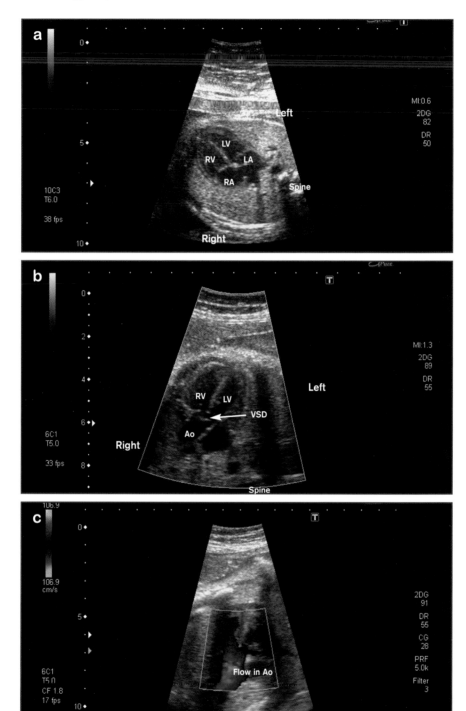

Figure 8.2. An example of tetralogy of Fallot with good sized pulmonary arteries. a) The four-chamber view appears normal. b) The aorta is overriding the crest of the ventricular septum and the ventricular septal defect. c) Colour flow shows flow from both ventricles in the aorta (shown in blue).

Figure continued overleaf.

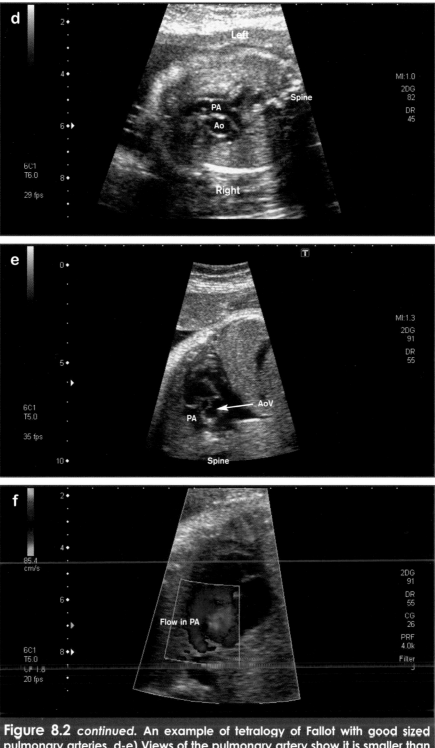

Figure 8.2 *continued.* **An example of tetralogy of Fallot with good sized pulmonary arteries. d-e) Views of the pulmonary artery show it is smaller than the aorta but it is still a good size. f) There is laminar forward flow across the pulmonary valve (shown in blue).**

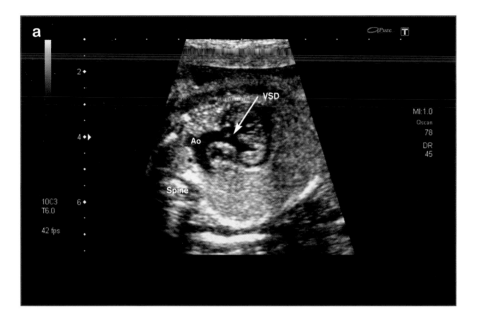

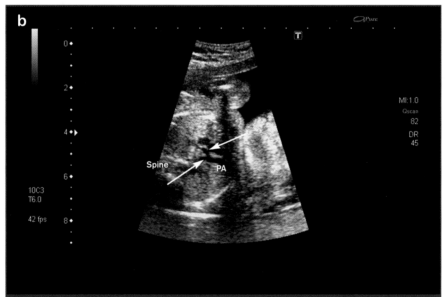

Figure 8.3. An example of tetralogy of Fallot with small pulmonary arteries. a) The aorta is seen overriding the crest of the ventricular septum and the ventricular septal defect. b) The pulmonary artery in this example is very small, though confluent branch pulmonary arteries can be seen (arrows).

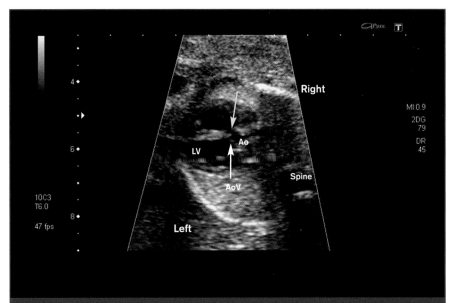

Figure 8.4. A view of the aorta arising from the left ventricle. In this view, there is the impression of override but the appearance of the defect (yellow arrow) is above the aortic valve and this is artefact.

Extracardiac associations

Tetralogy of Fallot can be associated with extracardiac abnormalities, which may be either structural or chromosomal. It can also be associated with other syndromes or structural malformations. These include midline defects, such as omphalocoele and pentalogy of Cantrell, central nervous abnormalities, diaphragmatic hernia and renal abnormalities. It can also occur in syndromes such as VACTERL or CHARGE, where there are multiple associated lesions. Tetralogy has also been associated with fetal hydantoin syndrome, fetal carbamazepine syndrome, fetal alcohol syndrome and maternal phenylketonuria. Chromosomal anomalies include trisomies 21, 13, 18 and various additions or deletions, particularly chromosome 22q11 deletions (DiGeorge and Shprintzen syndromes). In cases with an associated atrioventricular septal defect, 75-80% will have trisomy 21.

In our large fetal series, tetralogy of Fallot was associated with chromosomal abnormalities in 21% of cases. Of these, 32% were trisomy 21, 23% were 22q11 deletion, 19% were trisomy 18, 6% were trisomy 13 and 13% had various other chromosomal abnormalities including unbalanced translocations and deletions, a case of 47XXY, a case of 69XXX and a case of 92XXYY. A further 14% had an extracardiac anomaly (with a normal karyotype), which included anophthalmia, cleft lip and palate, cystic hygroma, Dandy Walker malformation, diaphragmatic hernia, duodenal atresia, ectopia, exomphalos, hemivertebrae, microcephaly, renal abnormalities, scoliosis and tracheo-oesophageal atresia.

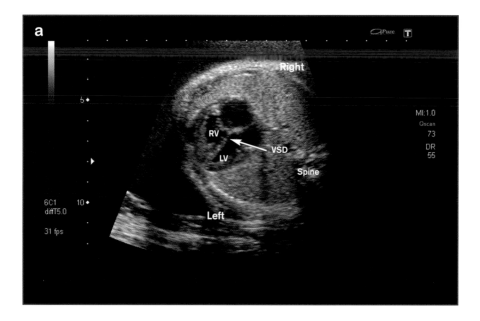

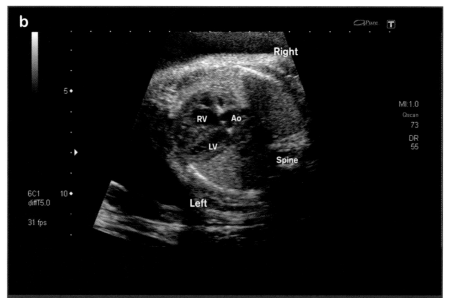

Figure 8.5. A further example of tetralogy with a moderate sized pulmonary artery. a) The four-chamber view appears essentially normal, though the ventricular septal defect is just visible. b) The aorta is overriding the crest of the ventricular septum and the ventricular septal defect.

Figure continued overleaf.

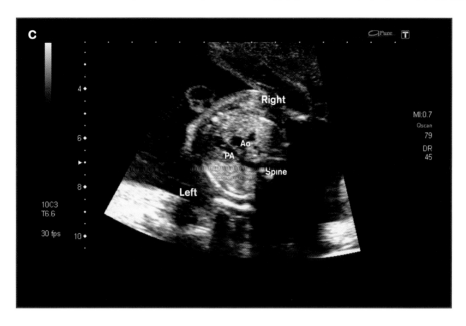

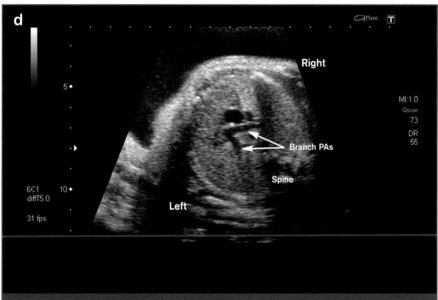

Figure 8.5 *continued*. **A further example of tetralogy with a moderate sized pulmonary artery. c) The pulmonary artery is slightly smaller than the aorta. d) Confluent branch pulmonary arteries of equal size are seen.**

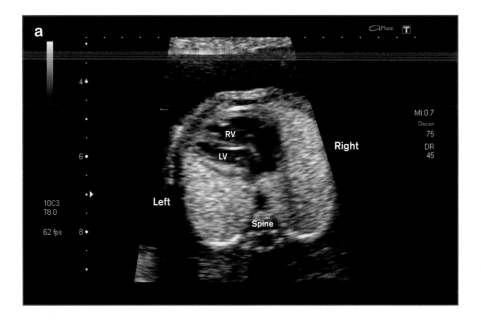

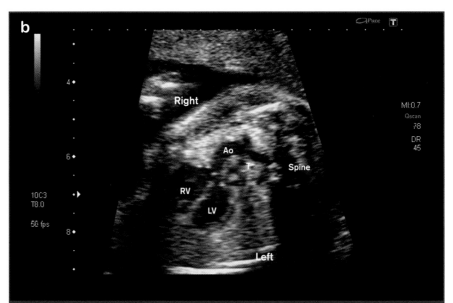

Figure 8.6. An example of tetralogy with a right-sided aortic arch. a) The four-chamber view appears normal, though there is some leftward deviation of the cardiac axis. b) The aorta is overriding the crest of the ventricular septum and the ventricular septal defect. In this view, the aorta can be seen to descend to the right of the trachea.

Figure continued overleaf.

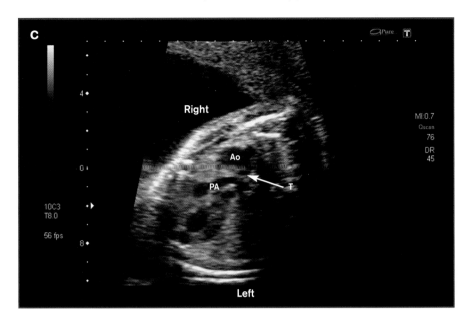

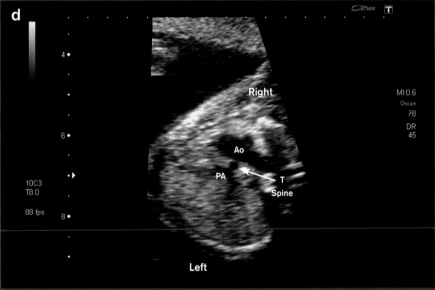

Figure 8.6 *continued*. An example of tetralogy with a right-sided aortic arch. c) The pulmonary artery is significantly smaller than the aorta. d) In the three-vessel view the pulmonary artery is much smaller than the aorta and the aortic arch is right-sided.

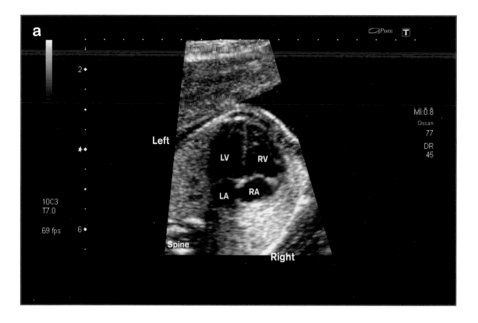

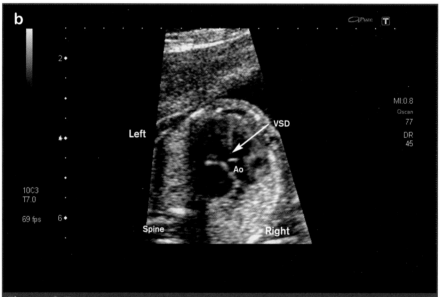

Figure 8.7. An example of tetralogy of Fallot with pulmonary atresia. a) The four-chamber view appears normal. b) The aorta is overriding the crest of the ventricular septum and the ventricular septal defect.

Figure continued overleaf.

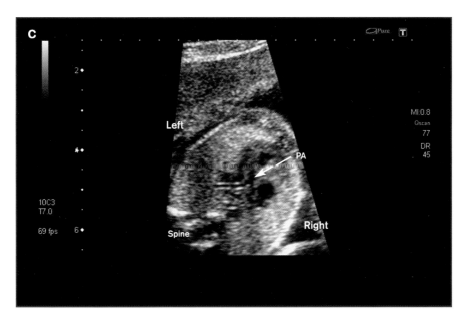

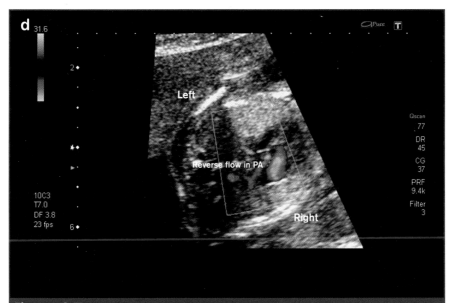

Figure 8.7 *continued*. An example of tetralogy of Fallot with pulmonary atresia. c) The pulmonary artery is tiny but tiny confluent branch pulmonary arteries can be seen. d) Colour flow mapping shows reverse filling (shown in red) of the tiny pulmonary arteries from the arterial duct.

Management and outcome

Most babies with tetralogy of Fallot will not need immediate neonatal intervention postnatally. The initial priority is to address the adequacy of pulmonary blood flow. If the pulmonary blood flow is inadequate then a systemic to pulmonary (Blalock-Taussig) shunt may be required. In cases with well-developed pulmonary arteries and adequate pulmonary blood flow, surgical repair may be undertaken as the first step and this is the preference where possible. The definitive repair is usually performed at around 6 months of age and consists of closure of the ventricular septal defect, relief of the right ventricular outflow tract obstruction and augmentation of the pulmonary arteries if required. The surgical repair itself carries a mortality of less than 5%, though there is also a risk associated with any initial procedure, for example, a shunt, required to establish adequate pulmonary blood flow prior to the definitive repair. Any associated anomalies, cardiac or extracardiac, will also affect the overall outcome. In the longer term, significant pulmonary regurgitation can occur, as can branch pulmonary artery stenosis, both of which will require further intervention.

Outcome in a large single-centre fetal series

Of 223 cases of tetralogy of Fallot diagnosed prenatally, 17% of pregnancies resulted in a termination of pregnancy. If the terminations are excluded then the outcome of the continuing pregnancies was: 7% resulting in spontaneous intrauterine death, 10% died in the neonatal period, 4% died in infancy and 77% were alive at last update. The outcome is unknown in 2% of the continuing pregnancies.

Of cases seen in the last 10 years, a termination of pregnancy took place in 10% of cases and 85% of the continuing pregnancies were alive at last follow-up.

Summary of fetal echocardiographic features associated with tetralogy.

- Leftward deviation of cardiac axis (sometimes)
- Normal four-chamber view (usually)
- Ventricular septal defect
- Aortic override
- Aorta may appear dilated
- Small pulmonary artery (pulmonary stenosis)
- Aortic arch may be right-sided

Summary of extracardiac associations in fetal tetralogy.

- Chromosomal
  - 21%
- Extracardiac abnormality (normal chromosomes)
  - 14%

Pulmonary atresia with a ventricular septal defect (PAT VSD)

Prevalence
The prevalence of pulmonary atresia with a ventricular septal defect in postnatal series is difficult to establish as there is no uniformity of classifiction of this diagnosis, due to the overlap with tetralogy of Fallot. In the Evelina fetal series, pulmonary atresia with a ventricular septal defect accounted for 2.2% of the total series and 2.3% of all cases of fetal congenital heart disease seen in the last 10 years.

Definition
In this condition there is a ventricular septal defect and anterior displacement of the aorta, as in tetralogy of Fallot, but the pulmonary valve or right ventricular outflow tract are atretic. Thus, there is no patent connection between the right ventricle and the main pulmonary artery.

Spectrum
There may be atresia of the pulmonary valve with the right ventricular outflow tract and main pulmonary artery identifiable, infundibular atresia, or long segment atresia, where the main pulmonary artery cannot be identified. The branch pulmonary arteries are often hypoplastic and may be confluent (join each other), or they may be discontinuous. The pulmonary blood flow is either via the arterial duct, or there may be collateral vessels arising directly from the aorta supplying the lungs. The aortic arch may be right-sided in some cases.

Fetal echocardiographic features
As with cases of tetralogy of Fallot, the cardiac position may be abnormal in some cases, with the apex directed more towards the left axilla than normal. The four-chamber view may be normal, though in some cases a ventricular septal defect may be seen (Figure 8.8a). Views of the great arteries will demonstrate a large vessel overriding the ventricular septal defect (Figure 8.8b). This large vessel is the aorta. In cases with pulmonary valvar atresia, the main pulmonary artery may be identified and this can be of varying size. However, there will be no forward flow detected in the main pulmonary artery and there will be retrograde flow from the arterial duct (Figures 8.7c-d). In cases with infundibular or long segment atresia, no main pulmonary artery can be identified, though confluent branch pulmonary arteries can often be seen (Figures 8.8c and Figure 8.9a). The pulmonary blood supply is either retrogradely from the arterial duct (Figure 8.8d), or from collateral vessels arising from the descending aorta (Figures 8.9b-c and 8.10). In some cases, the native pulmonary arteries may not be identified at all and blood supply to the lungs is from collateral vessels only.

Extracardiac associations
This form of congenital heart disease may be associated with chromosomal abnormalities, particularly chromosome 22q11 deletions. In our large fetal series, 17% of cases of pulmonary atresia with a ventricular septal defect had a proven chromosomal abnormality. Of these, 63% were 22q11 deletions and 19% were trisomy 13, with the remaining being a variety of chromosomal defects. A further 15% had extracardiac abnormalities, which included a CHARGE association, cleft lip, diaphragmatic hernia, duodenal atresia, renal abnormalities, scoliosis and talipes.

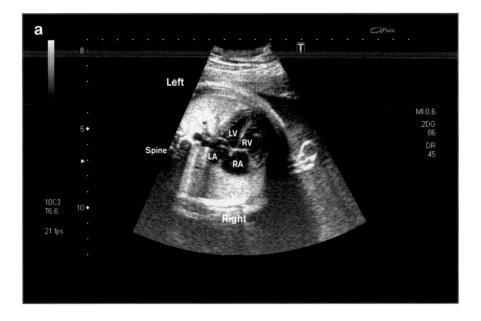

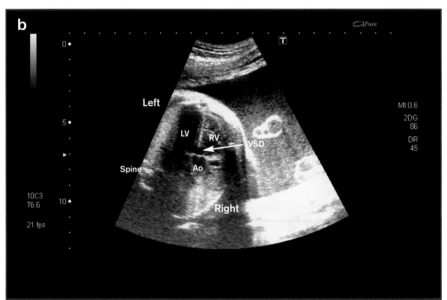

Figure 8.8. An example of pulmonary atresia with a ventricular septal defect. a) The four-chamber view appears normal. b) The aorta is overriding the crest of the ventricular septum and the ventricular septal defect. *Figure continued overleaf.*

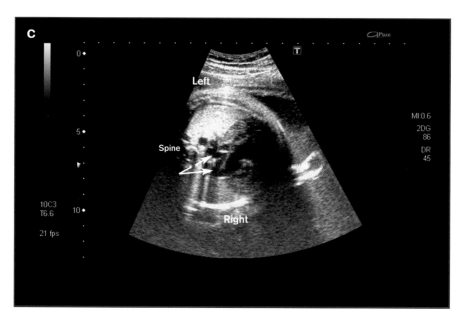

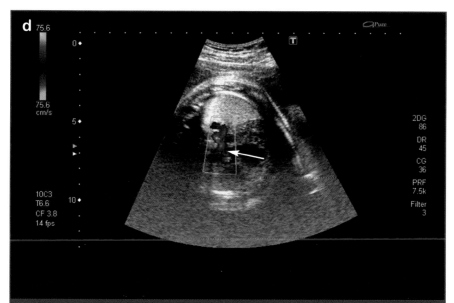

Figure 8.8 *continued*. An example of pulmonary atresia with a ventricular septal defect. c) No main pulmonary artery was identified in this example but confluent branch pulmonary arteries are seen (arrows). d) The confluent pulmonary arteries fill retrogradely from the arterial duct (shown in blue and arrow).

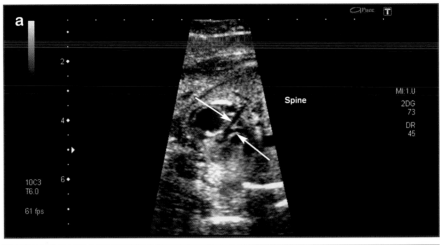

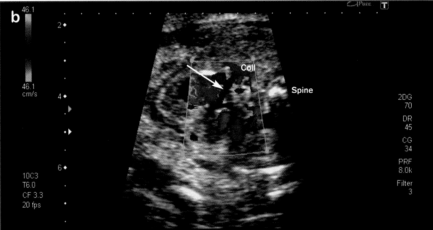

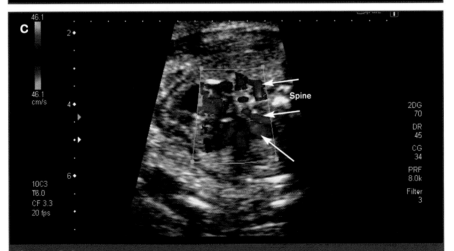

Figure 8.9. An example of pulmonary atresia with a ventricular septal defect with multiple collateral vessels. a) Tiny confluent branch pulmonary arteries are seen in this view (arrows). b) The tiny confluent branch pulmonary arteries fill retrogradely (shown in blue and arrow) from collateral vessels (shown in red). c) Multiple collateral vessels are seen (arrows).

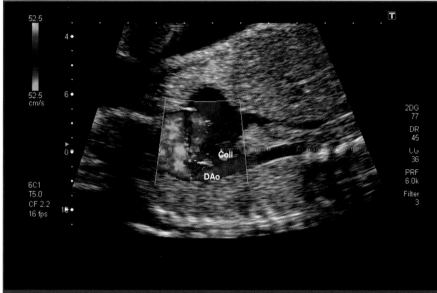

Figure 8.10. A collateral vessel (Coll) is seen arising from the descending aorta in a longitudinal view.

Management and outcome

This is a severe form of congenital heart disease. The management after birth will be dependent on whether there are confluent branch pulmonary arteries and the extent of any aortopulmonary collateral vessels.

Pulmonary blood flow will have to be established, most likely with a systemic to pulmonary artery shunt (Blalock-Taussig shunt), though if there are multiple aortopulmonary collateral arteries (MAPCAs) there may be sufficient pulmonary blood flow. Surgical repair, where possible, is typically undertaken at around a year of age. If there are confluent branch pulmonary arteries of adequate size, then repair consists of closure of the ventricular septal defect and insertion of a conduit between the right ventricle and the pulmonary arteries. Mortality for the shunt operation and later repair is around 5-10%, though the overall mortality by the age of 1 year is much higher. In the longer term further replacement of the right ventricle to pulmonary conduit will be required as the child grows.

If there are aortopulmonary collateral arteries, this will complicate management. In the most severe cases, no intervention may be possible. The feasibility of the surgical repair does depend on the growth and development of the branch pulmonary arteries.

Outcome in a large single-centre fetal series

Of 94 cases of pulmonary atresia with a ventricular septal defect diagnosed prenatally, 50% of pregnancies resulted in a termination of pregnancy. If the terminations are excluded then the outcome of the continuing pregnancies was: 6% resulting in spontaneous intrauterine death, 23% died in the neonatal period, 17% died in infancy and 49% were alive at last update. The outcome is unknown in 5% of the continuing pregnancies.

Of cases seen in the last 10 years, a termination of pregnancy took place in 33% of cases and 61% of the continuing pregnancies were alive at last follow-up.

Summary of fetal echocardiographic features associated with PAT VSD.

- Leftward deviation of cardiac axis (sometimes)
- Normal four-chamber view (often)
- Ventricular septal defect
- Aortic override
- No forward flow from the right ventricle to the pulmonary artery
- Main pulmonary artery is small or may not be identified
- Hypoplastic branch pulmonary arteries
- Retrograde flow in the arterial duct
- Collateral vessels in some cases
- Aortic arch may be right-sided

Summary of extracardiac associations in fetal PAT VSD.

- Chromosomal
  - 17%
- Extracardiac abnormality (normal chromosomes)
  - 15%

Common arterial trunk (CAT)

Prevalence
The prevalence of common arterial trunk is around 1-1.5% in postnatal series. In the Evelina fetal series, common arterial trunk accounted for 1.1% of the total series and 1.2% of cases of fetal congenital heart disease seen in the last 10 years.

Definition
This anomaly is characterised by a single great artery arising from the heart which gives rise to the systemic, pulmonary and coronary circulations. There is an associated ventricular septal defect.

Spectrum

This lesion is best categorised by describing the pattern of the pulmonary artery connection to the common trunk. This may be as a main pulmonary artery, which then divides into the two branch pulmonary arteries; or the two pulmonary artery branches may insert separately into the trunk, close to each other (which is the most common connection) or at some distance apart. The importance of this categorization is that this last connection is more difficult to repair surgically.

Common arterial trunk can be associated with interruption of the aortic arch, an atrioventricular septal defect, a single ventricle or a dominant ventricle, atrioventricular valve atresia, a right-sided aortic arch and a double aortic arch. The arterial duct is absent in about 50% of cases.

Fetal echocardiographic features

The cardiac position may be abnormal in some cases, with the apex directed more towards the left axilla compared to normal. The four-chamber view may be normal, though the ventricular septal defect may be evident (Figure 8.11a and 8.12a). Occasionally one of the ventricular chambers may be more dominant and rarely there may be atresia of either atrioventricular valve. A single arterial trunk will be identified arising from the heart and this gives rise to the aortic arch and the pulmonary arteries (Figures 8.11b-c). The truncal valve is often thickened and dysplastic and this may be associated with stenosis or regurgitation (Figures 8.12b-e). Turbulence detected on colour flow across the truncal valve and an increase in truncal velocity indicates truncal valve stenosis, the degree of which can vary (Figures 8.12c and 8.12e). Truncal valve regurgitation can also be detected with colour flow (Figure 8.12d). The aortic arch can be right-sided in some cases. Rarely, a common arterial trunk can be associated with an interrupted aortic arch and an example of this is shown in Figures 8.13a-b. In this case, a small vessel appears to arise from the side of the trunk and this has a 'pronged fork' appearance, which is a hallmark of an interrupted aortic arch (see Chapter 9).

Extracardiac associations

This condition can be associated with chromosomal anomalies particularly microdeletion of chromosome 22q11 and DiGeorge or Shprintzen syndromes.

In our large fetal series, common arterial trunk was associated with chromosomal abnormalities in 8% of cases, which included 22q11 deletion, trisomy 9, triploidy and an unbalanced translocation. A further 15% had an extracardiac anomaly, which included an absent arm, cleft lip, dolichocephaly, exomphalos and renal abnormalities.

Management and outcome

This is a major but repairable form of congenital heart disease. This lesion does not typically cause early compromise in the newborn period, unless there is significant truncal valve stenosis and regurgitation. Surgical repair is usually undertaken in the first few weeks after birth. This consists of closing the ventricular septal defect in a way which baffles the outflow from the left ventricle into the main trunk. The pulmonary arteries are disconnected

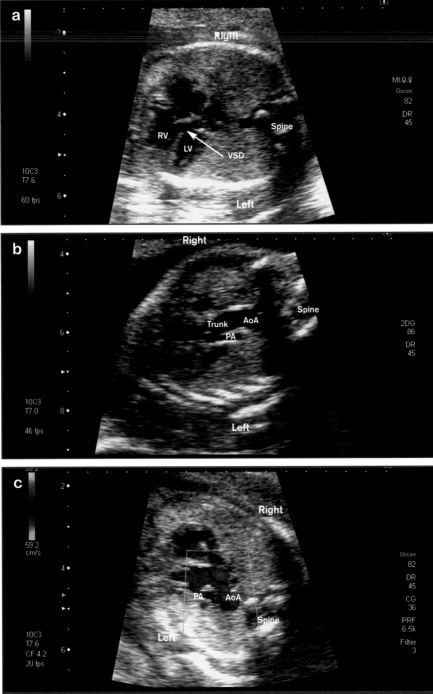

Figure 8.11. An example of a common arterial trunk. a) In the four-chamber view there is some leftward deviation of the cardiac axis. The left ventricle is slightly smaller than the right ventricle and a ventricular septal defect can be seen. b) A single arterial trunk is seen arising from the heart which gives rise to the aorta and the pulmonary artery. c) Colour flow shows the flow in the aorta and the pulmonary artery (both shown in blue).

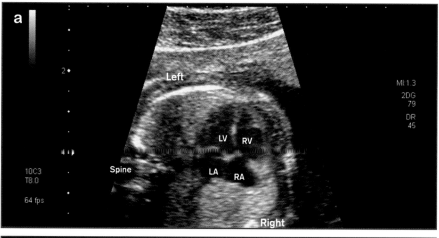

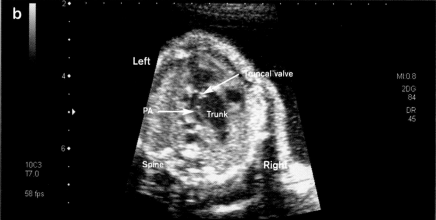

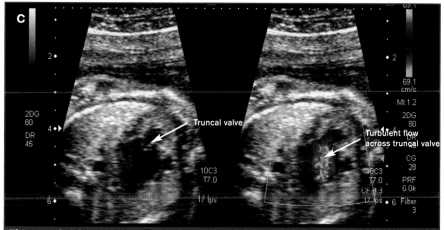

Figure 8.12. An example of a common arterial trunk associated with a dysplastic truncal valve, which was stenotic and regurgitant. a) In the four-chamber view the ventricular septal defect can be seen. b) A single arterial trunk arises from the heart and the truncal valve appears very dysplastic. The pulmonary artery can be seen arising from the side of the trunk. c) Turbulent flow is seen across the truncal valve with colour flow.

Figure continued overleaf.

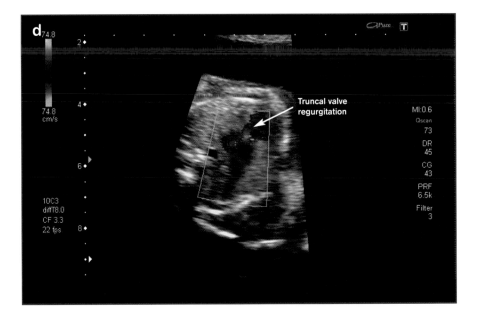

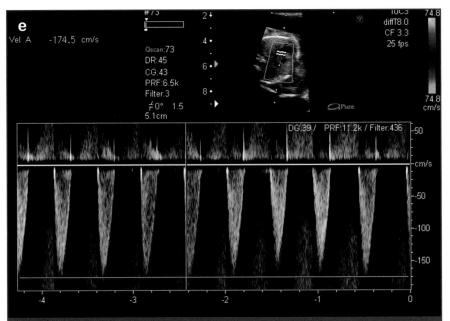

Figure 8.12 *continued.* **An example of a common arterial trunk associated with a dysplastic truncal valve, which was stenotic and regurgitant. d) There is also some truncal valve regurgitation seen with colour flow (seen in red). e) There is an increased Doppler velocity for the gestation across the truncal valve (1.74m/second) indicating some truncal valve stenosis.**

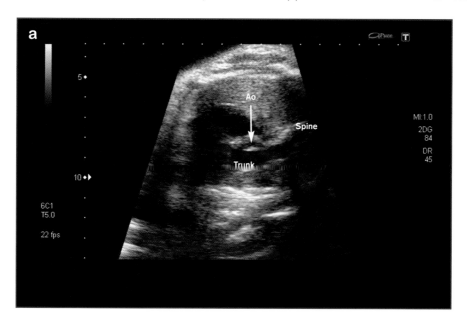

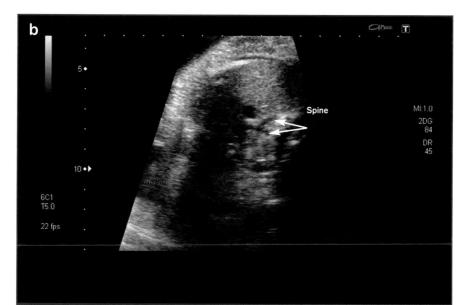

Figure 8.13. An example of a common arterial trunk with an interrupted aortic arch. a) A single arterial trunk is seen arising from the heart. A small vessel can be seen arising from the side of the trunk. b) The small vessel is the aorta and has a 'pronged fork' appearance (arrows) which is suggestive of an interrupted aortic arch.

from the trunk and connected to the right ventricle via a homograft. Surgical mortality is in the region of 5-10%, though the overall mortality by the age of 1 year is much higher. The risk is much higher if the truncal valve is stenotic or regurgitant. In the longer term the homograft between the right ventricle and pulmonary arteries will need to be replaced as the child grows. There can also be problems related to the function of the truncal valve and stenosis of the branch pulmonary arteries.

Outcome in a large single-centre fetal series

Of 48 cases of common arterial trunk diagnosed prenatally, 35% of pregnancies resulted in a termination of pregnancy. If the terminations are excluded then the outcome of the continuing pregnancies was: 26% died in the neonatal period, 19% died in infancy and 55% were alive at last update.

Of cases seen in the last 10 years, a termination of pregnancy took place in 33% of cases and 79% of the continuing pregnancies were alive at last follow-up.

Summary of fetal echocardiographic features associated with CAT.

- Leftward deviation of cardiac axis (sometimes)
- Four-chamber view may be normal
- Ventricular septal defect
- Single arterial trunk usually arising astride a ventricular septal defect, though it can arise predominantly from either ventricle
- Aortic arch arises from the main trunk
- Main pulmonary artery or branch pulmonary arteries arise from the main trunk
- Dysplastic truncal valve (sometimes)
- Stenotic truncal valve (sometimes)
- Regurgitant truncal valve (sometimes)
- Aortic arch may be right-sided

Summary of extracardiac associations in fetal CAT.

- Chromosomal
  - 8%
- Extracardiac abnormality (normal chromosomes)
  - 15%

Absent pulmonary valve syndrome (Abs PV)

Prevalence
This is a rare cardiac malformation. In a single-centre experience of over 4000 fetal cardiac abnormalities, an absent pulmonary valve accounted for 0.9% of the total.

Definition
This condition has some similarities to tetralogy of Fallot in that there is a ventricular septal defect, an overriding aorta and narrowing of the pulmonary valve. However, in this abnormality the pulmonary valve leaflets are rudimentary, appear dysplastic and are non-functional. Although the valve leaflets are very abnormal, they are not absent as the name suggests.

Spectrum
The abnormal pulmonary valve leaflets result in free pulmonary regurgitation and there may be associated pulmonary stenosis in some cases. A feature of this condition is massive dilatation of the main and, in particular, the branch pulmonary arteries, which can cause compression of the airway. The degree of pulmonary artery dilatation can be variable. The arterial duct is often absent in this lesion, though it may occasionally be present.

Fetal echocardiographic features
The four-chamber view of the fetal heart may be abnormal, as the right ventricle may be dilated and poorly functioning as a result of severe pulmonary regurgitation (Figure 8.14a and 8.15a). There is usually a ventricular septal defect most commonly with aortic override, as seen in tetralogy of Fallot. The pulmonary valve is rudimentary and dysplastic (Figures 8.14b and 8.15b). The pulmonary valve annulus may appear narrowed in some cases, though it may also be dilated. However, the main and branch pulmonary arteries are dilated, often massively dilated (Figures 8.14b-c and 8.15b). Colour flow will demonstrate to and fro flow in the region of the pulmonary valve and right ventricular outflow tract (Figures 8.14d-e and 8.15c). The forward flow into the pulmonary artery may be at high velocity indicating associated pulmonary stenosis.

Extracardiac associations
This form of congenital heart disease is associated with chromosomal abnormalities, particularly chromosome 22q11 deletions. It can also be associated with extracardiac structural malformations.

In our large fetal series, absent pulmonary valve syndrome was associated with chromosomal abnormalities in 11% of cases, of which two cases had 22q11 deletion, one case had trisomy 13, one case had trisomy 18 and two cases had various other chromosomal abnormalities. A further 18% of cases had other extracardiac abnormalities.

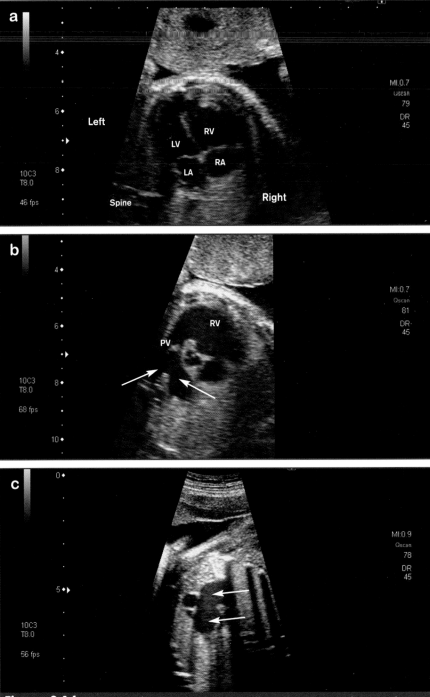

Figure 8.14 An example of absent/dysplastic pulmonary valve syndrome. a) In the four-chamber view the right atrium and right ventricle are slightly dilated compared to the left atrium and left ventricle. b) The pulmonary valve is dysplastic and the branch pulmonary arteries appear dilated (arrows). c) The branch pulmonary arteries appear very dilated in the thorax giving a cystic appearance (arrows).

Figure continued overleaf.

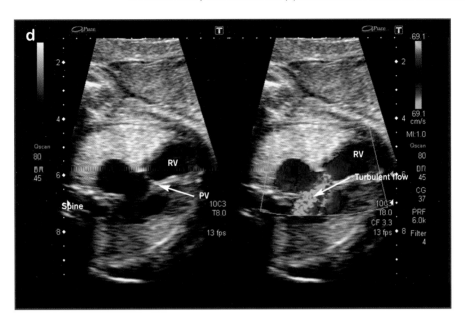

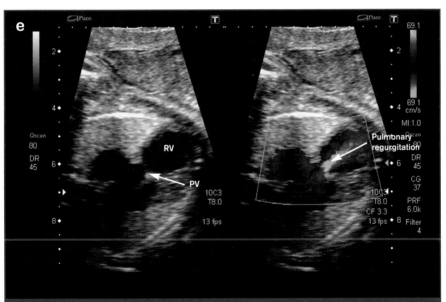

Figure 8.14 An example of absent/dysplastic pulmonary valve syndrome. d) There is turbulent flow indicating increased velocity across the pulmonary valve. e) There is also pulmonary regurgitation.

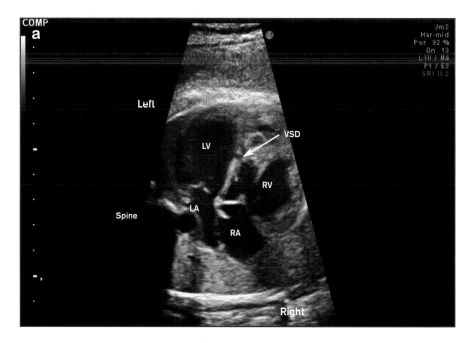

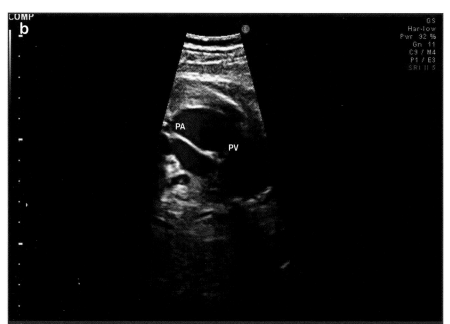

Figure 8.15. An example of absent/dysplastic pulmonary valve syndrome with a very dilated heart. a) In the four-chamber view there is marked cardiomegaly with the right ventricle appearing hypertrophied. As an incidental finding there is a small muscular ventricular septal defect. b) The pulmonary valve is rudimentary and dysplastic. The pulmonary artery is very dilated.

Figure continued overleaf.

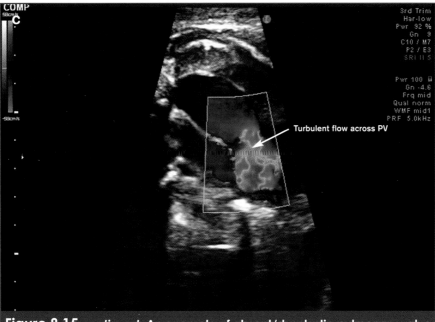

Turbulent flow across PV

Figure 8.15 *continued*. **An example of absent/dysplastic pulmonary valve syndrome with a very dilated heart. c) There is turbulent flow in the right ventricular outflow. There is also pulmonary regurgitation.**

Management and outcome

The prognosis in this condition is influenced by the degree of associated pulmonary compromise. In some babies the dilation of the pulmonary arteries is associated with severe compression of the airways or true bronchomalacia, which leads to early difficulties with respiration. In these cases, ventilation is required soon after birth and may be needed for several weeks or months even after surgical repair. The outlook for this group is very poor. If, however, there is no early respiratory distress, then surgical repair can be deferred and the prognosis is much better, with the vast majority of children surviving. Surgical repair consists of plication of the pulmonary arteries, insertion of a competent pulmonary valve and closure of the associated ventricular septal defect.

Outcome in a large single-centre fetal series

Of 38 cases of absent pulmonary valve syndrome diagnosed prenatally, 34% of pregnancies resulted in a termination of pregnancy. If the terminations are excluded then the outcome of the continuing pregnancies was: 20% resulting in spontaneous intrauterine death, 36% died in the neonatal period, 8% died in infancy and 36% were alive at last update.

Summary of fetal echocardiographic features associated with Abs PV.

- Abnormal four-chamber view
- Right ventricular dilatation
- Abnormal pulmonary valve leaflets
- Very dilated pulmonary arteries
- Marked pulmonary regurgitation (to and fro flow)
- Pulmonary stenosis (sometimes)
- Absent arterial duct (often)

Summary of extracardiac associations in fetal Abs PV.

- Chromosomal
  - 11%
- Extracardiac abnormality (normal chromosomes)
  - 18%

Aortic atresia with a ventricular septal defect (AoAt VSD)

Prevalence

This is a very rare cardiac malformation. In the Evelina fetal series, aortic atresia with a ventricular septal defect accounted for 0.2% of the total.

Definition

In this setting aortic atresia (see Chapter 6) occurs with a ventricular septal defect and two equal sized ventricles.

Fetal echocardiographic features

The four-chamber view may look essentially normal, apart from the ventricular septal defect (Figure 8.16a). Equal forward flow can be demonstrated into both ventricular chambers (Figure 8.16b), in contrast to cases with aortic atresia with hypoplastic left heart syndrome (Figures 6.4b and 6.5b). Views of the great arteries, however, will be abnormal. One large artery, the pulmonary artery, will be seen arising from the right ventricle and may be overriding the ventricular septal defect. The other great artery, the aorta, is tiny (Figure 8.16c) with no forward flow detected across the valve or in the ascending aorta. The aortic arch will appear very hypoplastic and there will be reverse flow from the arterial duct in the arch (Figure 8.16d).

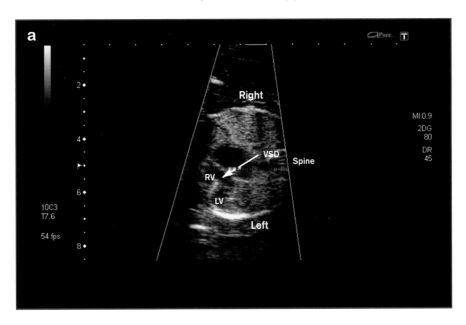

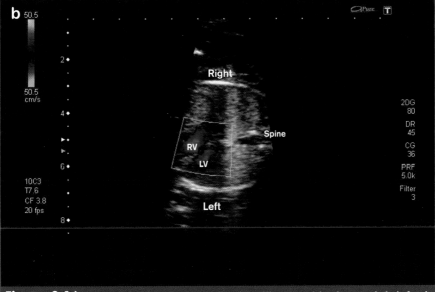

Figure 8.16. An example of aortic atresia with a ventricular septal defect. a) The four-chamber view shows balanced ventricles with a large ventricular septal defect. b) Colour flow shows forward flow into both ventricular chambers.

Figure continued overleaf.

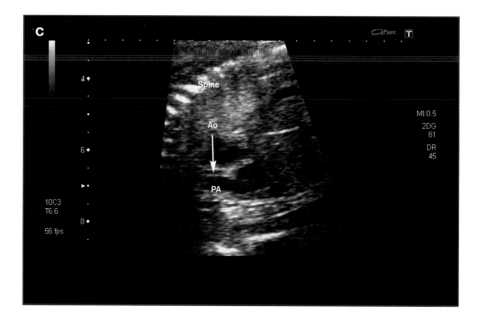

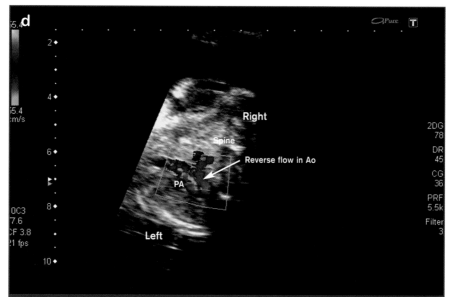

Figure 8.16 *continued*. An example of aortic atresia with a ventricular septal defect. c) A view of the great arteries shows a large pulmonary artery and a tiny aorta. d) In the three-vessel view there is reverse flow in the aortic arch (shown in red) confirming aortic atresia (see Chapter 6).

Extracardiac associations

As with other forms of aortic atresia, it is very unusual for this lesion to be associated with extracardiac abnormalities.

Management and outcome

Although there are two good sized ventricles, in this setting the surgical management is usually a modified Norwood approach (see section on aortic atresia and hypoplastic left heart syndrome, Chapter 6).

Outcome in a large single-centre fetal series

Of eight cases of aortic atresia with a ventricular septal defect diagnosed prenatally, five pregnancies resulted in a termination of pregnancy, one case resulted in a spontaneous intrauterine death, one case died in the neonatal period and one child was alive at last update.

Summary of fetal echocardiographic features associated with AoAt VSD.

- Equal sized ventricles in four-chamber view (often)
- Ventricular septal defect
- Pulmonary artery overrides ventricular septal defect
- Tiny ascending aorta and arch
- No forward flow in ascending aorta
- Reverse flow in aortic arch

Chapter 9

Aortic arch abnormalities

Summary

- Coarctation of the aorta
- Interrupted aortic arch
- Right aortic arch
  - Aberrant left subclavian artery
- Double aortic arch
- Aberrant right subclavian artery

Aortic arch abnormalities

Coarctation of the aorta (coarct)

Prevalence
Coarctation of the aorta accounts for 5-10% of congenital heart disease in postnatal series. In the Evelina fetal series, coarctation of the aorta accounted for 7.5% of the total series and 8.4% of all cases of fetal congenital heart disease seen in the last 10 years.

Definition
Coarctation of the aorta is a discrete area of narrowing in the aortic arch, usually in the juxtaductal region. More diffuse areas of narrowing in the arch, which can occur in association, are often termed tubular hypoplasia.

Spectrum
Coarctation can occur as an isolated defect or as a component of a complex cardiac malformation. In fetal life there is often additional hypoplasia of the isthmus and transverse arch. Associated cardiac lesions which are common include a ventricular septal defect, aortic stenosis and a bicuspid aortic valve. Coarctation can be part of Shone syndrome, which involves co-existing abnormalities of the mitral valve, aortic valve and the aortic arch. Coarctation can also occur in the context of complex cardiac abnormalities in association with other forms of congenital heart disease, including transposition of the great vessels, double-outlet right ventricle, congenitally corrected transposition, common arterial trunk, atrioventricular septal defect, double-inlet ventricle, tricuspid atresia and Ebstein's anomaly (see Chapters 4-8).

Fetal echocardiographic features

One of the difficulties with this diagnosis during fetal life is that the coarctation shelf lesion usually detected after birth cannot be seen before birth, so that the diagnosis is suspected on other suggestive features. These include asymmetry in the four-chamber view and a disparity between the sizes of the great arteries. Thus, in the four-chamber view, the right ventricle may appear dilated relative to the left ventricle (Figures 9.1a, 9.2a and 9.3a). There will be forward flow across the mitral valve (Figure 9.2b) and the left ventricle will reach the apex (Figures 9.1a, 9.2a and 9.3a). It is important to note that in some cases of fetal coarctation there may be no ventricular asymmetry and the two ventricles may appear of normal size (Figure 9.4a). This is particularly true in cases with an associated ventricular septal defect, but occasionally this may also be found in cases with an intact ventricular septum. The main clue to prenatal diagnosis of coarctation is a disparity in size between the two great arteries particularly in the three-vessel view and the transverse arch views. In these views, the pulmonary artery and duct will appear dilated compared with the aorta and arch, with the aortic isthmus appearing narrowed and hypoplastic (Figures 9.1b, 9.2c, 9.3b, 9.4b and 9.4c). It is important to follow the three-vessel view into the tracheal 'V' view to assess the aortic isthmus, as in some cases the aortic arch narrowing may only be evident in the region of the aortic isthmus (Figures 9.4b-c). The normal appearances of these views are shown in Chapter 2. Even though the aorta may appear quite hypoplastic in some cases of coarctation, there will be forward flow in the ascending aorta and arch (Figures 9.2d and 9.3c). Longitudinal views of the aortic arch do not always help in the diagnosis, but occasionally views very suggestive of a coarctation can be obtained (Figures 9.1c and 9.4d). Of note in these views is that the arch and isthmus appear hypoplastic and that there is an increased distance between the head and neck vessels (this may be between the second and third or, more rarely, the first and second).

Although the left heart structures can appear significantly smaller than those on the right in fetal coarctation, the majority of cases will maintain a biventricular circulation following arch repair after birth. In cases with a very tight coarctation with a very hypoplastic arch, distinction from an interrupted aortic arch can be difficult. In these cases, it is important to search for a complete arch and to demonstrate forward flow around the arch (Figures 9.5a-e)

Doppler studies are usually not helpful in making a correct diagnosis of coarctation of the aorta, the exception being that, occasionally in some cases, there may be a left to right shunt at atrial level. This is the reverse of the normal atrial shunt in the fetus and, if detected, raises the suspicion of a left heart obstructive lesion.

Other causes of right heart dominance should be excluded. An increase in the right ventricle to left ventricle ratio can be normal in late gestation, after about 26-28 weeks (Figures 2.35a-b in Chapter 2). Cardiac causes of asymmetery in the four-chamber view include total anomalous pulmonary venous drainage (Figure 4.2a in Chapter 4) and occasionally a ventricular septal defect can be associated with asymmetry in the absence of any other cardiac abnormality (Figure 9.6). A restricted arterial duct can result in the right ventricle appearing dilated (Figure 12.9 in Chapter 12). Cases with a direct connection of the umbilical vein to the right atrium can also result in right heart dominance (Figures 12.8a-c in

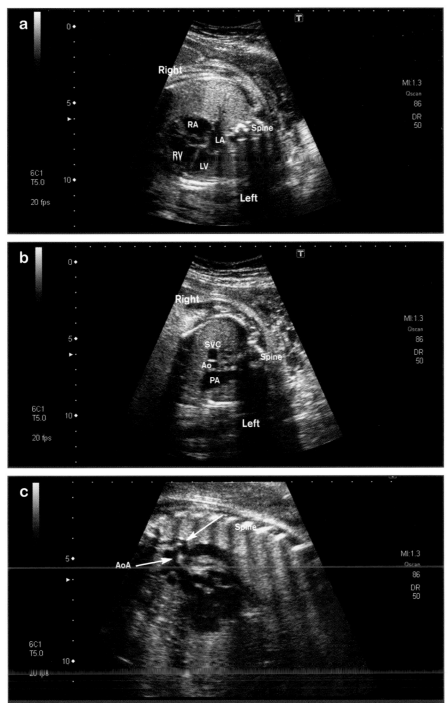

Figure 9.1. An example of coarctation with a hypoplastic and tortuous arch. (This baby had an arch repair after birth.) a) The four-chamber view shows asymmetry with the right atrium and right ventricle appearing dilated compared with the left atrium and left ventricle. The left ventricle reaches the apex of the heart. b) In the three-vessel view the aorta appears significantly smaller than the pulmonary artery. c) The aortic arch appears tortuous and kinked, with the third head and neck vessel (arrow) appearing to arise more distally than normal. There is a narrowing in the arch very suggestive of a coarctation.

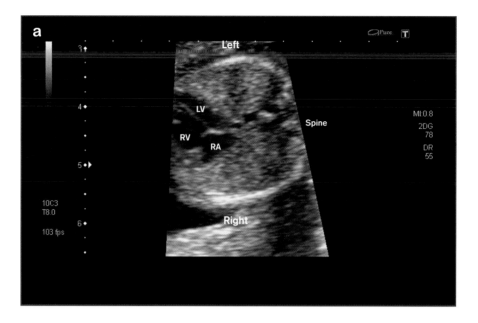

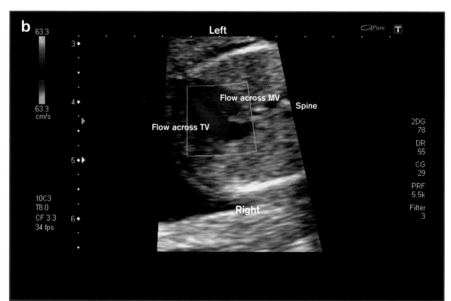

Figure 9.2. An example of coarctation with a small left ventricle. a) The four-chamber view shows marked asymmetry with the right atrium and right ventricle appearing dilated compared with the left atrium and left ventricle. The left ventricle reaches the apex of the heart. b) Colour flow shows flow across both atrioventricular valves (shown in red), though the mitral valve appears more narrow than the tricuspid valve.

Figure continued overleaf.

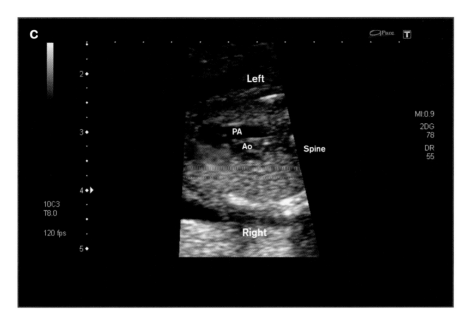

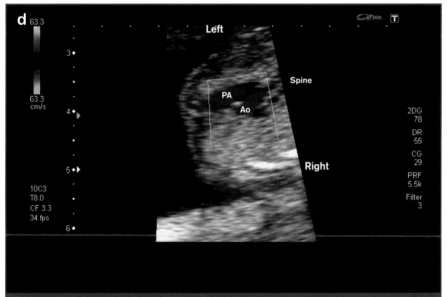

Figure 9.2 *continued.* **An example of coarctation with a small left ventricle. c) In the three-vessel view the aorta appears significantly smaller than the pulmonary artery. d) Colour flow in the three-vessel view shows there is forward flow in the aorta (seen in red).**

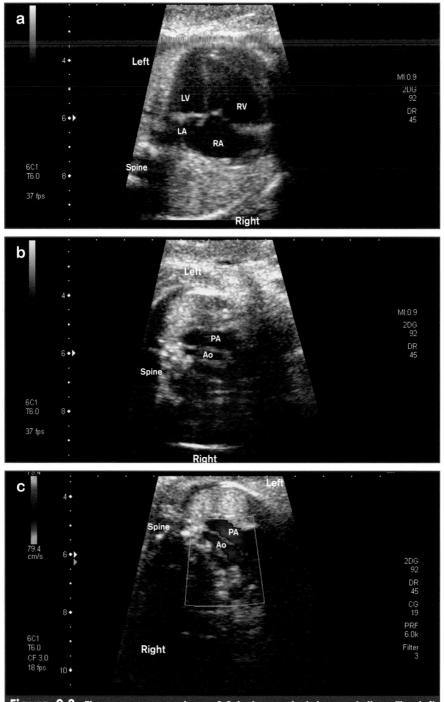

Figure 9.3. The same example as 9.2 but seen in later gestation. The left ventricle and aorta are small but there is still forward flow in the aorta and arch. (This baby had an arch repair after birth.) a) The four-chamber view shows marked asymmetry, but the left ventricle still reaches the apex of the heart. b) In the three-vessel view the aorta appears significantly smaller than the pulmonary artery. c) Colour flow in the three-vessel view shows there is forward flow in the aorta (seen in red).

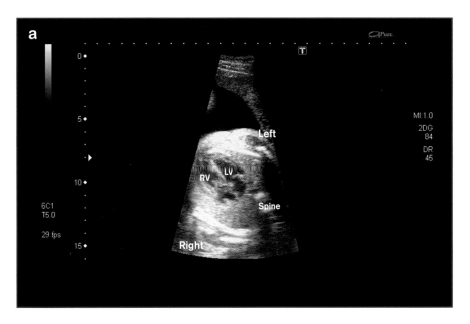

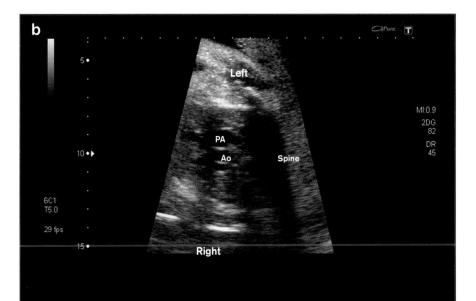

Figure 9.4. An example of coarctation with equal sized ventricles but with a hypoplastic isthmus and arch. (This baby required urgent arch repair on the first day of life.) a) In the four-chamber view the left and right ventricle are of approximately equal size. b) In the three-vessel view the aorta appears only slightly smaller than the pulmonary artery and in this view the level of suspicion for coarctation is not high.

Figure continued overleaf.

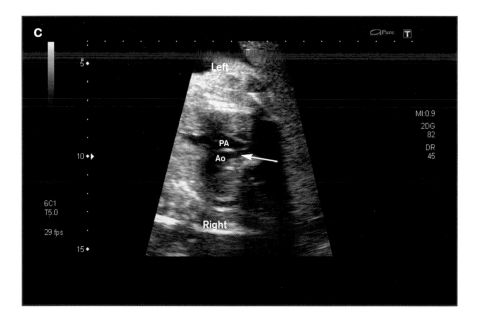

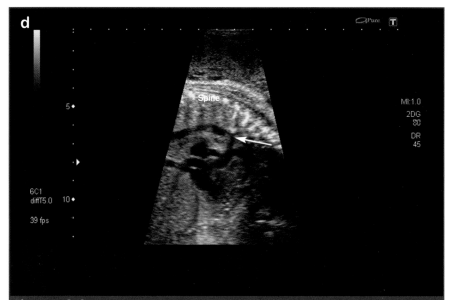

Figure 9.4 *continued.* An example of coarctation with equal sized ventricles but with a hypoplastic isthmus and arch. (This baby required urgent arch repair on the first day of life.) c) A view of the aortic isthmus in the tracheal 'V' view shows that the aortic isthmus does appear hypoplastic (arrow). d) A view of the aortic arch shows a hypoplastic region of the arch which is suggestive of coarctation (arrow).

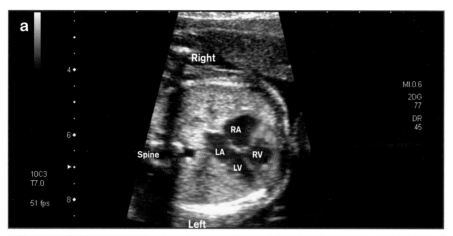

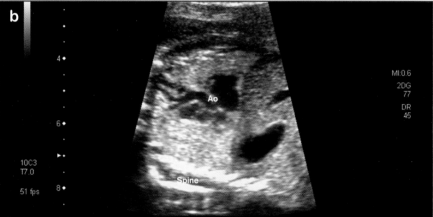

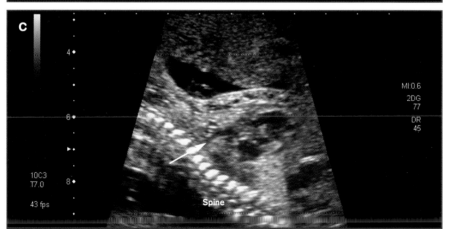

Figure 9.5. An example of a tight coarctation with a hypoplastic aortic arch that was difficult to distinguish from an interrupted aortic arch. (This baby had coarctation confirmed and an arch repair after birth.) a) The four-chamber view shows asymmetry with the right atrium and right ventricle appearing dilated compared with the left atrium and left ventricle. The left ventricle reaches the apex of the heart. b) A view of the ascending aorta going towards the arch has a 'pronged fork' (arrow) appearance suggesting an interrupted aortic arch. c) Careful searching revealed a very hypoplastic but complete aortic arch (arrow).
Figure continued overleaf.

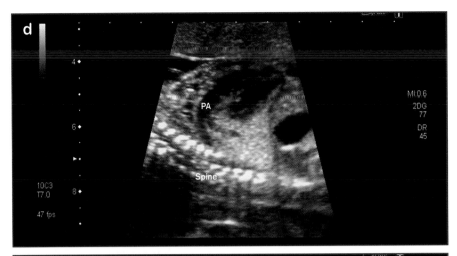

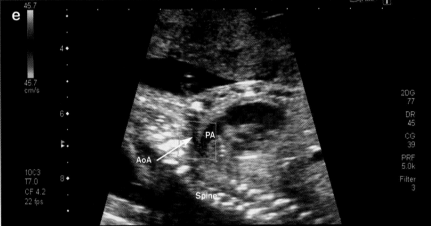

Figure 9.5 *continued.* **An example of a tight coarctation with a hypoplastic aortic arch that was difficult to distinguish from an interrupted aortic arch. (This baby had coarctation confirmed and an arch repair after birth.) d) A large pulmonary artery and duct are seen in this view. e) Colour flow shows forward flow in the large pulmonary artery and duct, and also in the hypoplastic aortic arch (both shown in blue).**

Chapter 12). Extracardiac anomalies can also sometimes result in right heart dominance. This appearance can be seen in babies with intrauterine growth retardation (Figure 9.7) and mild asymmetry is sometimes seen in babies with chromosomal anomalies. A left-sided diaphragmatic hernia can be associated with left heart compression and the appearance of right heart dominance (Figure 9.8). Some of these cases may have an associated coarctation of the aorta and this needs to be excluded as an additional diagnosis.

Extracardiac associations

Coarctation of the aorta can be associated with chromosomal abnormalities, in particular Turner's syndrome (45XO), but sometimes occurs with other chromosomal abnormalities,

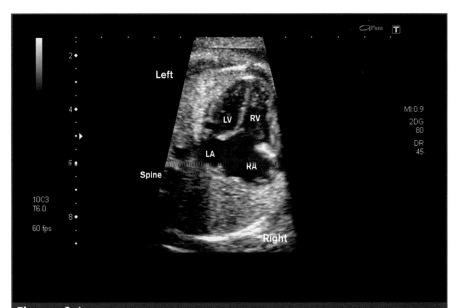

Figure 9.6. An example of asymmetry associated with multiple muscular ventricular septal defects. In the four-chamber view there is asymmetry with the right atrium and right ventricle appearing dilated compared with the left atrium and left ventricle. This baby had multiple small muscular ventricular septal defects but no other cardiac abnormality.

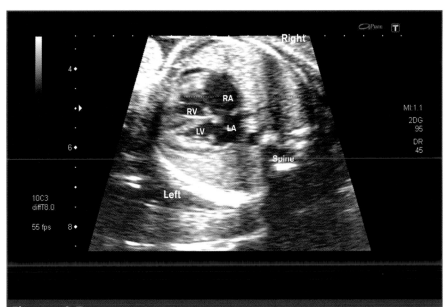

Figure 9.7. An example of the four-chamber view associated with intrauterine growth retardation showing cardiomegaly and mild asymmetry. There was no cardiac abnormality in this baby.

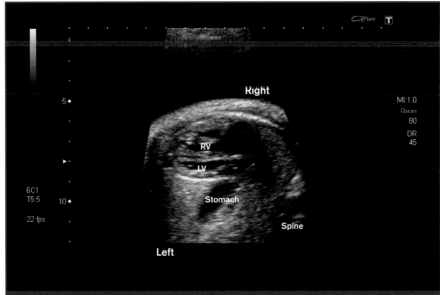

Figure 9.8. An example of a left-sided diaphragmatic hernia associated with mediastinal shift to the right, left heart compression and the appearance of right heart dominance.

including trisomy 18 and deletion of chromosome 22q11. It can also be associated with extracardiac structural abnormalities.

In our large fetal series, 19% of all cases of coarctation or coarctation with a ventricular septal defect had a chromosomal abnormality. Of these, 48% had Turner's syndrome, 8% had trisomy 18, 7% had trisomy 21 and 13% had trisomy 13. The remaining included cases of trisomy 22, 22q11 deletion and other translocations and deletions. An extracardiac abnormality in cases with normal chromosomes was associated in a further 14% of cases. These included cystic hygroma, Dandy Walker cysts, diaphragmatic hernia, encephalocoele, exomphalos, scoliosis, skeletal dysplasia and talipes.

Management and outcome

In view of ductal patency in fetal life, it is not possible to be absolutely categorical about the diagnosis of coarctation of the aorta before birth. The findings of ventricular and, more particularly, great artery asymmetry are a marker for this diagnosis, but not definitive. It is important to appreciate that some babies with these suggestive signs may prove to have a normal aortic arch after birth. If coarctation of the aorta is confirmed, then this will require surgical correction after birth, usually in the early neonatal period. For extensive narrowing of the aortic arch the approach is through a median sternotomy with the use of cardiopulmonary bypass. For less extensive narrowing of the aortic arch the surgical approach may be via a left thoracotomy, without cardiopulmonary bypass. The risk of such surgery ranges from 2-10%. If there is an associated ventricular septal defect this will make the repair more complicated. Some cases may require further intervention on the aortic arch at a later stage, either by repeat surgery or by catheter techniques. Lifelong cardiac review is indicated, to check for any obstruction in the left heart structures as the child grows and to maintain blood pressure control.

In cases of coarctation associated with other forms of heart disease, for example, an atrioventricular septal defect, transposition of the great arteries or a double-inlet ventricle, the outcome will be affected by the complexity of the repair and whether a biventricular repair is feasible or not.

Outcome in a large single-centre fetal series

Of 321 cases of definite coarctation of the aorta or coarctation with a ventricular septal defect diagnosed prenatally, 35% of pregnancies resulted in a termination of pregnancy. If the terminations are excluded then the outcome of the continuing pregnancies was: 10% resulting in spontaneous intrauterine death, 15% died in the neonatal period, 6% died in infancy and 68% were alive at last update. The outcome is not known in 1%.

Of cases seen in the last 10 years, a termination of pregnancy took place in 21% of cases and 71% of the continuing pregnancies were alive at last follow-up.

Associations in cases with asymmetry but no definite coarctation

As highlighted above, the diagnosis of coarctation of the aorta can be difficult to exclude in some babies with asymmetry in size between the left and right heart structures, even though coarctation is not strongly suspected. Many of these babies prove to be normal after birth, but of such cases seen in our large fetal series, approximately 13% had chromosomal abnormalities and a further 13% had extracardiac abnormalities with normal chromosomes. In 16% of cases there was a ventricular septal defect and in a further 9% there was either a persistent left superior vena cava or bilateral superior vena cava.

Summary of fetal echocardiographic features associated with coarct.

- **Right ventricle >left ventricle**
- **Pulmonary artery >aorta**
- **Arch hypoplasia**
- **Hypoplastic isthmus**
- **Left to right shunt at atrial level (occasionally)**

Summary of extracardiac associations in fetal coarct.

- **Chromosomal**
  - 19%
- **Extracardiac abnormality (normal chromosomes)**
  - 14%

Interrupted aortic arch (Int AA)

Prevalence

This is a rare condition. In the Evelina fetal series, an interrupted aortic arch accounted for 0.4% of the total.

Definition

Interruption of the aortic arch occurs when there is anatomical discontinuity between two adjacent parts of the aortic arch. More rarely this may be due to atresia in an area of the arch, where there may still be anatomical continuity via a solid cord.

Most commonly the interruption is between the left common carotid and the left subclavian artery, that is, the second and third head and neck vessels (also known as type B interruption). Less commonly the interruption is in the isthmus distal to the left subclavian artery (also known as type A interruption) or, least frequently, the interruption is between the brachiocephalic and left common carotid arteries, that is, the first and second head and neck vessels (also known as type C interruption).

Spectrum

An interrupted aortic arch is usually associated with a ventricular septal defect. It can also be found in association with other forms of congenital heart disease, such as transposition of the great vessels, double-outlet right ventricle, congenitally corrected transposition, aortopulmonary window, common arterial trunk, atrioventricular septal defect, double-inlet ventricle and tricuspid atresia.

Fetal echocardiographic features

In the four-chamber view there are often equal sized ventricles. However, there is usually an associated ventricular septal defect, which may be large and evident in the four-chamber view (Figures 9.9a-b). The aorta will appear significantly smaller than the pulmonary artery (Figures 9.9c-f) and there may be posterior deviation of the anterior wall of the aorta (Figure 9.9e). In type B interruption, the ascending aorta is small, being significantly smaller than the pulmonary artery. It will not be possible to demonstrate a complete aortic arch and in longitudinal views the ascending aorta forms a two-pronged fork appearance, which is typical of this diagnosis (Figure 9.9g-h). When the interruption is of type A, the features are similar to coarctation and it can be difficult to differentiate the two diagnoses. An example of a case

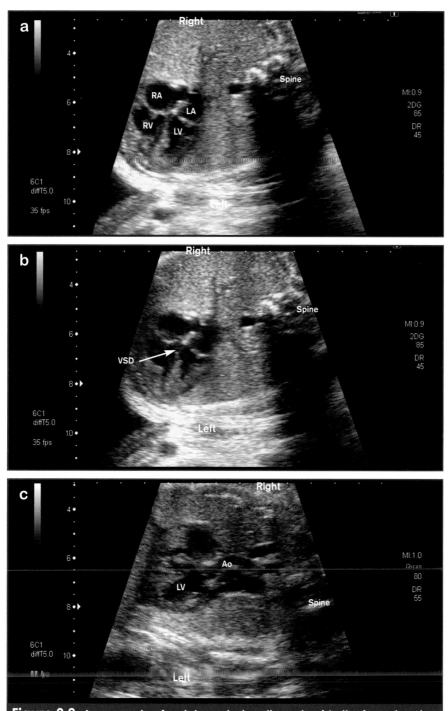

Figure 9.9. An example of an interrupted aortic arch. a) In the four-chamber view there are balanced ventricles (left ventricle same size as right ventricle). b) The associated ventricular septal defect is evident by angling the transducer towards the outlet septum. c) The aorta is seen arising from the left ventricle and it appears small.

Figure continued overleaf.

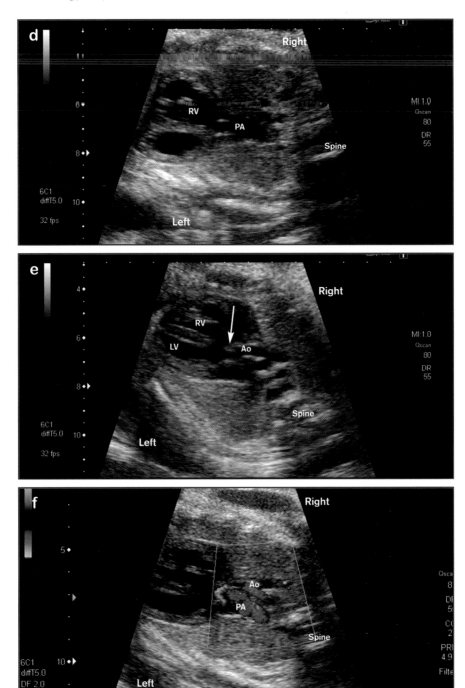

Figure 9.9 *continued*. **An example of an interrupted aortic arch. d) The pulmonary artery, which is larger than the aorta, is seen arising from the right ventricle. e) A view showing the ventricular septal defect and the aorta. The anterior wall of the aorta is deviated posteriorly (arrow). f) Colour flow shows forward flow in the small aorta and the larger pulmonary artery (shown in blue).**

Figure continued overleaf.

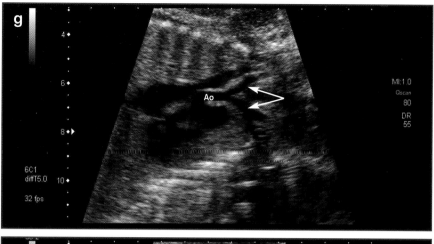

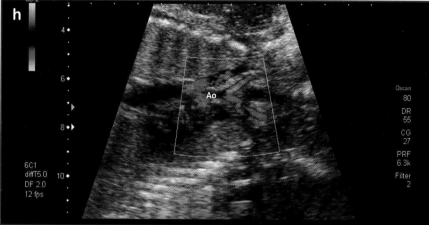

Figure 9.9 *continued*. **An example of an interrupted aortic arch. g) In longitudinal views the ascending aorta forms a two-pronged fork appearance (arrows), which is suggestive of the diagnosis of an interrupted aortic arch. h) Colour flow demonstrating the aorta in the same view as Figure 9.9g.**

of coarctation that was difficult to differentiate from an interrupted arch is shown in Figures 9.5a-e.

Extracardiac associations

An interrupted aortic arch, particularly the so called type B, is strongly associated with deletion of chromosome 22q11 and DiGeorge syndrome. It has also been associated with CHARGE syndrome.

In our large fetal series, 12% of cases of an interrupted aortic arch had a chromosomal abnormality, which were two cases with 22q11 deletion. An extracardiac abnormality was associated in a further 29% of cases. This included Cat Eye Syndrome, diaphragmatic hernia, exomphalos and hydrocephalus.

Management and outcome

As with coarctation of the aorta, surgical repair is usually undertaken in the neonatal period, though the repair for interruption is more complicated.

Outcome in a large single-centre fetal series

Of 17 cases of interrupted aortic arch (with a ventricular septal defect but no other cardiac lesion) diagnosed prenatally, 18% of pregnancies resulted in a termination of pregnancy. If the terminations are excluded then the outcome of the continuing pregnancies was: 7% resulting in spontaneous intrauterine death, 14% died in the neonatal period, 14% died in infancy and 65% were alive at last update.

Summary of fetal echocardiographic features associated with an Int AA.

- Right ventricle = left ventricle (often)
- Ventricular septal defect (often large)
- Small ascending aorta
- Complete arch not demonstrated
- Ascending aorta leads to two-pronged fork appearance

Summary of extracardiac associations in fetal Int AA.

- Chromosomal
  - 12%
- Extracardiac abnormality (normal chromosomes)
  - 29%

Right aortic arch

Definition

A left or right-sided aortic arch refers to the position of the aortic arch in relation to the trachea. The normal embryological development of the arch is from the primitive pharyngeal arch system consisting of six pairs of pharyngeal arch arteries and branchial pouches, some of which will regress and some of which will persist. The normal left aortic arch is formed from the left fourth arch and the left dorsal aorta. However, if either the left fourth arch or the left dorsal aorta regress and the right fourth arch or right dorsal aorta persists, then a right aortic arch will be formed.

Spectrum

A right aortic arch can be an isolated finding or can be associated with structural cardiac abnormalities, most commonly tetralogy of Fallot, common arterial trunk and pulmonary atresia with a ventricular septal defect. There are different branching patterns associated with a right aortic arch and some of these anomalies can create a vascular ring around the trachea and oesophagus, which may produce clinical symptoms. Others, however, are not associated with a vascular ring and may be asymptomatic. Most commonly the branching pattern is a mirror image (the first branch is the left brachiocephalic artery, giving rise to the left common carotid and left subclavian arteries, followed by the right common carotid and right subclavian arteries) and in these cases, there is unlikely to be a vascular ring, though there are occasional exceptions. The majority of cases of right aortic arch with mirror-image branching are associated with other heart defects. In some cases, the left subclavian artery may have an aberrant origin from a right aortic arch, usually distal to the right subclavian artery and an aberrant course of the artery, usually posterior to the oesophagus. If the duct is left-sided in these cases with a right arch and aberrant left subclavian artery, there is a risk of a vascular ring, which can cause compression of the trachea and oesophagus, and produce symptoms of respiratory obstruction and dysphagia. Cases of a right aortic arch with an aberrant left subclavian artery are much less commonly associated with other forms of congenital heart disease.

Fetal echocardiographic features

A right-sided aortic arch can be diagnosed in the three-vessel view. Normally, the aorta arises from the left ventricle and is directed initially towards the right shoulder. It then crosses the midline in front of the trachea and descends on the left. This left-sided arch forms a 'V' shape with the pulmonary artery and duct to join the descending aorta (Figures 2.9a and 2.17a in Chapter 2). If there is a right-sided aortic arch, the aorta stays to the right of the trachea and the normal 'V' is not seen as there is a gap between the pulmonary artery and aorta. The duct is usually left-sided and connects with the descending aorta behind the trachea in a 'U' shape (Figures 9.10a-b). An example of a right aortic arch with an aberrant left subclavian artery is shown in Figures 9.11a-b.

Extracardiac associations

A right aortic arch has been associated with chromosomal and extracardiac abnormalities, particularly when associated with other forms of congenital heart disease. The most common chromosomal abnormality is deletion of chromosome 22q11, though others can also occur. Extracardiac abnormalities include the VACTERL and CHARGE associations, as well as oesophageal atresia.

Management and outcome

The management and outcome will be governed by the extent of associated lesions, both cardiac and extracardiac, and the risk of a vascular ring. In the absence of any associated lesions usually no treatment is required.

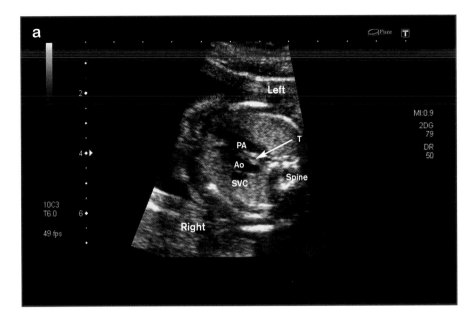

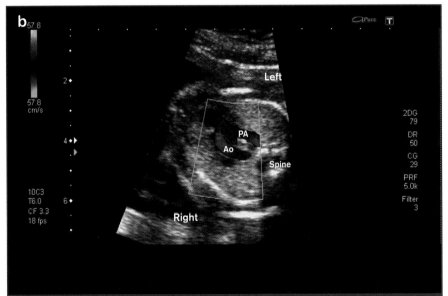

Figure 9.10. A right-sided aortic arch. a) In the three-vessel view the aortic arch is seen to descend to the right of the trachea. This forms a 'U' shape with the pulmonary artery and duct. b) Colour flow demonstrates the vessels seen in Figure 9.10a.

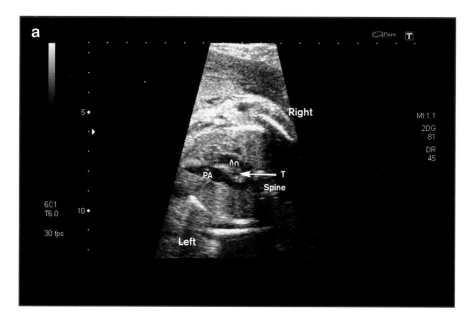

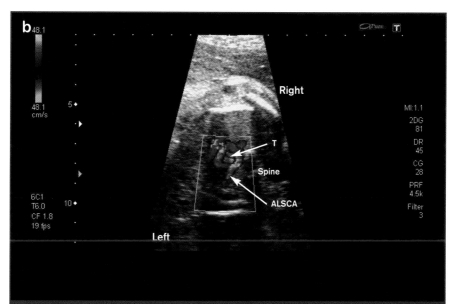

Figure 9.11. A right-sided aortic arch with an aberrant left subclavian artery (ALSCA). a) In the three-vessel view the aortic arch is seen to descend to the right of the trachea. This forms a 'U' shape with the pulmonary artery and duct as in Figure 9.10a. b) Colour flow demonstrates an aberrant left subclavian artery (ALSCA) and the potential for a vascular ring.

Double aortic arch

A double aortic arch is formed when both fourth arches and both dorsal aortas remain present, so that there are two aortic arches, one on either side of the trachea. A functioning double aortic arch forms a vascular ring around the trachea and oesophagus, which may cause respiratory obstruction and dysphagia. Most commonly there is a dominant right arch and a smaller left arch. In some cases, part of the left arch can become atretic and develop into a fibrous cord.

Aberrant right subclavian artery

The right subclavian artery usually arises above the level of the aortic arch as a branch of the innominate or brachiocephalic artery (first head and neck vessel) and courses to the right. An aberrant right subclavian artery arises anomalously as a fourth branch of the aortic arch. This vessel arises from the descending aorta behind the trachea and below the level of the aortic arch and passes towards the right and cranially (Figure 9.12). An aberrant right subclavian artery can occur in isolation as a normal variant or it can occur in association with other congenital heart disease. When occurring in isolation, this finding has been reported to be associated with an increased incidence of trisomy 21.

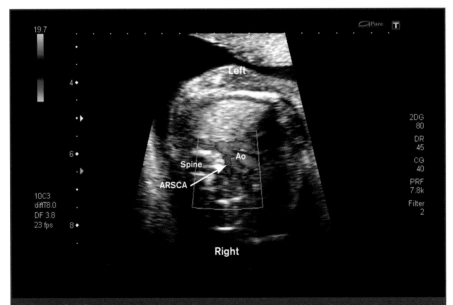

Figure 9.12. An example of an aberrant right subclavian (ARSCA) with a left-sided aortic arch. The aortic arch descends to the left of the trachea and an aberrant subclavian is seen with colour flow (shown in blue and arrow).

Chapter 10

Cardiomyopathies

Summary

- **Dilated cardiomyopathy**
- **Hypertrophic cardiomyopathy**

Cardiomyopathies

Prevalence

The prevalence of cardiomyopathy in postnatal series is around 1-2%. In the Evelina fetal series, cardiomyopathy accounted for 2.5% of the total series and 1.5% of all cases of fetal congenital heart disease seen in the last 10 years.

Definition

Cardiomyopathy is a term used for a range of heart muscle disease, unrelated to structural cardiac abnormalities. It can be primary and of unknown aetiology, or can be secondary to definable causes.

Spectrum

Cardiomyopathies can affect the left or right ventricle, or in some cases both ventricles. There are three main types of cardiomyopathy: dilated cardiomyopathy, hypertrophic cardiomyopathy and restricted cardiomyopathy.

Dilated cardiomyopathy

In dilated cardiomyopathy there is dilatation of either one or both ventricles, which in some cases may also be associated with ventricular hypertrophy. There is impaired cardiac function which may lead to the development of fetal hydrops. In fetal life dilated cardiomyopathy affects both ventricles in about 50% of cases, and either the right or left ventricle in the rest.

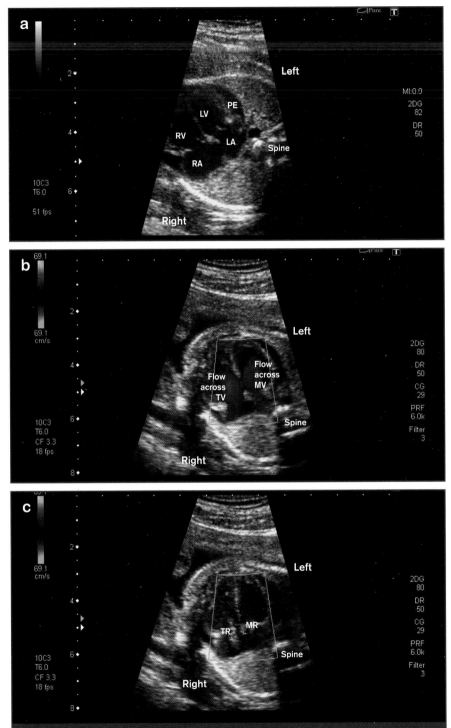

Figure 10.1. An example of a dilated cardiomyopathy. a) The four-chamber view shows a dilated heart. A pericardial effusion is also seen. b) Colour flow demonstrates flow across both atrioventricular valves (shown in red). c) Mitral and tricuspid regurgitation are seen on colour flow (shown in blue).

Hypertrophic cardiomyopathy

In hypertrophic cardiomyopathy there is abnormal hypertrophy of usually the left, or occasionally the right ventricle and sometimes both ventricles.

Restricted cardiomyopathy

In this group there is usually scarring of the muscle of either ventricle, as seen in endocardial fibroelastosis, but without any structural abnormality. This type is rarely seen in the fetus.

Fetal echocardiographic findings

Dilated cardiomyopathy

The cardiothoracic ratio will usually be increased (Figures 10.1a, 10.2a and 10.3a). The structure and connections of the heart will be normal. However, the left, right or both ventricles will appear dilated and appear poorly contracting with reduced function. There is likely to be atrioventricular valve regurgitation and though the inflow seen on colour flow may appear normal, the atrioventricular valve inflow Doppler traces may be abnormal, indicating reduced myocardial compliance (Figures 10.1b-c, 10.2b and 10.3b). The impaired function can also be demonstrated with M-mode echocardiography (Figure 10.2c). If there is severe ventricular dysfunction then there may be reduced outflow from the ventricle. An example of a right ventricular dilated cardiomyopathy with functional obstruction to the pulmonary outflow and reversed flow from the arterial duct is shown in Figures 10.3a-d.

Hypertrophic cardiomyopathy

There will be hypertrophy of either or both ventricles which is not associated with any structural cardiac abnormality, such as severe aortic or pulmonary stenosis (Figures 10.4a-c). There may be a decrease in the lumen size of the affected ventricle and the ventricular function will be impaired. As with dilated cardiomyopathy there is likely to be atrioventricular valve regurgitation (Figure 10.4b) and the atrioventricular valve inflow Doppler traces may be abnormal. There may also be associated fetal hydrops (Figure 10.4c).

Extracardiac associations

Cardiomyopathy can be associated with a pericardial effusion and with fetal hydrops. Although cardiomyopathy can be idiopathic with no identifiable cause, many cases are the result of some other disease process, as outlined below.

Causes of dilated cardiomyopathy

Dilated cardiomyopathy can be associated with metabolic disorders, genetic disorders, viral infections, fetal anaemia, renal disorders and immune-mediated disorders. Fetal tachycardias can also cause a dilated and poorly functioning heart, which may be seen even after the tachycardia has resolved, or in some cases with an intermittent tachycardia. A dilated dysfunctional right ventricle can be associated with a very restricted arterial duct (see Chapter 12). Other abnormalities that can result in dilation of the heart are congenital absence of the ductus venosus with direct connection of the umbilical vein to the heart (see Chapter 12), cerebral arteriovenous malformations and twin to twin transfusion syndrome.

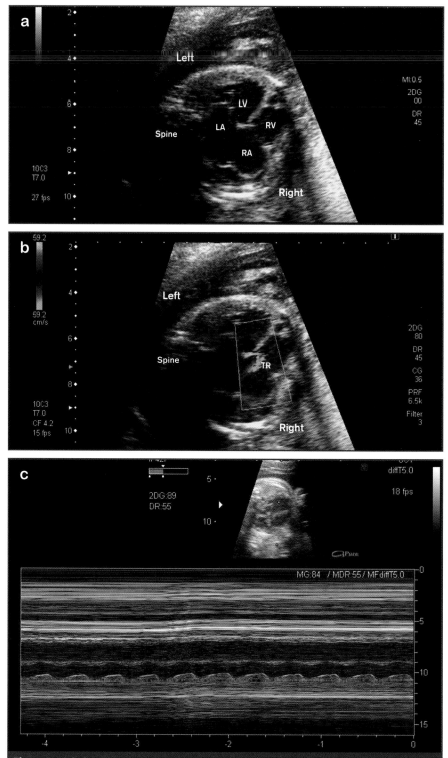

Figure 10.2. An example of a dilated cardiomyopathy. a) The four-chamber view shows a dilated heart with marked cardiomegaly. b) Colour flow demonstrates tricuspid regurgitation (shown in blue). c) M-mode echocardiography shows there is little ventricular or septal contraction.

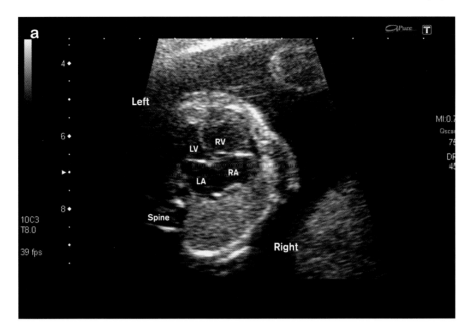

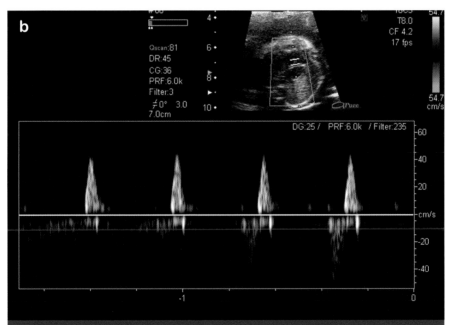

Figure 10.3. An example of a right ventricular cardiomyopathy associated with a dilated heart. a) The four-chamber view shows a dilated heart with cardiomegaly. b) The tricuspid valve inflow is abnormal with a single peak compared to the normal biphasic peak (see Chapter 2).

Figure continued overleaf.

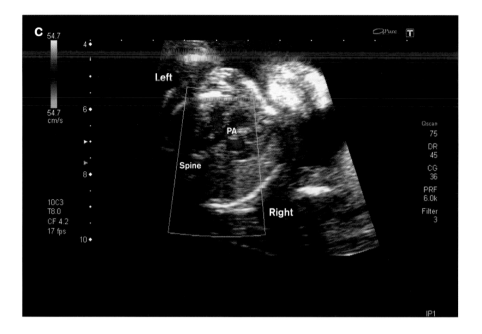

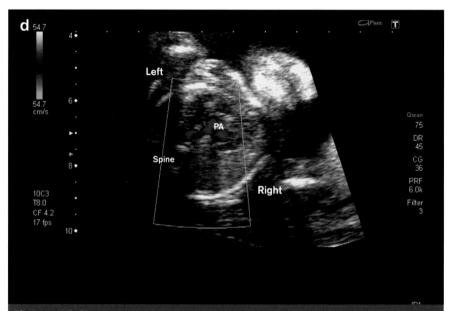

Figure 10.3 *continued.* **An example of a right ventricular cardiomyopathy associated with a dilated heart. c) A view of the pulmonary artery with colour flow showing some forward flow (shown in blue). d) Reverse flow in the pulmonary artery is also detected with colour flow (shown in red).**

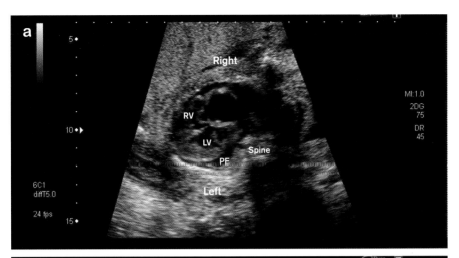

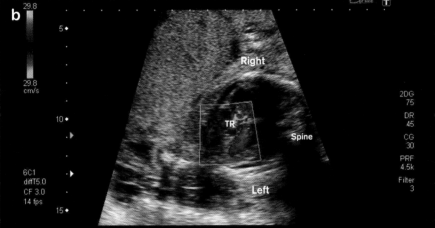

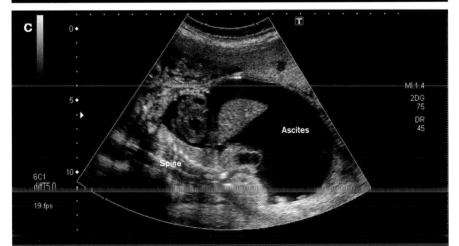

Figure 10.4. An example of a hypertrophic cardiomyopathy. a) In the four-chamber view the ventricular chambers, particularly the left ventricle, appear hypertrophied. There is some cardiomegaly and a pericardial effusion. b) There is tricuspid regurgitation seen on colour flow. c) There is associated fetal hydrops.

Causes of hypertrophic cardiomyopathy

Hypertrophic cardiomyopathy can be seen in infants of diabetic mothers. This is usually detected in the last trimester of pregnancy and typically will resolve spontaneously after birth. Familial hypertrophic cardiomyopathy can occasionally be detected prenatally, but most cases will not present until later. Thus, a normal fetal echocardiogram in those with a family history does not exclude the diagnosis. Non-compaction of the ventricular myocardium can be associated with poor ventricular function and can lead to fetal hydrops (Figures 10.5a-d).

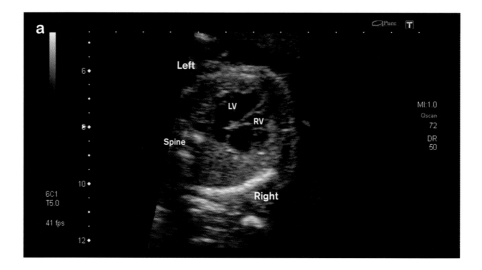

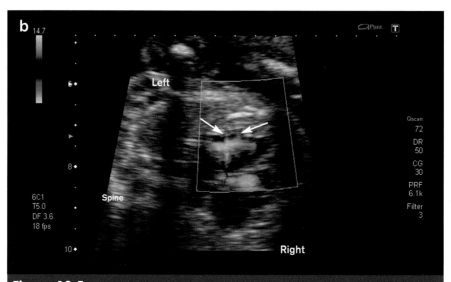

Figure 10.5. An example of non-compaction of the left ventricle associated with fetal hydrops. a) In the four-chamber view both ventricles appear slightly globular and hypertrophied. b) Colour flow demonstrates the characteristic echocardiographic feature of non-compaction, which is deep crypts within the myocardium (arrows), seen in the left ventricle in this example.
Figure continued overleaf.

The echocardiographic features of this condition are deep crypts within the myocardium of either ventricle.

Other causes of a hypertrophic cardiomyopathy include Noonan's syndrome, metabolic storage disorders, for example, Pompe's disease, renal agenesis, and twin to twin transfusion syndrome.

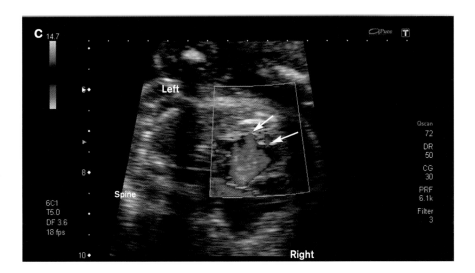

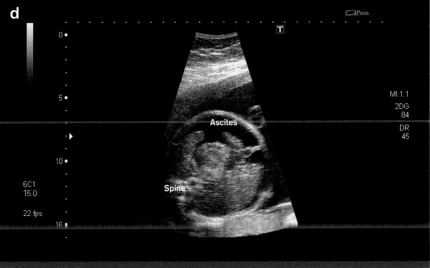

Figure 10.5 *continued*. **An example of non-compaction of the left ventricle associated with fetal hydrops. c) Colour flow demonstrates the characteristic echocardiographic feature of non-compaction, which is deep crypts within the myocardium (arrows), seen in the left ventricle in this example. d) There is associated fetal ascites.**

Echogenic appearance of cardiac chambers suggesting cardiomyopathy

Occasionally the cardiac chambers or septum may appear echogenic suggesting the possibility of a cardiomyopathy (Figure 10.6). These cases may be associated with a viral infection, or may be immune-mediated. Echogenicity associated with viral infections is likely to resolve. Cases that are immune-mediated may develop heart block and require further monitoring for this (see Chapter 13).

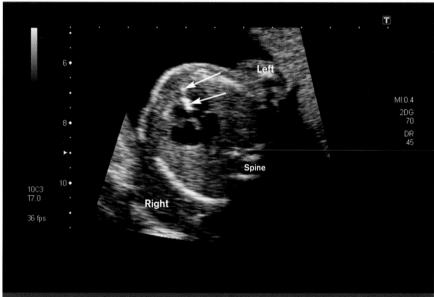

Figure 10.6. The ventricular septum appears very echogenic in this example (arrows). The cardiac function was normal and this appearance resolved after birth.

Progression

Cardiomyopathy can develop or progress in severity as pregnancy advances and an example of progression is shown in Figures 10.7a-c and 10.8a-b. In addition, a normal fetal echocardiogram does not preclude the possibility of a cardiomyopathy developing later in high-risk cases. If a cardiomyopathy is identified, sequential studies are important to monitor progression with advancing gestation.

Management and outcome

Assessment should be made to exclude any identifiable or known cause of cardiomyopathy. This includes a detailed fetal anomaly scan, maternal blood samples for viral studies (including TORCH screen and evidence of parvovirus infection that can be

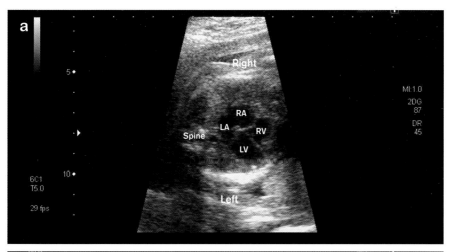

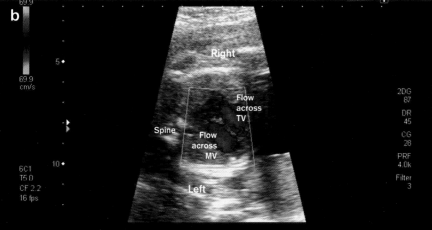

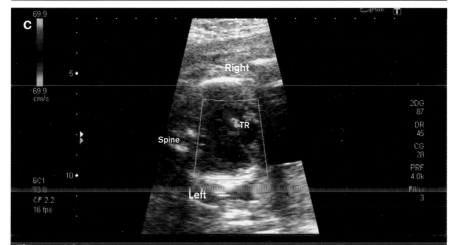

Figure 10.7. An example of a cardiomyopathy that progressed. a) In the four-chamber view the heart appears a normal size and the function was only minimally reduced. b) The inflow across the atrioventricular valves seen with colour flow is equal on both sides. c) Tricuspid regurgitation is seen with colour flow.

271

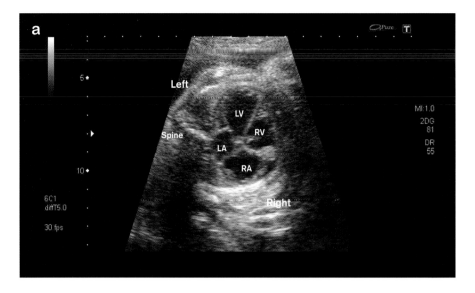

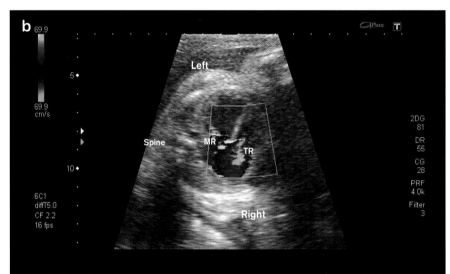

Figure 10.8. The same example as Figure 10.7 seen in later pregnancy. a) In the four-chamber view there is marked cardiomegaly with a markedly increased cardiothoracic ratio. The function of the heart was significantly impaired at this stage. b) There is mitral and tricuspid regurgitation seen with colour flow.

associated with fetal anaemia), and maternal anti-Ro and anti-La antibodies to exclude immune-mediated causes. Maternal diabetes mellitus should be excluded. Metabolic causes can be difficult to exclude before birth and further investigations for this may be indicated after birth. Taking parental consent for storage of blood or fetal tissue for later evaluation is appropriate, particularly in cases where no cause has been identified.

The prognosis and outcome will depend on the type of cardiomyopathy, the underlying cause, the degree of ventricular impairment and whether there is associated fetal hydrops.

Outcome in a large single-centre fetal series

Of 105 cases of cardiomyopathy with a structurally normal heart diagnosed prenatally, 28% of pregnancies resulted in a termination of pregnancy. If the terminations are excluded then the outcome of the continuing pregnancies was: 30% resulting in spontaneous intrauterine death, 21% died in the neonatal period, 4% died in infancy and 42% were alive at last update. The outcome is unknown in 3% of the continuing pregnancies.

Of cases seen in the last 10 years, a termination of pregnancy took place in 29% of cases and 70% of the continuing pregnancies were alive at last follow-up.

Of the 105 cases, 51% had a biventricular cardiomyopathy, 24% had a left ventricular cardiomyopathy, 22% had a right ventricular cardiomyopathy and 3% had a diabetic cardiomyopathy. The outcome was the worst for those with a left ventricular cardiomyopathy and best for those with a diabetic cardiomyopathy followed by those with a right ventricular cardiomyopathy. Of the continuing pregnancies, 27% of those with a left ventricular cardiomyopathy are surviving, compared with 100% of those with a diabetic cardiomyopathy, 58% of those with a right ventricular cardiomyopathy and 38% of those with a biventricular cardiomyopathy.

Summary of fetal echocardiographic features associated with cardiomyopathy.

- Increased cardiothoracic ratio
- Dilated cardiac ventricles
- Hypertrophied cardiac ventricles
- Echogenicity of cardiac ventricles
- Impaired ventricular function
- Atrioventricular valve regurgitation
- Associated pericardial effusion +/- fetal hydrops

Chapter 11

Cardiac tumours

Summary

- Rhabdomyoma
- Teratoma
- Fibroma
- Other

Cardiac tumours

Prevalence

Cardiac tumours are rare heart lesions, but are seen relatively frequently in the fetus. In the Evelina fetal series, cardiac tumours accounted for 1.1% of the total. Of these, 76% were rhabdomyomas, 15% were teratomas, 2% fibromas, 2% hamartomas and 5% of unknown type.

Rhabdomyoma

The most common type of tumour encountered are rhabdomyomas, which are homogeneous circumscribed tumours, that are usually multiple but rarely can be single. They are variable in size and site, occurring in the ventricular free walls, the ventricular septum or the atrial free walls (Figures 11.1a-d, 11.2 and 11.3). They do not normally cause any cardiac compromise, but occasionally can become obstructive, if they become very large, and can lead to fetal hydrops, or occasionally may cause arrhythmias. The natural history of rhabdomyomas is to appear in mid-gestation and increase in size through the pregnancy, but postnatally the tendency is for them to shrink and even eventually disappear completely.

The main concern following diagnosis is the strong association of multiple rhabdomyomas with the genetic condition, tuberous sclerosis. The clinical spectrum of tuberous sclerosis is very broad, developmental delay and epilepsy being the best known features. Genetic counselling is therefore important in all cases detected prenatally.

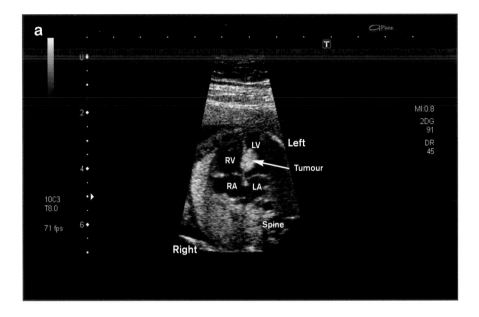

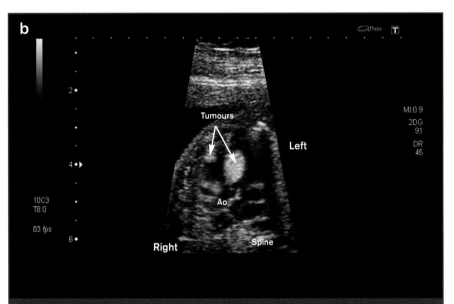

Figure 11.1. An example of multiple rhabdomyoma. a) There is a large homogeneous tumour in the left ventricle which appears to be attached to the ventricular septum. b) This tumour gives the impression of obstructing the left ventricular outflow, though the aorta is a normal size. In this view, a second smaller tumour is also seen in the right ventricle.

Figure continued overleaf.

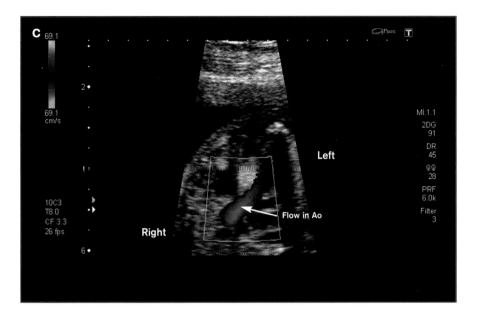

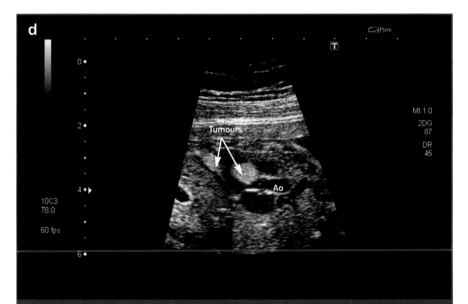

Figure 11.1 *continued.* **An example of multiple rhabdomyoma. c) Colour flow shows laminar flow in the left ventricular outflow (shown in blue); the Doppler velocity in the outflow was normal. d) A different view shows a further tumour at the apex.**

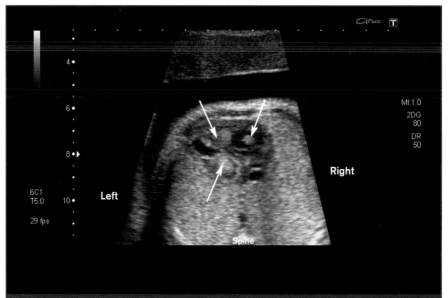

Figure 11.2. An example of multiple rhabdomyoma. Several tumours are seen affecting both ventricular chambers and the septum (arrows).

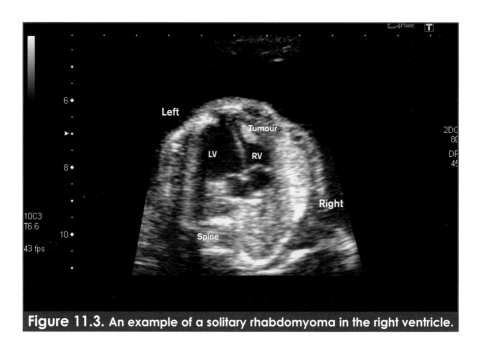

Figure 11.3. An example of a solitary rhabdomyoma in the right ventricle.

Of 35 cases of rhabdomyoma diagnosed prenatally, 37% resulted in a termination of pregnancy. If the terminations are excluded then the outcome of the continuing pregnancies was: 9% had a spontaneous intrauterine death and 86% were alive at last update, with the outcome unknown in 5%.

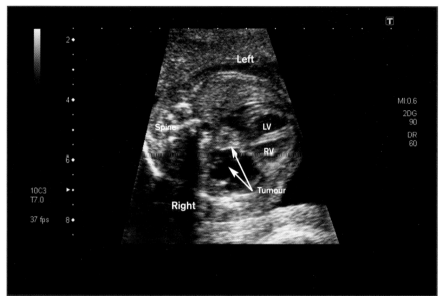

Figure 11.4. An example of a teratoma which appeared to be situated on top of the atria and the arterial roots. This tumour has a cystic appearance, in contrast to rhabdomyoma which are homogeneous.

Teratoma

Less commonly a teratoma may be seen. This is a cystic pericardial tumour which can be attached to the aortic root or pulmonary artery. It is usually single, multicystic and of mixed echogenicity and frequently associated with a pericardial effusion. The tumour may compress the heart and cause fetal hydrops and intrauterine death because of its size, though it is histologically benign. Teratomas can be successfully removed surgically after birth. Examples of teratoma are shown in Figures 11.4 and 11.5a-b.

Of seven cases of cardiac teratoma diagnosed prenatally, 29% of pregnancies resulted in a termination of pregnancy. Of the continuing pregnancies, 40% had a spontaneous intrauterine death, 20% died in the neonatal period and 40% are alive.

Fibroma

These are rare tumours which are usually single. They occur in the ventricular myocardium or the septum and can be difficult to distinguish from rhabdomyoma. However, they may degenerate centrally and form cysts. They can be associated with a pericardial effusion and are generally associated with a poor outlook.

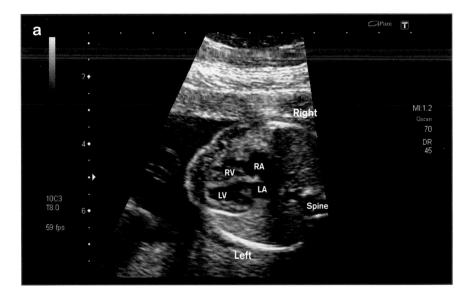

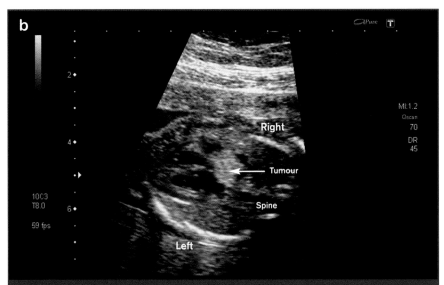

Figure 11.5. Another example of a teratoma. a) The four-chamber view in this example appears normal. b) There is a tumour mass, which has a cystic appearance arising near the origin of the arterial roots.

Other

Very rarely a tumour associated with the heart may prove to be a haemangioma or a hamartoma. Sometimes tumours are seen in unusual positions and the type may not be clearly identified before birth. An example of a tumour which appeared to be attached to the tricuspid valve and was causing right ventricular outflow tract obstruction is shown in Figures 11.6a-c.

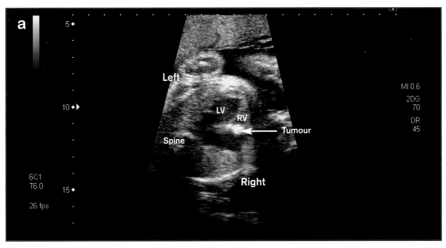

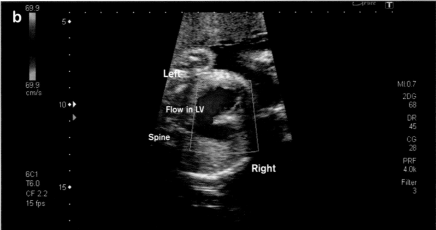

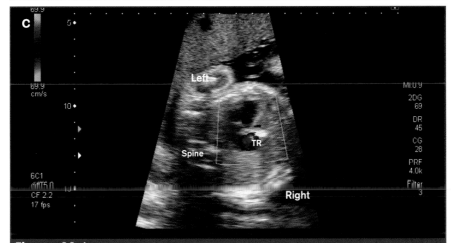

Figure 11.6. An example of a tumour that appeared to be attached to the tricuspid valve. a) In the four-chamber view a bright echogenic tumour is seen in the region of the tricuspid valve. b) Colour flow shows flow from the left atrium into the left ventricle (shown in red) but little flow is seen on the right side of the heart. c) Colour flow shows that there is tricuspid regurgitation.

Chapter 12

Other cardiac anomalies

Summary

- Coronary artery fistula
- Aortico-left ventricular tunnel
- Criss-cross heart
- Ventricular aneurysms and diverticula
- Aortopulmonary window
- Direct connection of the umbilical vein to the atrium (agenesis of ductus venosus)
- Ductal constriction
- Ectopia cordis
- Pericardial effusions

Other cardiac anomalies

Coronary artery fistula

Prevalence
This is a rare cardiac malformation accounting for 0.2% of congenital heart disease in postnatal series. In the Evelina fetal series, isolated artery fistula accounted for 0.14% of the total.

Definition
A coronary artery fistula is a vascular communication connecting one of the coronary arteries to either a cardiac chamber or a great vessel.

Spectrum
A coronary artery fistula can occur as an isolated lesion or can be associated with other congenital heart disease, in particular, pulmonary atresia with an intact interventricular septum and tetralogy of Fallot. A coronary artery fistula can affect either coronary artery or, rarely, both.

Fetal echocardiographic features
The fetal cardiac findings will depend on the site of the fistula and on its size. Examples of a fistula draining to the right atrium are shown in Figures 12.1a-e and 12.2a-g. Coronary

arteries are usually not easily identifiable in the fetus, but in instances where there is a fistula, the coronary artery may be easily seen or appear dilated (Figures 12.1b and 12.2b). If the fistula drains to either atrium, then the atrium may appear enlarged and there may be cardiomegaly (Figures 12.1a and 12.2a). If the drainage is to the ventricle, then the ventricle may appear dilated, though in some cases it may appear normal. An example of a fistula draining to the left ventricle, but with a normal sized left ventricle is shown in Figures 12.3a-c. Fistulas connecting with a great vessel will be detected because of abnormal flow patterns within the vessel. In all cases, the abnormal flow pathway from the dilated coronary artery to the site of drainage will help confirm the diagnosis (Figures 12.1c, 12.2c-d and 12.3c). There may be an increased velocity at the point of entry into the cardiac chamber indicating some degree of stenosis (Figure 12.2e). If there is significant flow in the fistula causing 'coronary steal' then reverse flow, or to and fro flow, will be seen in the aortic arch (Figures 12.1d-e and 12.2f-g).

Extracardiac associations
It is unusual for extracardiac abnormalities to occur with isolated cases of coronary artery fistula, though fetal hydrops may occur if there is cardiac compromise.

Management and outcome
If a coronary artery fistula is small it may not have any adverse effect and may not require treatment. However, coronary artery fistulas may enlarge over time and can eventually produce symptoms of cardiac ischaemia, heart failure or arrhythmias. Thus, larger fistulas, or those producing symptoms, will require closure. This can be achieved with the use of a coil or occlusion device introduced through a catheterisation procedure, or via a surgical approach.

Outcome in a large single-centre fetal series
Of six cases of coronary artery fistula diagnosed prenatally, a termination of pregnancy took place in one case, there was one death in infancy and the remaining cases were alive at last update.

Summary of fetal echocardiographic features associated with coronary artery fistula.

- Dilated atrium or ventricle depending on site of drainage
- Dilated coronary artery
- Abnormal flow pattern draining to atrium or ventricle, which may be high velocity flow

---

Aortico-left ventricular tunnel

Prevalence
This is an extremely rare cardiac malformation. In the Evelina fetal series, aortico-left ventricular tunnel accounted for 0.12% of the total.

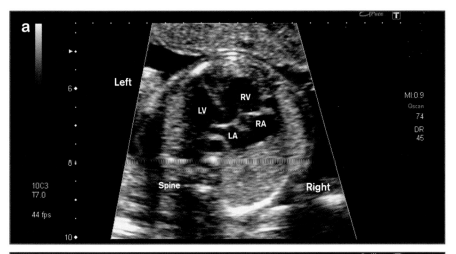

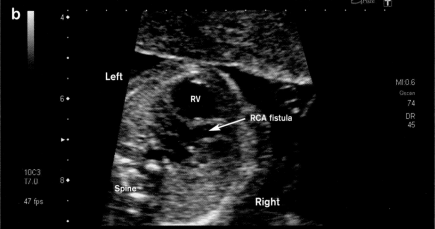

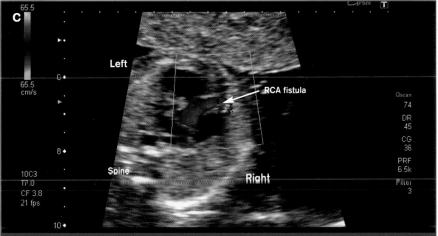

Figure 12.1. An example of a coronary artery fistula draining to the right atrium. a) In the four-chamber view there is cardiomegaly and the right heart structures appear dilated compared to the left. b) The right coronary artery is very dilated. c) The flow in the right coronary artery and fistula is seen with colour flow (shown in red).

Figure continued overleaf.

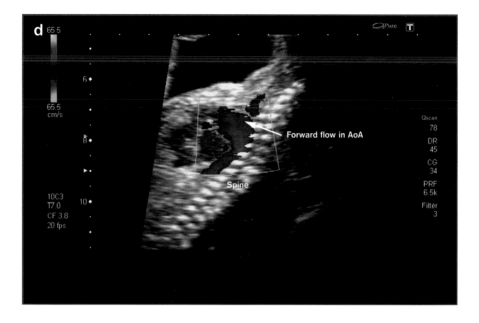

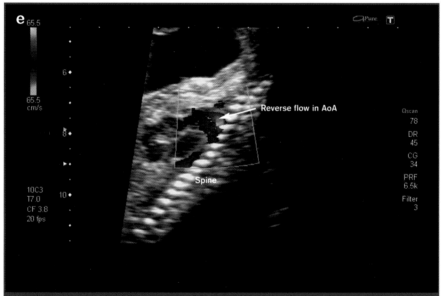

Figure 12.1 *continued.* **An example of a coronary artery fistula draining to the right atrium. d-e) To and fro flow is seen in the aortic arch, shown in a longitudinal view. The forward flow is seen in Figure 12.1d (shown in blue) and the reverse flow is seen in Figure 12.1e (shown in red).**

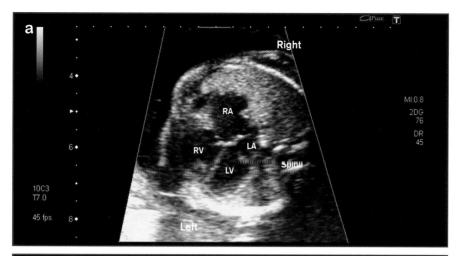

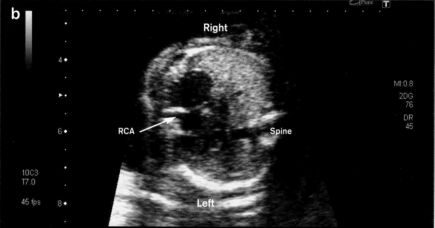

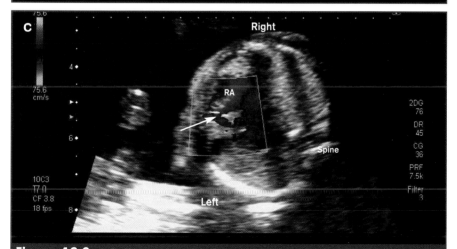

Figure 12.2. A further example of a coronary artery fistula draining to the right atrium. a) In the four-chamber view there is cardiomegaly and the right atrium in particular appears dilated. b) The right coronary artery is dilated. c) The flow in the right coronary artery is seen with colour flow (arrow) and the flow enters the right atrium (shown in red).

Figure continued overleaf.

287

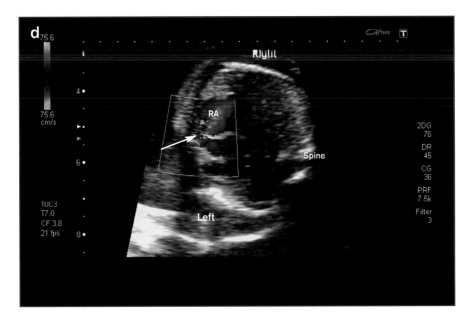

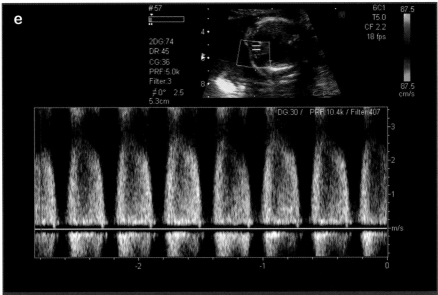

Figure 12.2 *continued.* A further example of a coronary artery fistula draining to the right atrium. d) A further view of the flow in the right coronary artery opening to the right atrium, seen with colour flow. There is turbulence at the point of entry into the right atrium (arrow). e) Pulsed Doppler confirms a high velocity of 3m/second at the point of entry.

Figure continued overleaf.

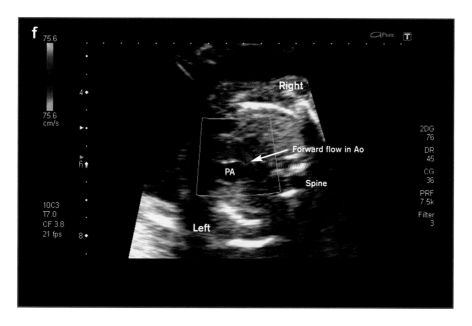

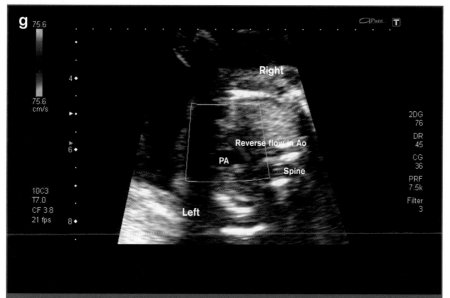

Figure 12.2 *continued.* A further example of a coronary artery fistula draining to the right atrium. f-g) To and fro flow is seen in the aorta in a three-vessel view. The forward flow is seen in Figure 12.2f (shown in blue) and the reverse flow is seen in Figure 12.2g (shown in red).

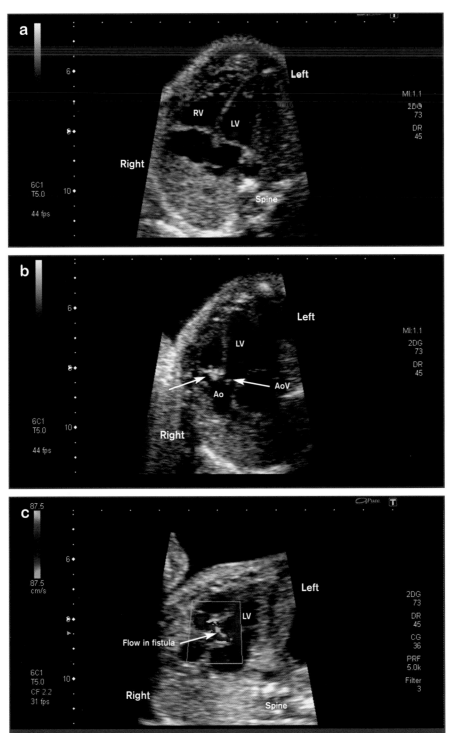

Figure 12.3. An example of a coronary artery fistula draining to the left ventricle. a) The four-chamber view appears normal. b) The right coronary artery appears dilated (arrow). c) There is a fistula from the right coronary artery which opens into the left ventricle just beneath the aortic valve (flow in fistula shown in blue).

Definition
In aortico-left ventricular tunnel there is an abnormal channel or communication that originates in the ascending aorta, bypasses the aortic valve and terminates in the left ventricle.

Spectrum
The features of this condition are aortic regurgitation, a dilated ascending aorta and a dilated left ventricle. Aortic stenosis can coexist in fetuses with aortico-left ventricular tunnel.

Fetal echocardiographic features
Aortic regurgitation is rare in the fetus and the detection of significant aortic regurgitation should raise the possibility of aortico-left ventricular tunnel. In some cases, the left ventricle may be dilated or dysfunctional. Colour flow will show the regurgitant flow into the left ventricle, which will not be across the aortic valve, but rather around the valve.

Differential diagnosis
The finding of a dilated poorly contracting left ventricle suggests the possibility of critical aortic stenosis and this diagnosis can be made in error. In some cases, aortic stenosis can coexist with aortico-left ventricular tunnel and the diagnosis of aortic stenosis with aortic regurgitation might be made with the tunnel being overlooked. Another mistaken diagnosis is tetralogy of Fallot, as the appearance of the bulbous aortic root can be misinterpreted as aortic override.

Extracardiac associations
This anomaly is not usually associated with extracardiac malformations.

Management and outcome
Although this lesion can be successfully repaired after birth, the cases seen before birth probably represent the more severe end of the spectrum. Thus, severe regurgitation can cause significant volume overload and lead to fetal hydrops.

Outcome in a large single-centre fetal series
Of five cases of aortico-left ventricular tunnel diagnosed prenatally, there were two terminations of pregnancy, two babies died in the neonatal period and there is one child alive at last update.

Summary of fetal echocardiographic features associated with aortico-left ventricular tunnel

- Dilated aortic root
- Dilated left ventricle
- Regurgitation from the aorta into the left ventricle
- Bulging of the ascending aorta into the right ventricular outflow tract
- Thickened aortic valve (occasionally)

Criss-cross heart

Prevalence
A criss-cross heart is a rare and complex cardiac abnormality accounting for less than 0.1% of all congenital heart disease. In the Evelina fetal series, criss-cross hearts accounted for 0.16% of the total.

Definition
In a criss-cross heart the ventricles are twisted causing the inflow streams across the two atrioventricular valves to cross each other, rather than be parallel as in a normal heart.

Spectrum
A criss-cross heart is usually associated with severe and complex forms of congenital heart disease.

Fetal echocardiographic features
The characteristic feature is the crossing of the axes or inflow streams of the atrioventricular valves. Normally the two inflow streams across the atrioventricular valves into the ventricles are parallel (see Figure 2.2c in Chapter 2). In a criss-cross heart the appearance is of each atrium draining to the opposite ventricle, though there is in fact atrioventricular concordance with the atrium draining to the correct ventricle, but the orientation is not normal. An example of a criss-cross heart with transposition of the great arteries is shown in Figures 12.4a-d.

Extracardiac associations
Extracardiac abnormalities can be associated depending on the exact cardiac anatomy and thus should be excluded.

Management and outcome
In the majority of cases of criss-cross heart, a biventricular repair is not possible and surgical management is aimed at a staged surgical palliation (Fontan type circulation).

Outcome in a large single-centre fetal series
Of seven cases of a criss-cross heart diagnosed prenatally, there were three terminations of pregnancy, one child died in infancy and three cases were alive at last update.

Summary of fetal echocardiographic features associated with criss-cross heart.

- **Direction of flow across the two atrioventricular valves crosses (normally the two inflows are parallel)**
- **May be associated with complex congenital heart disease**

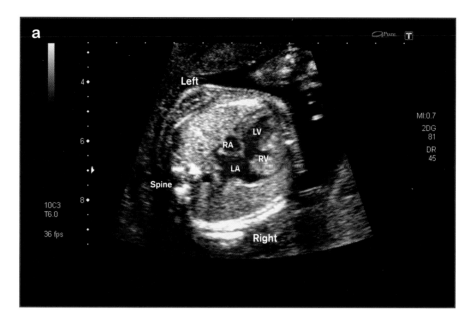

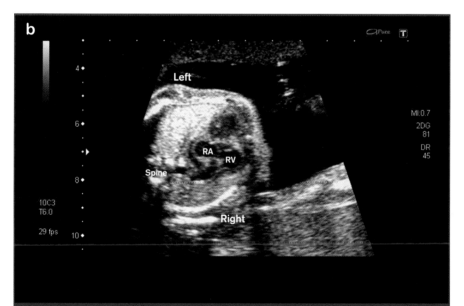

Figure 12.4. An example of a criss-cross heart with transposition of the great arteries. a) In the four-chamber view there is one large ventricular chamber and a smaller one anteriorly. The large ventricle appears to be the left ventricle. The atrium receiving the pulmonary veins (left atrium) appears to be connected to this left ventricle. The other atrium (right atrium) appears to lie to the left of the left atrium. b) A view in a different plane to that seen in 12.4a, shows the right atrium connected to the small right ventricle. The direction of the atrioventricular valves crosses in opposite directions (criss-cross).

Figure continued overleaf.

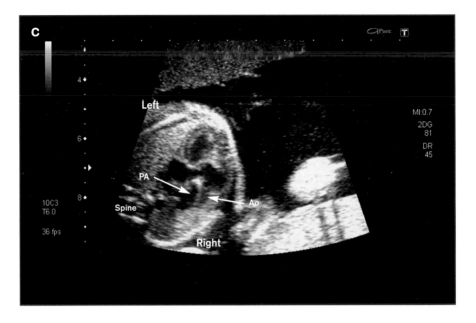

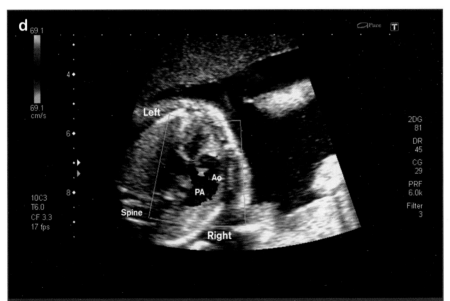

Figure 12.4 *continued*. An example of a criss-cross heart with transposition of the great arteries. c) The great arteries arise in parallel orientation, with the aorta arising from the smaller right ventricle and the pulmonary artery arising from the left ventricle. d) The flow in the great arteries is seen with colour Doppler (shown in blue).

Ventricular aneurysms and diverticula

Prevalence
These are very rare cardiac malformations. In the Evelina fetal series, ventricular aneurysms and diverticula accounted for 0.21% of the total.

Definition
Ventricular aneurysms and diverticula produce a pouching out of the ventricular wall. Diverticula have a narrow neck communicating with the ventricle, whereas aneurysms have a broad base communication with the ventricular cavity.

Spectrum
Ventricular aneurysms and diverticula can affect either ventricle, can be of varying size and can affect different parts of the ventricular wall. Some cases can be associated with other forms of congenital heart disease.

Fetal echocardiographic features
The four-chamber view usually appears abnormal, with the aneurysm or diverticulum distorting the appearance of the ventricular wall and the normal shape of the ventricular cavity. The ventricle will appear to be asymmetrically dilated and there may be marked cardiomegaly (Figures 12.5 and 12.6). Colour flow will demonstrate blood flowing between the aneurysm or diverticulum and the ventricular cavity.

Extracardiac associations
Extracardiac abnormalities can sometimes be present and this type of cardiac abnormality can be associated with pericardial effusions and fetal hydrops.

Management and outcome
Due to the rarity of this lesion and the different types of cases, the outcome is difficult to predict. The overall outcome can be good in isolated cases, though there have also been reports of adverse outcome.

Outcome in a large single-centre fetal series
Of nine cases of ventricular aneurysm diagnosed prenatally, there were two terminations of pregnancy, two cases had a spontaneous intrauterine death and five cases were alive at last update. Of the nine cases, an aneurysm or diverticulum was present in the left ventricle in five cases and in the right ventricle in four cases. There was associated congenital heart disease in three out of four cases affecting the right ventricle; one case with tricuspid atresia, one case with absent pulmonary valve syndrome and one case with a ventricular septal defect. Of those with the left ventricle affected, one case also had an interrupted aortic arch.

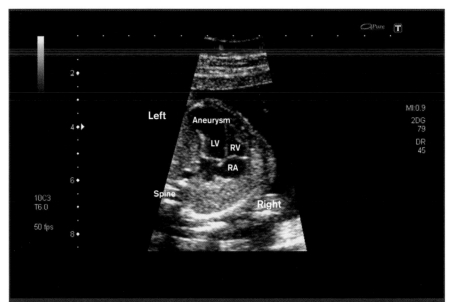

Figure 12.5. An example of a ventricular aneurysm. A bulge can be seen at the apex of the left ventricle.

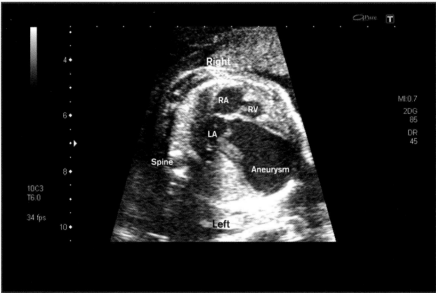

Figure 12.6. An example of a ventricular aneurysm associated with marked cardiomegaly.

> **Summary of fetal echocardiographic features associated with ventricular aneurysms and diverticula.**
>
> - **Cardiomegaly**
> - **Distortion of ventricular shape**
> - **Asymmetrical dilation of ventricle (left or right ventricle may be affected)**
> - **May be associated congenital heart disease**

Aortopulmonary window

Prevalence
Aortopulmonary window is a very rare lesion accounting for about 0.1% of all congenital heart defects. It is an extremely rare diagnosis in the fetus. In a series of over 4000 cardiac abnormalities, only one case of aortopulmonary window has been diagnosed.

Definition
In this lesion there is a hole in the wall between the aorta and pulmonary artery.

Spectrum
Aortopulmonary window may occur as an isolated lesion or can be associated with other forms of congenital heart disease.

Fetal echocardiographic findings
This is a very difficult diagnosis to make in fetal life. There is a hole in the wall between the aorta and pulmonary artery, above the level of the arterial valves (Figure 12.7).

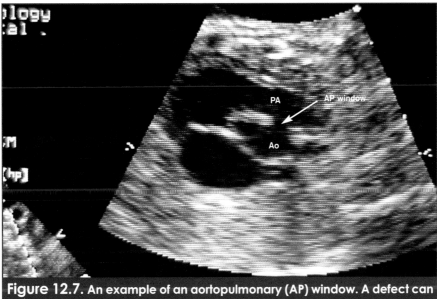

Figure 12.7. An example of an aortopulmonary (AP) window. A defect can be seen between the aorta and pulmonary artery.

Management and outcome

The haemodynamic effects of an aortopulmonary window are similar to that seen with a large unrestrictive ventricular septal defect. There is a large and usually unrestricted left-to-right shunt which gets worse as pulmonary vascular resistance falls during the newborn period. Volume overload and pulmonary over-circulation can lead to progressive left ventricular dysfunction and congestive heart failure.

Surgery to correct an aortopulmonary window is successful in most cases, but the mortality is higher in cases associated with other cardiac defects that complicate repair.

Summary of fetal echocardiographic features associated with an aortopulmonary window.

- **Defect in the wall between the aorta and pulmonary artery above the level of the arterial valves**
- **May be associated with other congenital disease**

Direct communication of the umbilical vein to the right or left atrium (agenesis of the ductus venosus)

This is a rare form of vascular malformation. The umbilical vein is normally directed through the ductus venosus, which has an important role in regulating flow back to the heart. If the ductus venosus is absent (agenesis of the ductus venosus), there will not be any regulation of flow, resulting in volume overload of the heart. This usually causes cardiomegaly, which is often observed with this anomaly, but in some instances can also result in fetal hydrops, which will have an adverse effect on the outcome. An example of the umbilical vein connecting directly to the right atrium is shown in Figures 12.8a-c.

A good outcome can generally be anticipated, provided there is no deterioration in cardiac function due to volume overload as pregnancy advances and there is no hydrops. Once the baby is born, then the umbilical vein will of course, be removed from the circulation, so that the volume loading of the heart is rectified. It is important to exclude any extracardiac abnormalities.

Ductal constriction

This is a rare problem, which may occur in late gestation. Although it can be related to maternal ingestion of non-steroidal anti-inflammatory medication, it can also occur without any identifiable cause. Ductal constriction can cause right ventricular dilation and dysfunction associated with tricuspid regurgitation in some cases (Figures 12.9). Although the right ventricular dysfunction can look dramatic, these findings usually resolve after delivery. Doppler studies in the duct will usually demonstrate an increased velocity with aliasing of the signal on colour flow.

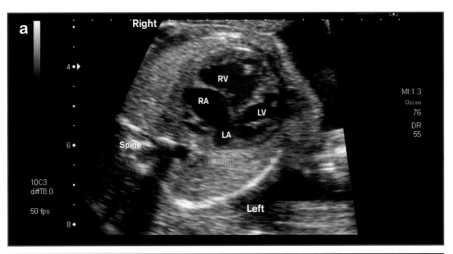

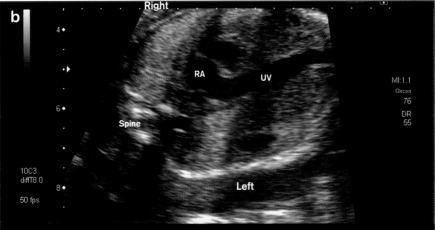

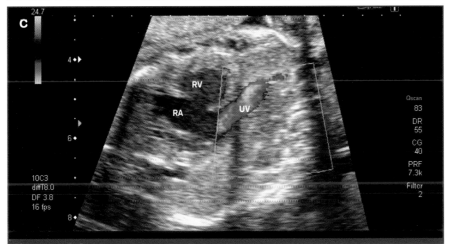

Figure 12.8. An example of the umbilical vein connecting directly to the right atrium. a) In the four-chamber view there is cardiomegaly and the right heart structures appear dilated compared to the left. b) A large umbilical vein (UV) can be seen draining to the right atrium. c) The flow in the umbilical vein towards the heart is seen with colour flow (shown in blue).

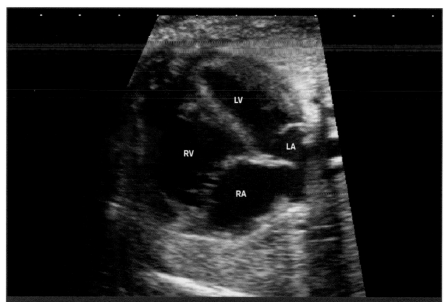

Figure 12.9. The four-chamber view in an example of ductal constriction. The right atrium and right ventricle are dilated and there was severe right ventricular dysfunction. This recovered after delivery.

Ectopia cordis

This occurs when the heart in its pericardial sac lies partially or completely outside the chest cavity (Figure 12.10). It is due to partial or complete absence of the sternum. Ectopia cordis can be associated with congenital heart malformations, but the heart structure can also be normal. There may or may not be skin covering the defect. If there is no skin cover, the heart appears to float freely in the amniotic fluid. The anterior abdominal wall must be examined for evidence of an associated gut protrusion. Outcome is generally poor as it is difficult to replace the heart within the chest cavity, which is often too small.

Pericardial effusions

It is common to see a rim of fluid around the ventricular chambers during fetal life (Figures 2.36 and 2.37 in Chapter 2). This should be distinguished from a true pericardial effusion, which usually extends around the atrioventricular groove and measures more than 2mm (Figures 12.11, 12.12 and 12.13). Pericardial effusions can be associated with other abnormalities and detailed evaluation of the fetus should be undertaken to exclude structural cardiac malformations, functional and rhythm disturbances of the heart, other indicators of fetal hydrops, extracardiac abnormalities and markers of chromosomal anomalies.

The outcome will be determined by the extent of associated abnormality. In isolated cases with no other abnormality detected, a good outcome is anticipated.

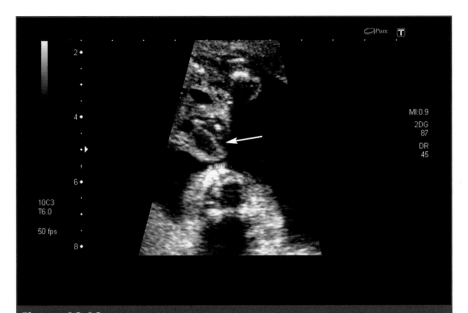

Figure 12.10. An example of ectopia cordis. Part of the heart protrudes out of the chest and lies outside the chest (arrow). The structure of the heart in this example was normal.

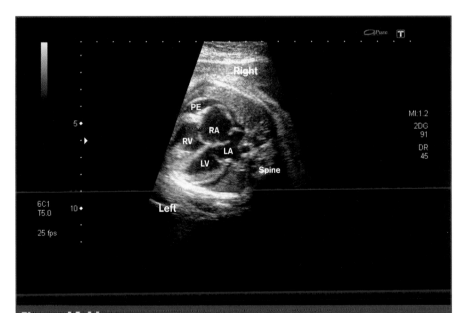

Figure 12.11. An example of a pericardial effusion with cardiomegaly. The structure and function of the heart were normal. These findings were due to fetal anaemia and recovered following a blood transfusion.

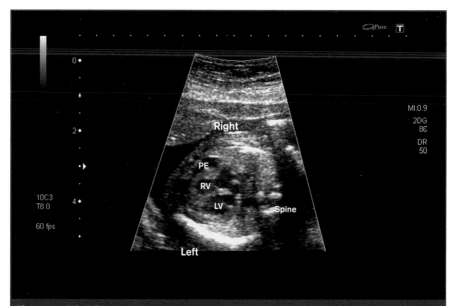

Figure 12.12. An example of a pericardial effusion which gave the impression of ventricular hypertrophy. The cardiac function was normal and no cardiac abnormality was detected after birth.

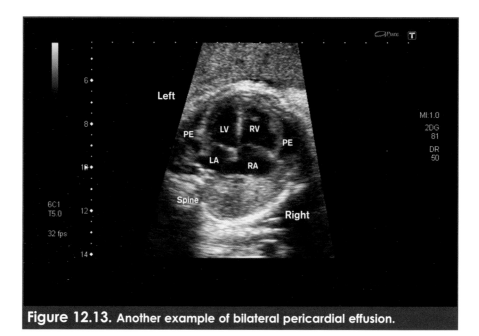

Figure 12.13. Another example of bilateral pericardial effusion.

Chapter 13

Rhythm disturbances in the fetus

Summary

- Normal rhythm and modes of assessment
- Irregular heart rhythms
- Fetal bradycardia
- Fetal tachycardia

Normal rhythm and modes of assessment

The normal heart rate in the mid-trimester fetus varies between 120-160 beats per minute. There are three main categories of fetal arrhythmia. These are:

- An irregular heart rhythm.
- A slow heart rhythm (bradycardia).
- A fast heart rhythm (tachycardia).

Assessment of rhythm disturbances in fetal life is aimed at establishing the relationship between the atrial and ventricular contractions. This is most commonly done by echocardiography using either M-mode echocardiography or Doppler techniques, or a combination of the two methods. Newer techniques include fetal electrocardiography, tissue Doppler echocardiography and fetal magnetocardiography.

M-mode echocardiography

M-mode echocardiography, though generally little used now in fetal cardiac assessment, is still a useful technique in the assessment fetal arrhythmias, as it allows atrial and ventricular activity to be recorded simultaneously. In order to do this the M-mode cursor line has to be positioned through either, an atrium and ventricle, or alternatively through the aortic valve and left atrium. A normal M-mode trace is shown in Figure 2.29 in Chapter 2.

Doppler techniques

Fetal heart rhythms can also be assessed using pulsed Doppler techniques. Different methods have been used including simultaneous recording of mitral valve inflow and aortic valve outflow traces, or ascending aorta and superior vena cava traces, or pulmonary artery and pulmonary vein traces. Any of these techniques may be used, but the important thing is that the operator should be familiar with the technique being used, in order to correctly interpret the traces obtained. To obtain a trace of mitral valve inflow and aortic valve outflow, the Doppler sample volume is positioned in the left ventricle to capture the inflow and outflow of the left ventricle simultaneously (Figure 13.1a). An example of a normal trace obtained from the aortic and mitral valves is shown in (Figure 13.1b). The Doppler tracing shows inflow across the mitral valve above the baseline and outflow in the left ventricular outflow tract below the baseline. Simultaneous recording of the ascending aorta and superior vena cava is illustrated in Figures 13.1c-d.

Other methods of assessing fetal heart rhythm

Direct electrocardiographic assessment of fetal heart rhythm (fetal ECG) can be performed via the maternal abdomen, though currently the use of this is limited. This is because of the poor quality traces obtained across the maternal abdomen, and the fact that although fetal QRS waves can be obtained, 'P' waves are not detected.

A newer technique using tissue Doppler imaging allows more accurate localisation of arrhythmias, but its use is also limited as it measures the mechanical consequence of the arrhythmia, rather than the conduction itself.

Another novel technique of fetal magnetocardiography does appear to be more promising in providing high quality electrophysiological signals for more accurate diagnosis of fetal arrhythmia. However, practical limitations are that fetal magnetocardiography is not widely available, requires a magnetically shielded room, and can take several hours to perform.

Irregular fetal heart rhythms

An irregular heart rhythm is the most common form of fetal arrhythmia. This type of rhythm disturbance can cause a great deal of anxiety to midwives, obstetricians and to the pregnant mother, but is usually benign. Irregular heart rhythms occur most commonly in the third trimester, though they can occur in earlier gestation. The irregular rhythm is most often the result of multiple atrial premature contractions (atrial ectopic beats), but ventricular extrasystoles (ventricular ectopic beats) are occasionally seen.

In a normal regular heart rhythm, for every atrial beat there is a ventricular response (Figures 2.27 and 2.29 in Chapter 2). When a premature atrial contraction occurs this can sometimes be transmitted to the ventricle causing an irregularity. Or, if it occurs very early in diastole it may not be conducted to the ventricle, which will still be in the refractory period

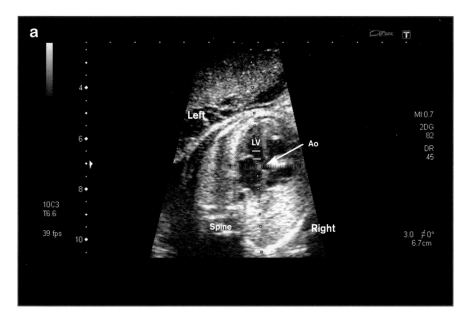

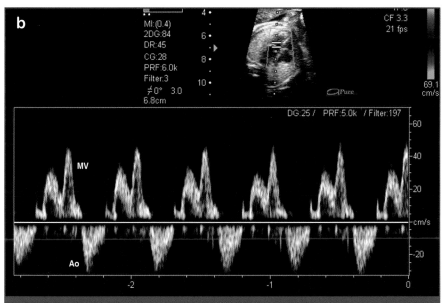

Figure 13.1. a) The Doppler sample volume is positioned in the left ventricle to capture the inflow and outflow of the left ventricle simultaneously. **b)** A normal Doppler trace recording the aortic outflow and the mitral valve inflow simultaneously.

Figure continued overleaf.

305

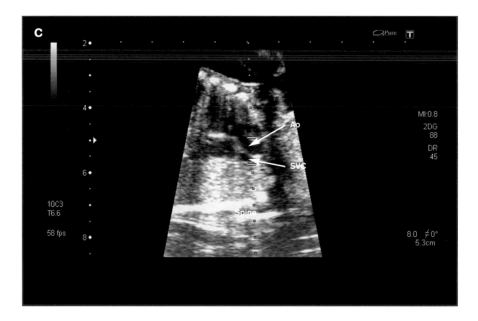

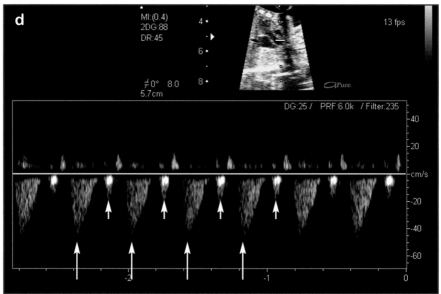

Figure 13.1 *continued. c)* The Doppler cursor is positioned to capture SVC and aortic flow simultaneously. *d)* A normal Doppler trace recording SVC and aortic flow simultaneously. The large arrows indicate aortic outflow and equate to ventricular contraction. The smaller arrows indicate reversal of flow in the SVC during atrial contraction and equate to this.

from the previous beat. This then appears as a missed beat (Figures 13.2a-b). Multiple blocked ectopics of this type can produce a slow heart rate of around 70-80 beats per minute (Figure 13.3). It is of great importance to distinguish this type of slow heart rate from complete heart block (see below), as the outcome and prognosis of the two conditions is very different. Blocked atrial premature contractions can be demonstrated on M-mode or pulsed Doppler traces. However, if every other beat is an atrial ectopic beat (atrial bigeminy) and alternate beats are not conducted, then this can potentially be misinterpreted as complete heart block. In atrial bigeminy, however, the time interval between all the atrial beats will not be regular as every other atrial beat, the ectopic beat, will occur earlier than the preceding beat (Figure 13.3). In heart block the atrial contractions are usually regular with the same time interval between them (see below). Whilst blocked atrial ectopic beats or atrial bigeminy can resolve back to normal sinus rhythm, or have periods of normal rhythm interspersed with the irregular rhythm, complete heart block usually causes a persistent irreversible bradycardia.

Ventricular ectopics are rare but can occur in fetal life. In these cases, M-mode or pulsed Doppler traces will demonstrate an irregular ventricular rhythm, but with a normal regular atrial rhythm (Figure 13.4a-b).

Management and outcome

Ectopic beats, whether atrial or ventricular, are generally regarded as being benign and in the majority of cases will resolve spontaneously, either before delivery or early in the neonatal period. Ectopic beats are not a sign of fetal distress and therefore premature delivery is not indicated. However, in 1-2% of fetuses with premature atrial contractions, a fetal tachycardia may develop, which may then require treatment (see below). Those particularly at risk of developing a tachycardia are those with multiple blocked atrial ectopic beats associated with a bradycardia. In the newborn period, premature atrial contractions have been noted to be associated with a re-entry circuit with the potential of developing tachycardias.

Evidence of structural heart disease should be excluded in all cases. If ectopic beats are infrequent (less than one for every 10 sinus beats) then no further action or investigation is required. If they are more frequent, then follow-up should be arranged, which may be in the form of fetal heart auscultation every 1-2 weeks, to monitor for the development of a fetal tachycardia. If the ectopics resolve prior to delivery then no further investigation is usually required. However, if the heart rate is still irregular at the time of delivery, a postnatal electrocardiogram (ECG) is recommended to exclude pre-excitation. An irregular heart rate at the time of labour, though not a cause of distress to the baby, can cause problems for the obstetric team in terms of using the fetal heart rate as a means of monitoring for fetal well being.

The majority of babies with an irregular heart rhythm will have an uneventful outcome with spontaneous resolution of the arrhythmia.

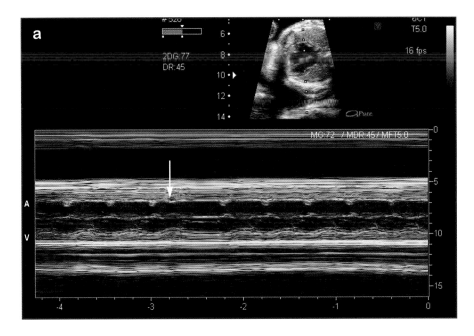

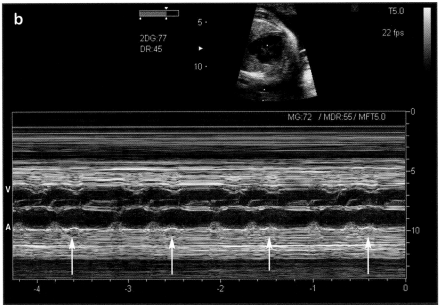

Figure 13.2. a) An example of a single atrial ectopic beat (arrow) seen with M-mode. b) An M-mode trace showing multiple atrial ectopic beats (arrows).

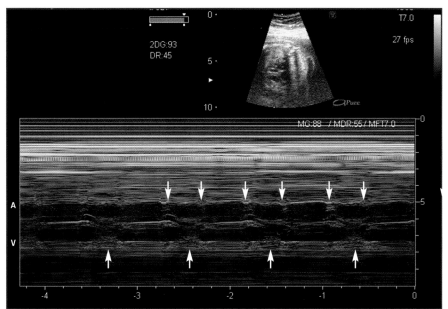

Figure 13.3. An M-mode trace showing multiple coupled (bigeminy) blocked ectopic beats producing bradycardia. There is a ventricular response to every other atrial beat. However, for the atrial beats that are arrowed, the distance between the first two beats is shorter than the distance between the second and third beat. Similarly, the distance between the third and fourth beats is shorter than the distance between the fourth and fifth beat. This helps to distinguish this example from complete heart block where the distance between the atrial beats remains the same.

Fetal bradycardia

A fetal bradycardia is defined as a heart rate of less than 120 beats per minute.

Sinus bradycardia

A transient sinus bradycardia, with 1:1 atrioventricular conduction is commonly observed in the mid-trimester fetus and is usually of no consequence. However, a sustained bradycardia needs further evaluation. A persistent bradycardia of between 90-120 beats per minute with 1:1 atrioventricular conduction can be an indication of long QT syndrome (Figure 13.5). It may also be associated with maternal anti-Ro and anti-La antibodies and is sometimes seen in fetuses with left atrial isomerism, where there is no sinus node. A prolonged sinus bradycardia is occasionally seen in a sick or pre-terminal fetus with other pathologies.

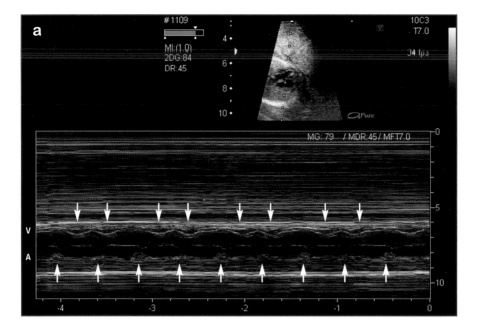

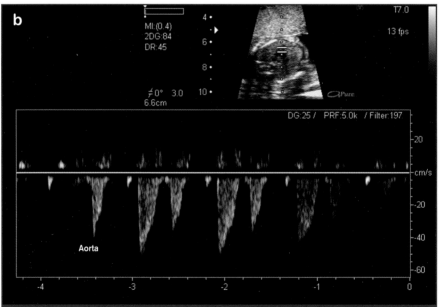

Figure 13.4. a) An M-mode trace showing ventricular ectopic beats. The atrial rate is regular but there are coupled ventricular beats (ventricular bigeminy). b) The aortic Doppler trace shows coupled ventricular beats.

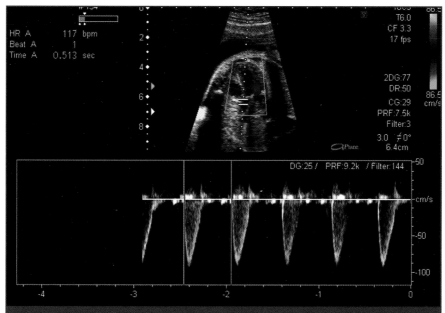

Figure 13.5. Doppler tracing showing a slightly slow heart rate in a mid-trimester fetus (117 beats per minute). A persistent sinus bradycardia should raise the possibility of long QT syndrome as part of the differential diagnosis.

Multiple blocked ectopics producing a bradycardia

A bradycardia can be produced by multiple blocked atrial ectopic beats, but in these cases there will not be 1:1 atrioventricular conduction (see above). As described above, some of these cases can be difficult to distinguish from congenital heart block (see below), but careful assessment with M-mode or Doppler echocardiography should allow the distinction to be made. It is important to note that the majority of these cases will usually resolve spontaneously and no treatment is required, though in a small minority there is a risk of a tachycardia developing.

Congenital heart block

The diagnosis of concern in fetuses with a persistent bradycardia of less than 70-80 beats per minute is congenital complete heart block.

Congenital heart block can be classified as first degree, second degree or third degree. In general, first- and second-degree heart block do not produce symptoms, though progression to complete heart block can occur, which may cause symptoms.

First-degree heart block

In first-degree heart block there is slowed conduction through the atrioventricular node but there is still regular 1:1 conduction from the atrium to the ventricle. This is detected in postnatal life by a prolonged PR interval on an electrocardiogram tracing (ECG). This is not generally possible in the fetus, where instead a prolonged atrioventricular (AV) time interval is assessed on pulsed Doppler echocardiography, though this is not always easy (Figures 13.6a-b). Recent reports have also described the use of fetal electrocardiograms to measure cardiac time intervals in normal fetuses and for the detection of prolonged PR intervals in fetuses of mothers carrying anti-Ro and anti-La antibodies.

Second-degree heart block

In second-degree heart block only some of the impulses from the atrium are conducted to the ventricle, but there is often a regular ratio of atrioventricular conduction. Thus, for example, in 2:1 block, every other atrial beat is conducted so that there will be a ventricular contraction after every other atrial beat, producing a bradycardia (Figure 13.7). There can also be a progressive prolongation of the PR interval until an atrial beat is dropped (Wenckebach phenomenon).

Third-degree heart block (complete heart block)

Complete heart block occurs where there is complete dissociation between atrial and ventricular contractions. There is no electrical communication between the atria and the ventricles, so they contract independently of each other with no fixed relationship between them (Figures 13.8a-c). Congenital heart block can occur with a structurally normal heart, when it is termed isolated congenital heart block, or it can occur with structural congenital heart disease. The majority of cases, though not all, of complete heart block with structural heart disease are associated with left atrial isomerism (see Chapter 3).

Isolated congenital complete heart block

The vast majority (approximately 90%) of cases of isolated congenital heart block are associated with maternal autoimmune antibodies (anti-Ro and anti-La antibodies). Some mothers may have evidence of an autoimmune connective tissue disease, such as systemic lupus erythematosus or Sjögren's syndrome, but most of the mothers are asymptomatic and unaware that they carry the antibodies, until they have a baby with heart block. Of note is that about 2% of mothers with anti-Ro or anti-La antibodies (SSA/Ro or SSB/La) will have a baby with heart block. The risk of recurrence when a previous baby has been affected with heart block is about 20%. It is thought that the antibodies cross the placenta after 16-18 weeks of gestation and damage the atrioventricular node. This can result in first-degree, second-degree or complete heart block. First- and second-degree heart block may be reversible in some cases and intrauterine treatment with dexamethasone has been advocated for such cases, with reports of successful regression in a few, but not all cases. Complete heart block, however, is considered to be irreversible.

There are a small number of cases of complete heart block of unknown aetiology where the maternal antibody status is negative.

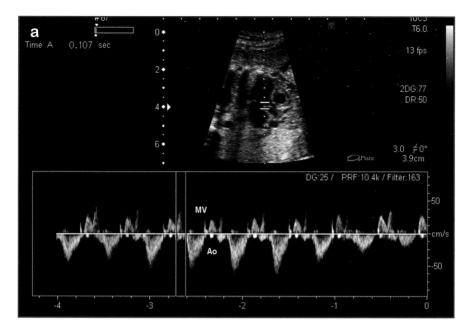

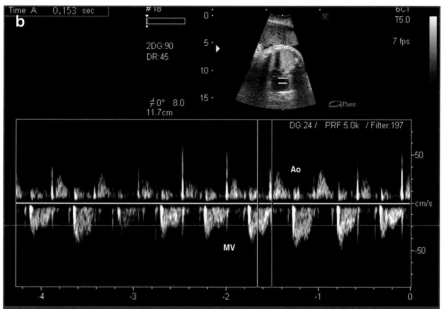

Figure 13.6. a) A normal AV time interval (0.107 seconds) measured with Doppler. b) The AV time interval measured with Doppler in this example was just above the normal range at 0.153 seconds. In cases associated with maternal autoantibodies, it is important to follow this sequentially in case heart block is developing.

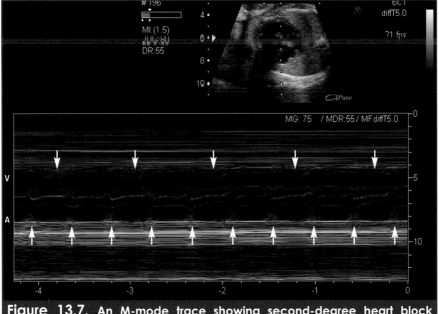

Figure 13.7. An M-mode trace showing second-degree heart block resulting in bradycardia. In this example there is a constant atrial rate and a ventricular response to every other atrial beat. This is different from the example shown in 13.3, where there are blocked atrial ectopics producing a bradycardia.

Fetal echocardiographic features of isolated complete heart block

The structure of the heart will be normal, though in the majority of cases there is some cardiomegaly and the ventricular chambers may appear hypertrophied (Figures 13.9a and 13.10). The heart rate (ventricular rate) is very slow, usually between 45-75 beats per minute with many cases having a rate between 55-65 beats per minute at presentation. This can be measured with Doppler or M-mode traces (Figures 13.8b-c and 13.11b-c). The atrial rate can also easily be measured on M-mode traces (Figures 13.8a and 13.11a). The atrial rate is usually within the normal limits of 120-160 beats per minute, most often around 130-140 beats per minute. There may be some impairment of ventricular function and atrioventricular valve regurgitation may be detected (Figure 13.9b).

A pericardial effusion is often seen with complete heart block (Figure 13.9a), but in the absence of any other signs of hydrops, this can be associated with a good outcome. However, complete heart block may lead to the development of fetal hydrops and this is associated with a poorer outcome. Echogenicity in areas of the myocardium or atrial walls (Figure 13.12) can be seen in some cases, a feature which may be associated with a poor long-term prognosis, particularly if affecting the ventricles and associated with impaired ventricular function. Occasionally, ascites alone is seen without any other features of hydrops (Figure 13.13). This can be immune-mediated in cases where there are maternal antibodies and some of these cases will respond to dexamethasone therapy (see below).

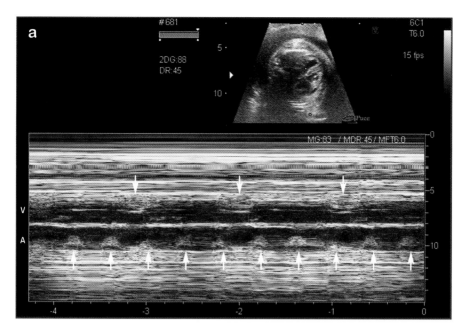

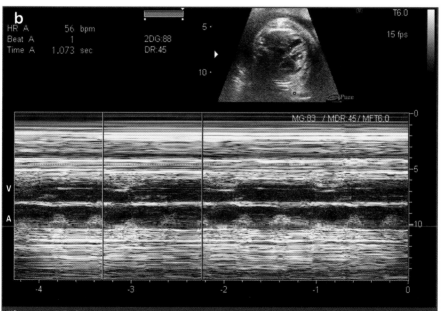

Figure 13.8. An example of complete heart block. a) The M-mode trace shows a normal and regular atrial rate. The ventricular rate is much slower and there is no fixed relationship between atrial and ventricular contractions. b) The ventricular rate measured on M-mode is 56 beats per minute.

Figure continued overleaf.

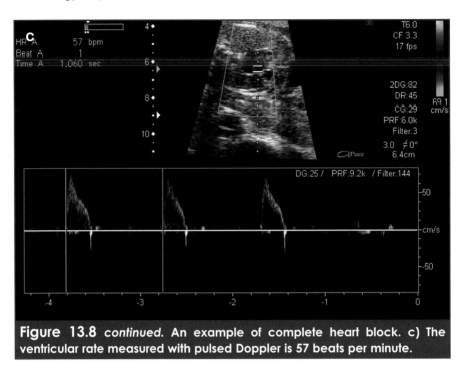

Figure 13.8 *continued*. **An example of complete heart block. c) The ventricular rate measured with pulsed Doppler is 57 beats per minute.**

Fetal echocardiographic features of complete heart block associated with structural heart disease

The echocardiographic features will be determined by the associated structural abnormality. Most commonly this will be in association with left atrial isomerism, though not in all cases. The heart will usually appear enlarged with ventricular hypertrophy. The heart rate will be slow and heart block can be confirmed with M-mode or Doppler echocardiography as described above. Some cases of left atrial isomerism may be associated with a sinus bradycardia rather than complete heart block. An example of complete heart block associated with an atrioventricular septal defect and left atrial isomerism is shown in Figures 4.16a-d in Chapter 4.

Management and outcome

Intrauterine therapy has been tried in selective cases of isolated congenital heart block. Beta-agonists such as salbutamol and terbutaline have been used to try and increase the heart rate in fetuses where the heart rate is less than 50-55 beats per minute, or in fetuses with associated hydrops. While this can increase the heart rate in some cases, the treatment is not effective in all cases and has not been proven to improve the overall outcome. Steroids have also been advocated in the management of heart block in the fetus, though this remains controversial, particularly for first-degree and third-degree heart block. Using steroids for second-degree heart block is probably the least controversial, but further studies are required to evaluate the benefits against the concerns regarding growth restriction and maternal side

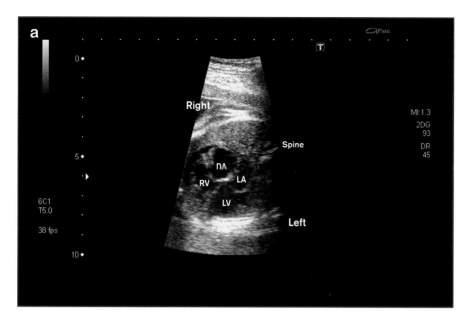

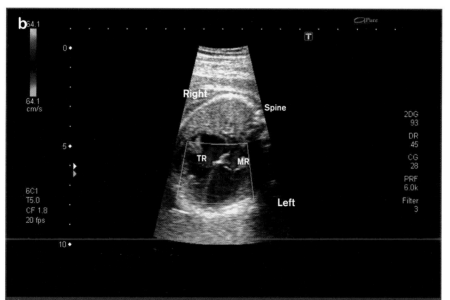

Figure 13.9. a) The four-chamber view of an example of complete heart block associated with cardiomegaly and a pericardial effusion. b) Colour flow shows both mitral and tricuspid regurgitation (shown in red).

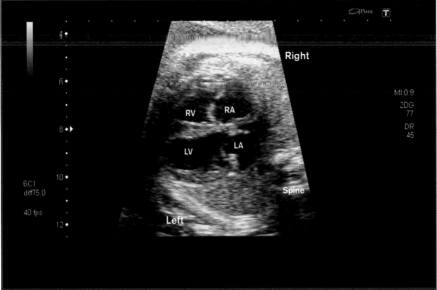

Figure 13.10. The four-chamber view of an example of complete heart block showing cardiomegaly and hypertrophy of the ventricular chambers.

effects. Although fetal pacing has been attempted, to date there are no survivors of intrauterine pacing.

Delivery at or near term is usually recommended, as managing heart block in premature babies can present huge difficulties. However, early delivery should be considered if there is clear evidence of deterioration in cardiac function, or a fall in heart rate resulting in development of early hydrops. The mode of delivery is usually a Caesarean section due to difficulties in monitoring for fetal well-being.

The prognosis for complete heart block associated with structural heart disease is poor and these cases are associated with a high mortality with very few long-term survivors. The outlook for isolated complete heart block is much better, but this does not universally carry a good prognosis. Adverse prognostic factors are fetal hydrops, a heart rate less than 50 beats per minute at presentation and a negative maternal anti-RO antibody status.

Outcome in a large single-centre fetal series

Isolated complete heart block

Of 88 cases of isolated complete heart block, one pregnancy resulted in a termination of pregnancy. Of the remaining, 9% resulted in spontaneous intrauterine death, 10% died in the neonatal period, 6% died in infancy and 75% were alive at last update. Fetal hydrops was associated in 17 cases, of which there are five survivors.

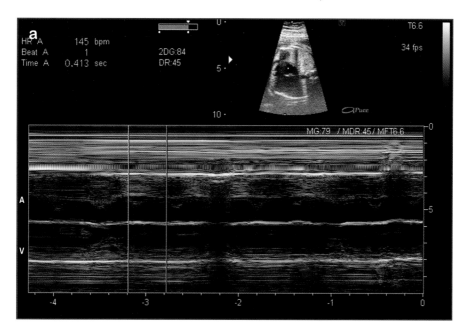

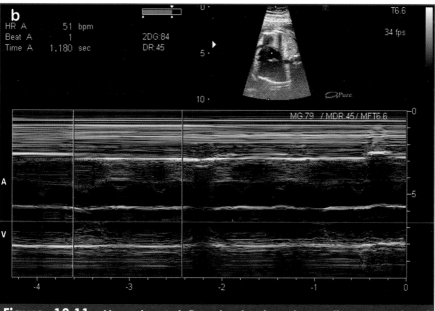

Figure 13.11. M-mode and Doppler tracings in another example of complete heart block with a heart rate of 48-51 beats per minute. a) The atrial rate measured on M-mode is 145 beats per minute. b) The ventricular rate measured on M-mode is 51 beats per minute.

Figure continued overleaf.

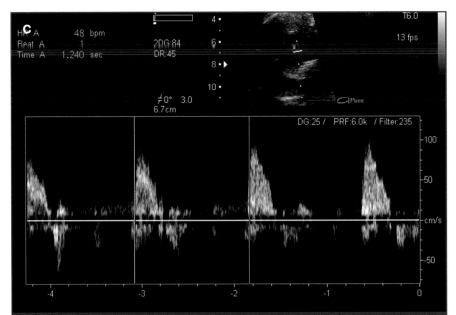

Figure 13.11 *continued.* M-mode and Doppler tracings in another example of complete heart block with a heart rate of 48-51 beats per minute. c) The ventricular rate measured with pulsed Doppler is 48 beats per minute.

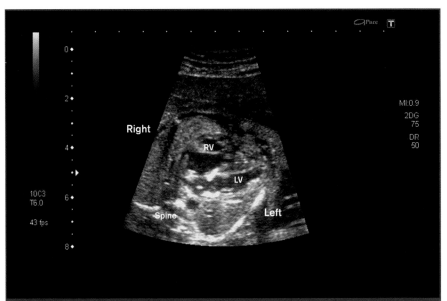

Figure 13.12. An example of complete heart block where there was increased echogenicity seen in the region of the atrial septum and ventricular walls.

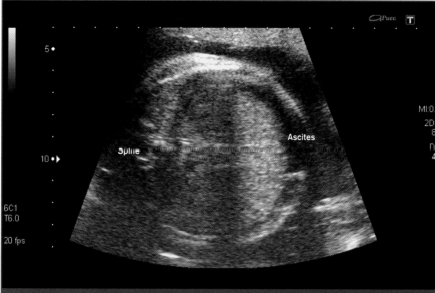

Figure 13.13. An example of complete heart block where there was immune-mediated ascites with no other evidence of fetal hydrops. This resolved after a short course of maternal dexamethasone therapy.

Complete heart block with structural congenital heart disease

Of 81 cases of complete heart block associated with structural heart disease, 54% of pregnancies resulted in a termination of pregnancy. If the terminations are excluded then the outcome of the continuing pregnancies was: 43% resulting in spontaneous intrauterine death, 32% died in the neonatal period, 9% died in infancy and 16% were alive at last follow-up. Left atrial isomerism was associated in 80% of the cases.

Fetal tachycardia

A tachycardia in the fetus is defined as a heart rate above 180 beats per minute, though a significant fetal tachycardia from a cardiac perspective is defined as a heart rate of greater than 200 beats per minute. The commonest significant tachycardias are re-entry tachycardias. Less commonly the tachycardia is an atrial tachycardia, as in atrial flutter. Much more rarely there may be atrial fibrillation, chaotic atrial tachycardia or a ventricular tachycardia.

Types of tachycardia seen in the fetus

Sinus tachycardia

A sinus tachycardia with a heart rate of 170-190 beats per minute is sometimes seen, but this is not usually an indication for treatment. It is important to exclude any other abnormalities

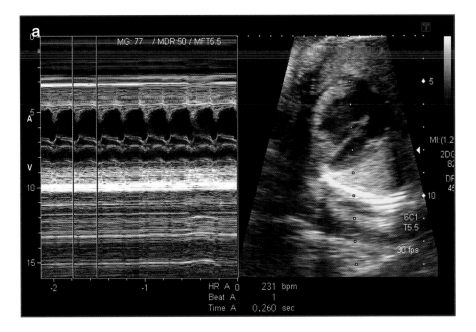

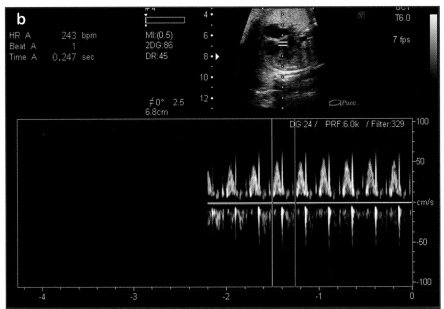

Figure 13.14. An example of supraventricular tachycardia shown with M-mode and pulsed Doppler. a) The heart rate measured on M-mode is 231 beats per minute. There is 1:1 atrial to ventricular contraction. b) The heart rate measured on Doppler later in the same study is 243 beats per minute.

Figure continued overleaf.

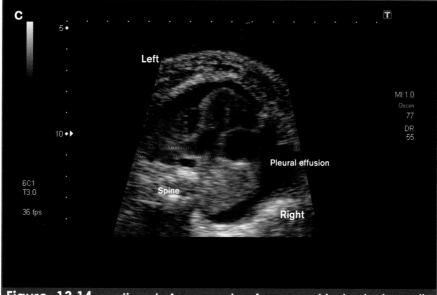

Figure 13.14 *continued.* **An example of supraventricular tachycardia shown with M-mode and pulsed Doppler. c) There was associated fetal hydrops, pleural effusion and ascites.**

in the baby and in particular to ensure there is no evidence of any anomaly that would result in a high output state.

Supraventricular tachycardia

In re-entry tachycardia there is a 1:1 ratio of atrial and ventricular contractions, which can be documented with M-Mode or Doppler echocardiography in the fetus (Figures 13.14a-b). Other less common tachycardias, such as ectopic atrial tachycardia and permanent junctional reciprocating tachycardia, can also be associated with 1:1 atrial to ventricular contraction. Differentiation of the type of supraventricular tachycardia in the fetus can be made to some extent, by examining time intervals between atrial and ventricular contractions. If there is a short time interval between the ventricular and atrial contraction (short VA tachycardia), the most likely mechanism is re-entry via an accessory pathway, which is the most common type of fetal tachycardia. The heart rate in these cases is typically around 240 beats per minute. In cases with a long time interval (long VA tachycardia), the mechanism is more likely to be ectopic atrial tachycardia or junctional reciprocating tachycardia. In these rarer forms of supraventricular tachycardia the heart rate is often around 200-220 beats per minute.

Atrial flutter

In atrial flutter the atrial rate is usually between 300-500 beats per minute, and often is much faster than the ventricular rate, due to a variable degree of atrioventricular block (Figures 13.15a-e).

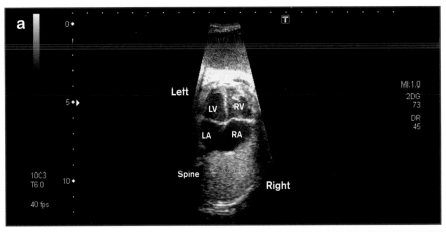

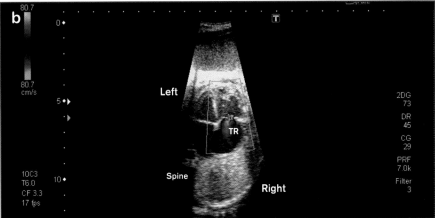

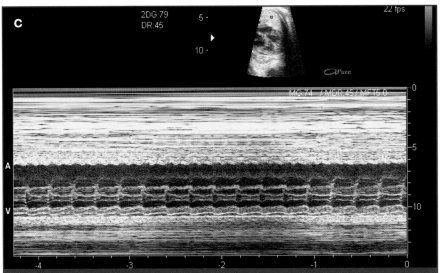

Figure 13.15. An example of atrial flutter. a) In the four-chamber view there is cardiomegaly, with the right heart structures appearing more dilated than the left-sided structures. b) Colour flow shows tricuspid regurgitation (shown in blue). c) The M-mode trace shows that the atrial rate is faster than the ventricular rate.

Figure continued overleaf.

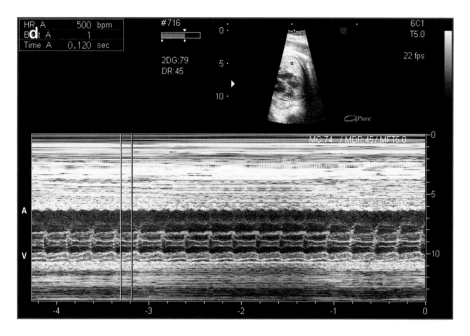

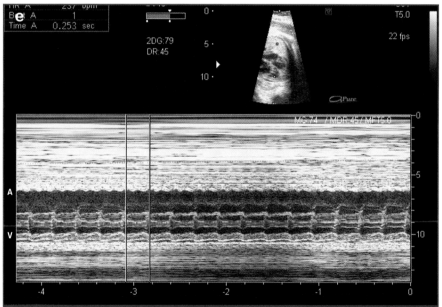

Figure 13.15 *continued.* **An example of atrial flutter. d) The atrial rate measured on M-mode is 500 beats per minute. e) The ventricular rate measured on M-mode is 237 beats per minute.**

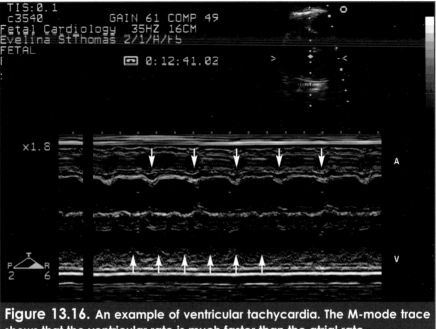

Figure 13.16. An example of ventricular tachycardia. The M-mode trace shows that the ventricular rate is much faster than the atrial rate.

Atrial fibrillation
Although extremely rare in the fetus, atrial fibrillation has been documented during fetal life.

Ventricular tachycardia
In ventricular tachycardia the ventricular rate will be higher than the atrial rate (Figure 13.16). However, sometimes there can be retrograde conduction producing a tachycardia with 1:1 conduction that can be difficult to distinguish from supraventricular tachycardia.

Fetal echocardiographic features in tachycardia

The structure of the fetal heart is normal in most cases, though occasionally a structural abnormality can be associated. The heart rate will be fast, with a significant tachycardia having a heart rate of over 200 beats per minute. There may be cardiomegaly and the cardiac function may be impaired. There may also be associated fetal hydrops (Figure 13.14c). Assessment of the type of tachycardia as described above will need to be made before deciding on the management strategy.

Management and outcome

The prenatal management of fetal tachycardias remains controversial and varies from centre to centre. There is controversy about whether all cases should be treated, and in the cases that are treated, controversy extends to the optimal timing of treatment, the types of drugs used, the doses and route of administration of drugs.

The options when faced with a fetus with a tachycardia are: observation only, early delivery and prenatal drug therapy.

Observation only

This approach is reasonable in a minority of fetuses, where the pregnancy is near term, the episodes of tachycardia are short-lived and there is no evidence of intrauterine cardiac failure.

Early delivery

This depends on the gestational age and whether there is intrauterine cardiac failure. In general the results of premature delivery have been disappointing because of the added complications of prematurity. Where possible, it is better to control the arrhythmia in utero, rather than deliver early.

Prenatal drug therapy

Drug treatment has been advocated prenatally to control the rhythm disturbance before delivery, in order to prevent or treat cardiac failure. However, there have been no controlled trials of therapy. The decision to treat a tachycardia will depend on the gestational age of the fetus, signs of cardiac failure, duration of the tachycardic episodes and parental wishes. The choice of drug depends on the type of tachycardia, the anti-arrhythmic drugs available and the experience of those involved.

The optimum treatment for fetal tachycardias is contentious and various drugs have been used, though many have been reported as single cases or in a handful of patients. Most of the larger reported series are retrospective studies, where treatment has been biased by physician and institutional preferences. There have been no randomised controlled trials to date and no single agent is universally effective, though some drugs may be more effective in certain situations. The presence of hydrops makes treatment and conversion more imperative but also more difficult.

The most common first-line drugs that are currently used are digoxin, flecainide and sotalol. The doses used for control of fetal tachycardia are outlined in Table 13.1. Reported conversion rates for digoxin, flecainide and sotalol drugs are shown in Table 13.2. In some countries where flecainide is not available or not widely used, sotalol has been used more commonly, though some units have chosen amiodarone for first-line therapy as an alternative to sotalol.

For fetuses with atrial flutter or re-entry supraventricular tachycardia and no signs of fetal hydrops, maternal digoxin therapy has been used widely. Several more recent reports have suggested that sotalol therapy may be more effective in the treatment of atrial flutter. Digoxin therapy alone is not very effective in fetuses with hydrops due to poor placental transfer. In these cases, therapies widely used have included flecainide, sotalol and amiodarone. Other drugs that have also been used include adenosine, procainamide, propranolol, propafenone,

Table 13.1. Three commonly used drugs for the treatment of fetal tachycardia.

Drug	Mechanism	Dose	Comments
Digoxin	Slows atrioventricular nodal conduction	0.25mg three times a day given to the mother	Most often given orally to the mother Not effective in hydropic fetuses Can take up to 2-3 weeks to have an effect Monitor blood levels and maternal ECG
Flecainide	Sodium channel blocker Does not slow atrioventricular nodal conduction Effective in blocking accessory pathway	100mg three times a day given to the mother	Rapid effect often in 48 hours, though may take up to one week Effective in fetal hydrops Monitor blood levels and maternal ECG
Sotalol	Potassium channel blocker and beta blocker Slows atrioventricular nodal conduction and accessory pathway conduction	80mg twice daily given to the mother	Often used for atrial flutter with hydrops Monitor maternal ECG

Table 13.2. Reported conversion rates of the three most commonly used drugs for fetal tachycardia.

Drug	Conversion in non-hydropic fetus	Conversion in hydropic fetus
Digoxin	50-100%	0-20%
Flecainide	58-100%	43-59%
Sotalol	40-100%	50%

Note: The conversion rate for flecainide used in hydropic fetuses seen at Evelina Children's Hospital in the last 10 years is 74%

and quinidine. Various routes of administration have also been selected, which include transplacental therapy by giving maternal oral or intravenous doses of drugs, or direct fetal therapy via the umbilical vein, intramuscular, intraperitoneal, or intra-amniotic routes. However, in general, most centres will now elect to treat with maternal oral therapy for the majority of cases. Despite the various forms and route of therapy, the overall results in the larger reported series are similar. Our preference for first-line therapy has been digoxin for non-hydropic fetuses and flecainide for hydropic fetuses. In both instances the drugs are administered orally to the mother.

The most important prognostic factor is the presence of fetal hydrops when mortality is much higher. However, the outcome in this group is significantly improved if the rhythm is controlled prior to delivery.

Outcome in a large single-centre fetal series
A fetal tachycardia was diagnosed in 230 cases, of which 74% were supraventricular tachycardia (44% were intermittent), 23% were atrial flutter (39% were intermittent) and the remaining were rare types of tachycardia. Of all cases of fetal tachycardia, 1% of pregnancies resulted in a termination of pregnancy. If the terminations are excluded then the outcome of the continuing pregnancies was: 4% resulting in spontaneous intrauterine death, 3% died in the neonatal period, 2% died in infancy and 91% were alive at last update.

Of cases seen in the last 10 years, one pregnancy resulted in a termination and 96% of the continuing pregnancies were alive at last follow-up.

Chapter 14

Counselling and outcome following prenatal diagnosis of congenital heart disease

Summary

- Approach before, during and after the scan
- Information to parents
- Choices after prenatal diagnosis of congenital heart disease
- Associated anomalies
- Further follow-up and care
- Outcome of fetal congenital heart disease

Counselling following antenatal detection of congenital heart disease is a complex process, which encompasses the time before the fetal heart scan, what happens during the scan and what happens afterwards. At all times it is vital to appreciate the distress and anxiety the parents and family may be feeling, so as to deal with the situation in a sympathetic and respectful manner. It is also important that all information given to the parents is provided in a way that they can understand. This information also needs to be disseminated to all those involved in the care of the pregnant woman and her baby. Management after the initial diagnosis and counselling involves a range of personnel from different sub-specialties, both at the tertiary centre and at the pregnant woman's local hospital. A multidisciplinary team taking a holistic approach will be able to provide optimum care for mother and baby.

Before the scan

Before the scan, information should be provided about the purpose of the scan and its implications. Explanation should be given of how the scan will be conducted, by whom and who else may be present in the scan room. The parents should be made aware that the scan may take time and that there may be silences in order to allow the operator to concentrate. They should be advised that they will be given all the information regarding their baby's heart at the end of the scan. The parents should also be made aware of the types of congenital heart disease that cannot be detected before birth and those that are difficult to diagnose during fetal life.

During the scan

During the scan it is important to ascertain the details of the heart findings as quickly as possible, though accuracy of diagnosis is paramount. If there are trainees or observers present, there must be no discussion or questions asked during the scan, if the parents are as yet unaware of the problem. The operator should avoid pointing out and talking about the findings whilst scanning. This can be very upsetting for the parents, who may already be very anxious and frightened. The scan can be reviewed and discussed separately after the parents have been counselled regarding the findings.

After the scan

After the scan is complete and all the necessary information has been obtained, the parents can be appropriately counselled. Ideally this should be done in a quiet room separate from the scan room. The aim of the counselling session is to provide the parents with complete information, or as complete as possible, regarding their baby's heart problem and any related abnormalities. This includes details of the cardiac diagnosis, the extent of possible associations – both cardiac and extracardiac, the risk of intrauterine loss and the likely postnatal management and outcome (see below).

Information to parents at time of initial counselling

Following the diagnosis of fetal congenital heart disease, the parents should be given adequate and appropriate information regarding the abnormality, as described above. Diagrams should be used to explain the normal heart and these compared with the specific problem in their baby. These can also be used to explain the treatment strategies available after birth. Some types of cardiac anatomy will be suitable for a 'corrective' procedure to restore near normal anatomy. However, many of the cardiac abnormalities detected prenatally may not be suitable for a biventricular repair and the surgical strategy is palliative, being aimed at achieving a single-ventricle circulation. Information regarding the number of procedures and the timing of them should be provided, as well as the current available outcomes.

Although information about early outcome from both surgical and interventional procedures is usually available, the longer-term outcome and morbidity are less clearly defined and harder to provide. In all cases, the best and worst outcome should be addressed as well as the most likely outcome. The outcome from fetal life should also be discussed, as the overall outlook from prenatal diagnosis is still worse than for cases where the diagnosis is made after birth. Data from fetal series will take into account those cases that result in spontaneous intrauterine loss, as well as those that are born alive but do not make it to surgery or intervention. Another factor to consider is whether the lesion can progress during fetal life and this possibility needs to be raised and discussed at the time of counselling, if appropriate. There is a recurrence risk for congenital heart disease, which is higher in some lesions such as left heart disease and isomerism, than others. This can be discussed with the parents with appropriate information being given about screening future pregnancies and in some select cases involving a geneticist.

All information should be provided in a non-directive manner and all management options available for their particular circumstances should be discussed with the parents. Written information should also be provided, as well as contact details for parent support groups and relevant information regarding suitable websites. Parents often find it beneficial to speak with other parents, who have or have had a child affected by a similar heart problem. This helps them to gauge aspects, such as quality of life, which are extremely important but often difficult to quantify. Parents should therefore be offered the option of speaking with other parents, if they wish. In some cases, where early neonatal intervention is anticipated, the parents may find it very helpful to speak with either a paediatric cardiac surgeon or, in cases where a catheter intervention is likely, with a paediatric cardiologist specialising in interventional techniques.

Benefits of having a health professional in a supportive role present at the time of counselling

It is very beneficial to have a nurse counsellor, specialist nurse practitioner or an equivalent health professional present at the time of initial counselling. A named individual in this supportive role, who is present at the time of initial counselling, can reinforce the information that was given and ensure that the parents' interpretation of the information given is correct. They can also provide support for the parents afterwards, as well as acting as a point of contact for them. Parents and families may not take in all the information they are given initially, as it is quite common for individuals to not remember everything they are told, nor to remember things accurately, when they are given bad news. It is therefore very important to make sure that ongoing support is available for the parents, to allow them to ask any further questions and to help them to understand the nature of the problem and all its implications.

Choices after prenatal diagnosis of congenital heart disease

There is no doubt that great distress can be caused by an antenatal diagnosis and the decision-making that follows. Diagnosis during pregnancy of cardiac anomalies associated with significant morbidity and mortality, allows choices for parents, even though these choices may be difficult and not always welcome. However, extra distress can be limited if the parents are provided with all the support and information that they need in order to make the right decision for them. Based on the information they are given, in some cases the parents will elect to terminate the pregnancy. Although decision-making regarding termination of pregnancy is a complex process, there are some consistent themes. Influencing factors include the perceived severity of the condition, the predicted quality of life for the child and the impact on the family. Additional factors are chosen lifestyles and financial situation, as well as cultural and religious beliefs. Parents who choose to proceed with the pregnancy make an active choice to do so and in a sense have self-selected to cope with what lies ahead. This is particularly significant in cases where single-ventricle palliation is the treatment strategy. In some instances of severe and complex heart malformations or those cases associated with multiple abnormalities, compassionate care after birth may be an option for the parents to consider. This option should be discussed with the parents and all the relevant health professionals involved in the care of the pregnant woman and her baby.

Associated abnormalities

Many forms of congenital heart disease are associated with extracardiac abnormalities, including chromosomal abnormalities and it is important to look for and exclude other abnormalities, with the option of fetal karyotyping being discussed where appropriate. This may influence parents' decision-making regarding termination of pregnancy, but it is also important in cases where parents wish to continue with the pregnancy, as any associated lesions may influence the overall outcome and the parents must be made aware of this. The presence of other significant abnormalities may influence the perinatal management so that this information is also of value for medical personnel. The extent and implications of possible associated abnormalities will need to be taken into account when counselling parents. Thus, the working relationship between a fetal cardiology specialist and a fetal medicine specialist is very important in the management of prenatal congenital heart disease, though local practices will govern how this is achieved.

Further follow-up and care

Prenatal diagnosis allows time to prepare families for the likely course of events after delivery and to optimise care for the baby at birth. The parents can meet with a member of the surgical team, as well as appropriate members of the other postnatal teams who will be involved in the postnatal care of the baby. It is paramount to provide continuing support for parents throughout the pregnancy and a named individual in a supportive role can play a key part in this. Although there have been concerns about the anxiety caused by prenatal diagnosis, in most instances the parents who are aware of a problem before birth and have been appropriately counselled, will be better informed and prepared at the time of initial surgical or interventional treatment after birth. Where appropriate, depending on the type of cardiac lesion and the need for early postnatal cardiac intervention, delivery can be planned at or near a centre with paediatric cardiology and paediatric cardiac surgical facilities. Whilst treatment for the vast majority of cases will take place after birth, prenatal treatment may be considered in a few select cases.

In cases where a termination of pregnancy takes place or an intrauterine death has occurred, permission for autopsy should be requested in appropriate cases. This should be performed by a pathologist experienced in congenital heart disease. The women and their partners should be offered further counselling after a termination or intrauterine loss. This is usually 6 weeks later and can be provided by the local obstetrician, tertiary specialists or both.

Outcome of fetal congenital heart disease

The outcome of congenital heart disease diagnosed from fetal life tends to be less good than that predicted from postnatal series. This can be seen from the outcome data for individual cardiac abnormalities provided throughout this book. A fetal series will note outcome from the time of diagnosis in fetal life. Thus, outcomes will reflect cases that have resulted in spontaneous intrauterine death or in early neonatal death without having any treatment, as well as those that go on to receive treatment. Postnatal series usually reflect the outcome of cases that have reached a tertiary centre for treatment after birth.

Cases of congenital heart disease in a fetal series will also be associated with a higher proportion of extracardiac and chromosomal abnormalities, which may adversely affect the outcome. In the early part of our large fetal series there was a notably high proportion of associated abnormality, though in latter years the proportion with associated abnormalities has decreased. This is partly related to improvement in obstetric screening, so that more isolated cardiac abnormalities are detected, and is partly attributable to the introduction of the nuchal translucency screening in the first trimester for the detection of chromosomal abnormalities. This latter method has led to the detection of trisomies earlier in pregnancy and although a significant number of these may be associated with heart disease, many may no longer be referred to tertiary fetal cardiology services for detailed evaluation of the fetal heart.

The types of cardiac abnormality seen in a fetal cardiac series are skewed towards the severe end of the spectrum, with the majority of abnormalities being associated with an abnormal four-chamber view. This bias is a reflection of four-chamber view screening, which has been used in routine obstetric anomaly scanning for over 25 years. As a result there has been a predisposition towards lesions that will result in single-ventricle palliation rather than a corrective procedure. However, over the last 10 years there has been some improvement in the proportion of great artery abnormalities being detected by screening (see Figure 1.1 in Chapter 1). The percentage of some individual cardiac lesions in the total fetal cardiac series at Evelina Children's Hospital compared to the percentage of the same lesions seen in the last 10 years of the series is shown in Table 14.1. Alongside improving detection rates of more isolated and repairable forms of congenital heart disease, there have also been improvements in surgical techniques, so that there has been significant improvement in overall outcome in recent years. The change in the last 10 years of the proportion of continuing pregnancies that are surviving is shown in Table 14.2.

The overall outcome for over 4000 fetal cardiac structural abnormalities diagnosed between 1980 and 2010 in the fetal cardiology unit at Evelina Children's Hospital is shown in Figure 14.1. This figure also shows the outcome as a percentage of the continuing pregnancies. The overall outcome, however, has changed with time and this is illustrated in Figure 14.2, where the percentage of terminations of pregnancy and the percentage of survivors of continuing pregnancies are shown by decade. The proportion of pregnancies resulting in a termination over the three decades fell from an average of 58% in the first decade, to 44% in the second decade, to 26% in the third decade. However, across the decades, the proportion resulting in termination is higher for complex lesions and those that will result in single-ventricle palliation. There has also been an improvement in survival, both as a percentage of the total series and as a percentage of the continuing pregnancies (Figure 14.2).

Table 14.1. The percentage of some individual cardiac lesions in the total fetal cardiac series at Evelina Children's Hospital compared to the percentage of the same lesions seen in the last 10 years of the series.

Lesion	Percentage of total fetal series	Percentage of fetal series seen in last 10 years
HLH	15.5%	12.4%
AVSD	16.0%	13.2%
Coarct	7.5%	8.4%
TAT	3.4%	3.0%
PAT IVS	3.2%	2.5%
Tetralogy	5.2%	7.2%
PAT VSD	2.2%	2.3%
CAT	1.1%	1.2%
TGA simple	2.0%	2.9%
TGA VSD	1.7%	2.4%
CCTGA	1.4%	1.6%
DIV	2.0%	2.0%
DORV	5.2%	3.3%
Ebstein's	1.9%	1.2%
TVD	1.5%	0.7%

HLH = hypoplastic left heart syndrome; AVSD = atrioventricular septal defect; Coarct = coarctation of the aorta; TAT = tricuspid atresia; PAT IVS = pulmonary atresia with an intact interventricular septum; Tetralogy = tetralogy of Fallot; PAT VSD = pulmonary atresia with a ventricular septal defect; CAT = common arterial trunk; TGA = transposition of the great arteries; TGA VSD = transposition of the great arteries with a ventricular septal defect; CCTGA = congenitally corrected transposition of the great arteries; DIV = double-inlet ventricle; DORV = double-outlet right ventricle; Ebstein's = Ebstein's anomaly; TVD = tricuspid valve dysplasia

Table 14.2. The change in the last 10 years of the proportion of continuing pregnancies that are surviving.

Lesion	TOP total series	TOP in last 10 years	Survivors of continuing pregnancies total series	Survivors of continuing pregnancies in last 10 years
HLH	62%	45%	37%	49%
AVSD	48%	40%	53%	60%
Coarct	35%	21%	68%	71%
TAT	59%	48%	70%	70%
PAT IVS	56%	46%	53%	64%
Tetralogy	17%	10%	77%	85%
PAT VSD	50%	33%	49%	61%
CAT	35%	33%	55%	79%
TGA simple	8%	5%	90%	94%
TGA VSD	23%	13%	87%	90%
CCTGA	37%	43%	76%	83%
DIV	55%	51%	75%	84%
DORV	56%	31%	51%	59%
Ebstein's	44%	23%	50%	65%
TVD	44%	46%	36%	71%

HLH = hypoplastic left heart syndrome; AVSD = atrioventricular septal defect; Coarct = coarctation of the aorta; TAT = tricuspid atresia; PAT IVS = pulmonary atresia with an intact interventricular septum; Tetralogy = tetralogy of Fallot; PAT VSD = pulmonary atresia with a ventricular septal defect; CAT = common arterial trunk; TGA = transposition of the great arteries; TGA VSD = transposition of the great arteries with a ventricular septal defect; CCTGA = congenitally corrected transposition of the great arteries; DIV = double-inlet ventricle; DORV = double-outlet right ventricle; Ebstein's = Ebstein's anomaly; TVD = tricuspid valve dysplasia

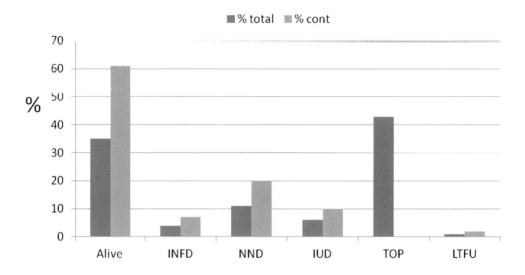

Figure 14.1. The outcome of over 4000 fetal structural abnormalities seen as a percentage of the total and as a percentage of continuing pregnancies where the terminations of pregnancy are excluded. INFD = death in infancy; NND = death in neonatal period; IUD = intrauterine death; TOP = termination of pregnancy; LTFU = lost to follow-up.

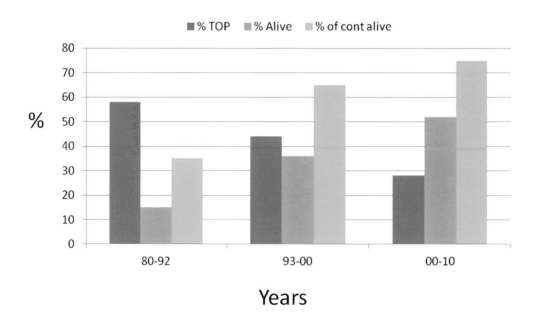

Figure 14.2. Change in percentage of pregnancies resulting in termination and improvement in survival rates over three different time eras. The percentage of survivors is shown as a percentage of the total and a percentage of the continuing pregnancies.

Chapter 15
What could cardiac findings mean?

Finding	Possible diagnosis	Features to help make diagnosis
Abnormal position		
Dextrocardia		
	No other abnormality	Cardiac apex to right and heart in right chest
		Normal cardiac structure
	Abnormal situs (see below)	Normal relation descending aorta and inferior vena cava not seen in abdomen
	Complex CHD	Abnormal heart structure
Dextroposition		
	Left diaphragmatic hernia	Heart shifted into right side of chest
		Appearance of heart being pushed across
		Fetal stomach or liver may be seen in chest
	Hypoplastic right lung	Heart shifted to right
		Apex may point towards right axilla or even more posteriorly
		Right lung appears hypoplastic
	Scimitar syndrome	Heart shifted to midline or into right chest
		Right lung hypoplastic
		Right-sided pulmonary veins difficult to visualise
	Congenital cystic adenomatoid malformation left lung	Mediastinal shift towards right
		Bright echogenic areas of lung that may be cystic

Finding	Possible diagnosis	Features to help make diagnosis
Abnormal position		
Midline heart		
	Abnormal situs (see below)	Normal relation descending aorta and inferior vena cava not seen in abdomen
	Complex CHD	Abnormal heart structure
	Hypoplastic right lung	Heart shifted to right
		Right lung appears hypoplastic
	Scimitar syndrome	Heart shifted to midline or into right chest
		Right lung hypoplastic
		Right-sided pulmonary veins difficult to visualise
Levoposition		
	Conotruncal malformations:	Apex of heart may point more towards left axilla
	• tetralogy of Fallot • pulmonary atresia with ventricular septal defect • common arterial trunk	Ventricular septal defect with great artery override
	Complex CHD	Abnormal heart structure
	Right diaphragmatic hernia	Mediastinal shift to left
	Congenital cystic adenomatoid malformation right lung	Mediastinal shift towards left
		Bright echogenic areas of lung that may be cystic
Abnormal situs		
	Situs inversus	Mirror image of normal situs
		Descending aorta to right of spine and inferior vena cava to left of spine
		Liver and gall bladder on the left, with spleen and stomach on right
		If total situs inversus will also have dextrocardia

Finding	Possible diagnosis	Features to help make diagnosis
Abnormal situs		
	Left atrial isomerism	Interrupted inferior vena cava (IVC not seen in normal position in upper abdomen)
		Vascular channel behind descending aorta (azygos continuation)
		Associated CHD (often atrioventricular septal defect)
		Bradycardia (often complete heart block)
		Heart position may be abnormal
	Right atrial isomerism	Inferior vena cava and descending aorta lie on same side of spine in abdomen
		Inferior vena cava lies directly anterior to the aorta in abdomen
		Usually associated with complex cardiac malformations
		Heart position may be abnormal
Abnormal size – large heart		
General		
	Cardiomyopathy	Dilated ventricular chamber(s)
		Ventricular chamber(s) may be hypertrophied
		Poorly functioning ventricular chamber(s)
		Either or both ventricles may be affected
		May have tricuspid regurgitation
		May have mitral regurgitation
	Complete heart block	Persistent bradycardia
		Complete atrioventricular dissociation on M-mode or Doppler tracings

Finding	Possible diagnosis	Features to help make diagnosis
Abnormal size – large heart		
General		
	High output states	Fetal anaemia
		Arteriovenous malformations
		Sacrococcygeal teratoma
	Twin to twin transfusion syndrome	Monochorionic-diamniotic twin pregnancy
		Recipient twin may have cardiomegaly, ventricular hypertrophy, impaired ventricular function and atrioventricular valve regurgitation
		Usually the right heart is affected
Right atrium dilated		
	Tricuspid regurgitation (severe)	
	Ebstein's anomaly	Tricuspid valve leaflets displaced apically
	Tricuspid valve dysplasia	Tricuspid valve leaflets appear dysplastic
	Coronary artery fistula to right atrium	Abnormal jet seen on colour Doppler entering right atrium and not related to tricuspid valve
	Direct communication umbilical vein to right atrium	Dilated umbilical vein seen to connect directly to right atrium
Left atrium dilated		
	Mitral regurgitation (severe)	
	Critical aortic stenosis with intact or restricted atrial septum	Dilated poorly functioning left ventricle
		Abnormal mitral valve
		No flow or very restricted flow across atrial septum
	Coronary artery fistula draining to left atrium	Abnormal jet of blood seen entering left atrium
	Direct communication umbilical vein to left atrium	Dilated umbilical vein seen to connect directly to left atrium

Finding	Possible diagnosis	Features to help make diagnosis
Abnormal size – large heart		
Right ventricle dilated		
	Absent pulmonary valve syndrome	Dilated pulmonary artery and, in particular, dilated branch pulmonary arteries
		Dysplastic rudimentary pulmonary valve
		To and fro flow in pulmonary artery
		May be pulmonary stenosis
	Some cases critical pulmonary stenosis	Restricted tricuspid valve motion
		Pulmonary artery may be small for the gestational age
		Pulmonary artery may be dilated
		Thickened restricted pulmonary valve
		Velocity of forward flow across pulmonary valve may be low, within normal range or increased
		Reverse flow from arterial duct in main pulmonary artery
	Some cases pulmonary atresia with intact septum if associated with tricuspid valve abnormalities	Features of Ebstein's anomaly or of tricuspid valve dysplasia
		Small pulmonary artery
		Reverse flow in pulmonary artery
	Right ventricular aneurysm or diverticulum	Out-pouching of right ventricular wall
		Right ventricle will appear to be asymmetrically dilated
	Coronary artery fistula draining to right ventricle	Abnormal jet of blood seen entering right ventricle
	Right ventricular cardiomyopathy	Poorly functioning right ventricle
		Tricuspid regurgitation

343

Finding	Possible diagnosis	Features to help make diagnosis
Abnormal size – large heart		
Left ventricle dilated		
	Critical aortic stenosis	Dilated, poorly contracting left ventricle
		Increased echogenicity of left ventricular walls
		Hypertrophied left ventricle
		Restricted mitral valve motion
		Mitral regurgitation
		Reversal of interatrial shunt
		Small aortic root and ascending aorta
		Thickened and restricted aortic valve
	Aortico-left ventricular tunnel	Dilated poorly contracting left ventricle
		Dilated aortic root
		Regurgitation from aorta into left ventricle
		Thickened aortic valve (occasionally)
	Left ventricular aneurysm or diverticulum	Out-pouching of left ventricular wall often at apex
		Left ventricle will appear to be asymmetrically dilated
	Coronary artery fistula draining to left ventricle	Abnormal jet of blood seen entering left ventricle
	Left ventricular cardiomyopathy	Poorly functioning left ventricle
		Mitral regurgitation
Abnormal size – small heart		
General		
	Bilateral pleural effusion	
	Tracheal atresia	

Finding	Possible diagnosis	Features to help make diagnosis
Abnormal size – small heart		
Right atrium small		
	Tricuspid atresia	Hypoplastic right ventricle
		No opening tricuspid valve
		No flow from right atrium to right ventricle
		Ventricular septal defect
Left atrium small		
	Total anomalous pulmonary venous drainage	Pulmonary veins not seen draining to left atrium with colour flow
		Right heart dominance (sometimes)
		Dilated coronary sinus (possibly)
		Confluence behind left atrium
	Coarctation of aorta	Right ventricle > left ventricle
		Pulmonary artery > aorta
		Arch hypoplasia
		Hypoplastic isthmus
		Left to right shunt at atrial level (sometimes)
	Hypoplastic left heart syndrome	Mitral atresia:
		• no opening mitral valve
		• no flow from left atrium to left ventricle
		• small left atrium and left ventricle
		Aortic atresia:
		• globular hypoplastic left ventricle
		• hypoplastic aorta
		• no forward flow across aortic valve
		• retrograde flow in aortic arch

345

Finding	Possible diagnosis	Features to help make diagnosis
Abnormal size – small heart		
Right ventricle small		
	Tricuspid atresia	Hypoplastic right ventricle
		No opening tricuspid valve
		No flow from right atrium to right ventricle
		Ventricular septal defect
	Pulmonary atresia with intact ventricular septum	Hypertrophied right ventricle
		Poorly contracting right ventricle
		Restricted tricuspid valve motion
		Tricuspid regurgitation jet (high velocity)
		Small pulmonary artery (rarely may be normal size)
		No forward flow in pulmonary artery
		Reverse flow in arterial duct
	Some cases critical pulmonary stenosis	Similar to pulmonary atresia with intact ventricular septum
		Restricted tricuspid valve motion
		Pulmonary artery may be small for the gestational age
		Thickened restricted pulmonary valve
		Velocity of forward flow across pulmonary valve may be low or within normal range
		Reverse flow from arterial duct in main pulmonary artery

Finding	Possible diagnosis	Features to help make diagnosis
Abnormal size – small heart		
Right ventricle small		
	Unbalanced atrioventricular septal defect	Atrioventricular septal defect with right ventricle smaller than left ventricle
		May be part of more complex CHD, e.g. isomerism
	Double-inlet left ventricle	Both atrioventricular valves drain into dominant left ventricle
		Right ventricle very hypoplastic
	Right ventricular cardiomyopathy	Poorly functioning right ventricle
Left ventricle small		
	Mitral atresia	No opening mitral valve
		No flow from left atrium to left ventricle
		Small left atrium
		Slit-like left ventricle
	Aortic atresia	Echogenic hypoplastic left ventricle
		Hypoplastic aorta
		No forward flow across aortic valve
		Retrograde flow in aortic arch
	Hypoplastic left heart syndrome	As above for mitral and aortic atresia
		Left to right shunt at atrial level
	Some cases critical aortic stenosis	Similar to aortic atresia
		Echogenic globular left ventricle
		Small aorta
		Aortic valve patent
		Reverse flow in aortic arch

Finding	Possible diagnosis	Features to help make diagnosis
Abnormal size – small heart		
Left ventricle small		
	Coarctation	Right ventricle > left ventricle
		Pulmonary artery > aorta
		Arch hypoplasia
		Hypoplastic isthmus
		Left to right shunt at atrial level (sometimes)
	Total anomalous pulmonary venous drainage	Left atrium and left ventricle may appear smaller than right atrium and right ventricle in some cases
		Pulmonary veins not seen draining to left atrium
		Dilated coronary sinus (possibly)
		Confluence behind left atrium (possibly)
		Identification of ascending or descending vein
	Unbalanced atrioventricular septal defect	Atrioventricular septal defect with left ventricle smaller than right ventricle
		Need to exclude coarctation of the aorta (see above)
		May be part of more complex CHD, e.g. isomerism
	Double-inlet right ventricle	Very rare
		Both atrioventricular valves drain into dominant right ventricle
Asymmetry with left heart smaller than right		
	Coarctation	See above
	Total anomalous pulmonary venous drainage	See above

Finding	Possible diagnosis	Features to help make diagnosis
Asymmetry with left heart smaller than right		
	Chromosomal anomalies (with normal heart)	Normal cardiac connections
		Right ventricle slightly > left ventricle
		Right atrium slightly > left atrium
		Aorta = pulmonary artery
	Normal in late gestation	Right atrium > left atrium
		Right ventricle > left ventricle
		Often seen after 28 weeks
		Need to exclude coarct (see above)
Abnormalities at crux		
No differential insertion		
	Atrioventricular septal defect	Common atrioventricular junction
		No offset cross at crux (loss of differential insertion)
		Atrial and ventricular components of varying sizes
		Atrioventricular valve regurgitation (some cases)
	Large inlet ventricular septal defect	Discontinuity in ventricular septum suggesting defect
		Colour flow demonstrated across defect
Both AV valves to one ventricle		
	Double-inlet ventricle	Usually double-inlet left ventricle
		Colour flow from both atrioventricular valves to dominant ventricle
		Other ventricle usually very hypoplastic
		Ventricular septal defect
		Great arteries may be transposed (discordant arterial connection)

Finding	Possible diagnosis	Features to help make diagnosis
Abnormalities at crux		
Exaggerated atrioventricular valve offsetting		
	Ebstein's anomaly	Downward displacement tricuspid valve leaflets (septal and mural) into right ventricle
		Right atrial enlargement
		Tricuspid regurgitation
		Increased cardiothoracic ratio
		Right ventricular outflow tract obstruction
Dysplastic tricuspid valve		
	Tricuspid valve dysplasia	Dysplastic but normally positioned tricuspid valve leaflets
		Right atrial enlargement
		Right ventricular enlargement
		Tricuspid regurgitation
		Increased cardiothoracic ratio
		Right ventricular outflow tract obstruction
Reversed atrioventricular valve offsetting		
	Corrected transposition (atrioventricular and ventriculo-arterial discordance)	Centrally positioned heart
		'Reversed' differential insertion of atrioventricular valves
		Moderator band in left-sided posterior ventricle (which is right ventricle)
		Pulmonary veins can be seen to drain to atrium that is connected to right ventricle (has moderator band)
		Parallel great arteries

Finding	Possible diagnosis	Features to help make diagnosis
Ventricle thick or poor function		
Left ventricle thick or poor function		
	Aortic stenosis (particularly critical forms of aortic stenosis)	Aortic valve dysplastic with restriction in its opening
		May have turbulent flow across the aortic valve at increased Doppler velocity
		May have low velocity flow across aortic valve
		May have reverse flow in aortic arch in critical cases
	Left ventricular cardiomyopathy	Left ventricle poorly contracting
		Left ventricle hypertrophied
		Left ventricle may be dilated
		May be mitral regurgitation
	Aortico-left ventricular tunnel	Dilated poorly contracting left ventricle
		Dilated aortic root
		Regurgitation from aorta into left ventricle
		Thickened aortic valve (occasionally)
Right ventricle thick or poor function		
	Pulmonary atresia with intact ventricular septum	Hypertrophied right ventricle
		Poorly contracting right ventricle
		Restricted tricuspid valve motion
		Tricuspid regurgitation jet (high velocity)
		Small pulmonary artery (rarely may be normal size)
		No forward flow in pulmonary artery
		Reverse flow in arterial duct

Finding	Possible diagnosis	Features to help make diagnosis
Ventricle thick or poor function		
Right ventricle thick or poor function		
	Pulmonary stenosis	Small or normal size pulmonary artery
		Pulmonary artery may be dilated (occasionally)
		Thickened restricted pulmonary valve leaflets
		Turbulent flow across pulmonary valve
		Pulmonary artery Doppler flow velocity increased above normal
	Right ventricular cardiomyopathy	Right ventricle poorly contracting
		Right ventricle hypertrophied
		Right ventricle may be dilated
		May be tricuspid regurgitation
Both ventricles thick or poor function		
	Cardiomyopathy	Ventricular chambers may be hypertrophied
		Poorly functioning ventricular chambers
		May have tricuspid regurgitation
		May have mitral regurgitation
	Diabetic cardiomyopathy	Both ventricle and septum appear hypertrophied
		Function usually preserved
	Noonan's syndrome	

Finding	Possible diagnosis	Features to help make diagnosis
Great arteries		
Aorta small		
	Aortic atresia	Hypoplastic aorta and arch
		No forward flow across aortic valve
		Reverse flow in aortic arch
	Aortic stenosis (particularly critical forms of aortic stenosis)	Aortic valve dysplastic with restriction in its opening
		May have turbulent flow across the aortic valve at increased Doppler velocity
		May have low velocity flow across aortic valve
		May have reverse flow in aortic arch in critical cases
	Coarctation	Right ventricle > left ventricle
		Pulmonary artery > aorta
		Arch hypoplasia
		Hypoplastic isthmus
		Left to right shunt at atrial level (sometimes)
	Interrupted aortic arch	Right ventricle = left ventricle (often)
		Ventricular septal defect (often large)
		Small ascending aorta
		Complete arch not demonstrated
		Ascending aorta leads to two-pronged fork appearance

Finding	Possible diagnosis	Features to help make diagnosis
Great arteries		
Aorta large		
	Aortico-left ventricular tunnel	Dilated poorly contracting left ventricle
		Dilated aortic root
		Regurgitation from aorta into left ventricle
		Thickened aortic valve (occasionally)
	Tetralogy of Fallot	Ventricular septal defect
		Aortic override
		Small pulmonary artery (pulmonary stenosis)
	Pulmonary atresia with ventricular septal defect	Ventricular septal defect
		Aortic override
		No forward flow from right ventricle to pulmonary artery
		Main pulmonary artery small or may not be identified
		Hypoplastic branch pulmonary arteries
		Retrograde flow in arterial duct
		Collateral vessels in some cases
	Common arterial trunk (a single large artery rather than large aorta, but may be mistaken for an aorta)	Ventricular septal defect
		Single arterial trunk usually arising astride ventricular septal defect
		Trunk gives rise to aortic arch and pulmonary arteries
Aortic valve dysplastic		
	Aortic stenosis	Aortic valve dysplastic with restriction in its opening
		Turbulent flow across the aortic valve usually with increased Doppler velocity
	Aortico-left ventricular tunnel	See above

Finding	Possible diagnosis	Features to help make diagnosis
Great arteries		
Pulmonary artery small		
	Pulmonary atresia	No forward flow from right ventricle to pulmonary artery
		Main pulmonary artery small or may not be identified
		Hypoplastic branch pulmonary arteries
		Retrograde flow in arterial duct
	Pulmonary stenosis	Small pulmonary artery
		Thickened restricted pulmonary valve leaflets
		Turbulent flow across pulmonary valve
		Pulmonary artery Doppler flow velocity increased above normal or may be normal
	Tetralogy of Fallot	See facing page
Pulmonary artery large		
	Absent pulmonary valve	Right ventricular dilatation
		Abnormal pulmonary valve leaflets
		Very dilated branch pulmonary arteries
		Marked pulmonary regurgitation (to and fro flow)
	Pulmonary stenosis	Dilated pulmonary artery
		Dysplastic pulmonary valve with increased Doppler velocity
Pulmonary valve dysplastic		
	Pulmonary stenosis	See above
	Absent pulmonary valve	See above
	Noonan's syndrome	

Finding	Possible diagnosis	Features to help make diagnosis
Great arteries		
Parallel great arteries		
	Transposition of the great arteries	Atrioventricular concordance: • left atrium connected to left ventricle • right atrium connected to right ventricle Ventriculo-arterial discordance: • aorta arises from right ventricle • pulmonary artery arises from left ventricle Parallel arrangement of great arteries Aorta arises anterior and to right of pulmonary artery Wide sweeping aortic arch
	Double-outlet right ventricle with aorta anterior	Ventricular septal defect Both great arteries arise predominantly from right ventricle Pulmonary override and parallel great arteries if ventricular septal defect is subpulmonary
	Corrected transposition	Centrally positioned heart Atrioventricular discordance: • left atrium connected to right ventricle • right atrium connected to left ventricle 'Reversed' differential insertion of atrioventricular valves Moderator band in left-sided ventricle Ventriculo-arterial discordance: • aorta arises from right ventricle • pulmonary artery arises from left ventricle Parallel arrangement of great arteries Aorta arises to left of pulmonary artery

Finding	Possible diagnosis	Features to help make diagnosis
Great arteries		
First artery seen moving cranially from four-chamber view is pulmonary artery		
	Transposition of the great arteries	See facing page
	Corrected transposition of the great arteries	See facing page
	Double-outlet right ventricle with aorta anterior	Both great arteries arise from right ventricle in a transposed arrangement
Great artery override		
	Malalignment ventricular septal defect	Ventricular septal defect
		Aortic override
		Normal size pulmonary artery from right ventricle
	Tetralogy of Fallot	Ventricular septal defect
		Aortic override
		Small pulmonary artery (pulmonary stenosis)
	Pulmonary atresia with ventricular septal defect	Ventricular septal defect
		Aortic override
		No forward flow from right ventricle to pulmonary artery
		Main pulmonary artery small or may not be identified
		Hypoplastic branch pulmonary arteries
		Retrograde flow in arterial duct
		Collateral vessels in some cases

Finding	Possible diagnosis	Features to help make diagnosis
Great arteries		
Great artery override		
	Common arterial trunk	Ventricular septal defect
		Single arterial trunk usually arising astride ventricular septal defect
		Trunk gives rise to aortic arch and pulmonary arteries
	Aortic atresia with ventricular septal defect	Ventricular septal defect
		Equal sized ventricles
		Pulmonary artery overriding ventricular septal defect
		Hypoplastic aorta
		Reverse flow in aorta and aortic arch
Abnormal three-vessel/tracheal view		
Small aorta		
	Aortic atresia	Hypoplastic aorta and arch
		Reverse flow in aorta
	Coarctation of the aorta	Aorta < pulmonary artery
		Isthmal hypoplasia
		Forward flow in arch
	Critical aortic stenosis	Aortic valve small
		Aortic valve dysplastic with restriction in its opening
		May have low velocity flow across aortic valve
		May have reverse flow in aortic arch

Finding	Possible diagnosis	Features to help make diagnosis
Abnormal three-vessel/tracheal view		
Small pulmonary artery		
	Tetralogy of Fallot	Ventricular septal defect
		Aortic override
		Pulmonary artery < aorta
		Forward flow in main pulmonary artery and duct
	Pulmonary atresia	Hypoplastic pulmonary artery
		Reverse flow in pulmonary artery
	Pulmonary stenosis	Small pulmonary artery
		Thickened restricted pulmonary valve leaflets
		Turbulent flow across pulmonary valve
		Pulmonary artery Doppler flow velocity increased above normal
Forward flow only seen in one great artery		
	Aortic atresia	Reverse flow in aortic arch
	Pulmonary atresia	Reverse flow in pulmonary artery
	Common arterial trunk	Ventricular septal defect
		Single arterial trunk usually arising astride ventricular septal defect
		Trunk gives rise to aortic arch and pulmonary arteries

Finding	Possible diagnosis	Features to help make diagnosis
Abnormal three-vessel/tracheal view		
'Two'-vessel view		
	Transposition of the great arteries	Atrioventricular concordance: • left atrium connected to left ventricle • right atrium connected to right ventricle Ventriculo-arterial discordance: • aorta arises from right ventricle • pulmonary artery arises from left ventricle Parallel arrangement of great arteries Aorta arises anterior and to right of pulmonary artery Wide sweeping aortic arch Aorta and SVC seen in three-vessel view but pulmonary artery not easily seen
'Four-vessel' view		
	Bilateral superior vena cava	A persistent left SVC is seen in addition to the right SVC
'U' shape not 'V' shape of vessels meeting descending aorta		
	Right-sided aortic arch	Aortic arch descends to the right of the trachea
Other		
Polyvalvar dysplasia		
	Chromosomal abnormality, particularly trisomy 18	Other features of chromosomal abnormality

Further reading

Books

Allan L, Hornberger L, Sharland G. *Textbook of Fetal Cardiology*. Greenwich Medical Media Limited: London, 2000.

Anderson RH, Baker EJ, Penny DJ, Redington AN, Rigby ML, Wernovsky G. *Paediatric Cardiology*, 3rd Edition. Churchill Livingstone/Elsevier: Philadelphia, PA, 2009.

Journals

Allan LD. A practical approach to fetal heart scanning. *Semin Perinatol* 2000; 24: 324-30.

Allan LD. Rationale for and current status of prenatal cardiac intervention. *Early Hum Dev* 2012; 88: 287-20.

Allan LD, Chita SK, Al-Ghazali W, *et al*. Doppler echocardiographic evaluation of the normal human fetal heart. *Br Heart J* 1987; 57: 528-33.

Allan LD, Chita SK, Sharland GK, *et al*. The use of flecainide in fetal tachycardias. *Br Heart J* 1991; 65: 46-8.

Allan LD, Crawford DC, Chita SK, *et al*. Familial recurrence of congenital heart disease in a prospective series of mothers referred for fetal echocardiography. *Am J Cardiol* 1986; 58: 334-7.

Allan L, Dangel J, Fesslova V, *et al*; Fetal Cardiology Working Group; Association for European Paediatric Cardiology. Recommendations for the practice of fetal cardiology in Europe. *Cardiol Young* 2004; 14: 109-14

Allan LD, Joseph MD, Boyd EGCA, *et al*. M-mode echocardiography in the developing human fetus. *Br Heart J* 1982; 47: 573-84.

Allan LD, Sharland GK. Prognosis in fetal tetralogy of Fallot. *Pediatr Cardiol* 1992; 13: 1-4.

Allan LD, Sharland GK. The echocardiographic diagnosis of totally anomalous pulmonary venous connection in the fetus. *Heart* 2001; 85: 433-7.

Allan LD, Sharland GK, Lockhart SM, *et al*. Chromosomal anomalies and congenital heart disease in the fetus. *Ultrasound Obstet Gynecol* 1991; 1: 8-11.

Allan LD, Sharland GK, Milburn A, *et al*. Prospective diagnosis of 1006 consecutive cases of congenital heart disease in the fetus. *J Am Coll Cardiol* 1994; 23: 1452-8.

Allan LD, Sharland GK, Tynan MJ. The natural history of the hypoplastic left heart syndrome. *Int J Cardiol* 1989; 25: 341-3.

Andrews RE, Tibby SM, Sharland GK, *et al.* Prediction of outcome of tricuspid valve malformations diagnosed during fetal life. *Am J Cardiol* 2008; 101: 1046-50.

Andrews R, Tulloh R, Sharland G, *et al.* Outcome of staged reconstructive surgery for hypoplastic left heart syndrome following antenatal diagnosis. *Arch Dis Child* 2001; 85: 474-7.

Arunamata A, Punn R, Cuneo B, *et al.* Echocardiographic diagnosis and prognosis of fetal left ventricular noncompaction. *J Am Soc Echocardiogr* 2012; 25: 112-20.

Arzt W, Tulzer G. Fetal surgery for cardiac lesions. *Prenat Diagn* 2011; 31: 695-8.

Atz AM, Travison TG, Williams IA, *et al.* For the Pediatric Heart Network Investigators. Prenatal diagnosis and risk factors for preoperative death in neonates with single right ventricle and systemic outflow obstruction: screening data from the Pediatric Heart Network Single Ventricle Reconstruction Trial. *J Thorac Cardiovasc Surg* 2010; 140: 1245-50.

Axt-Fleidner R, Schwarze A, Smrcek J, *et al.* Isolated ventricular septal defects detected by colour Doppler imaging: evolution during fetal and first year of postnatal life. *Ultrasound Obstet Gynecol* 2006; 27: 266-73.

Bader R, Hornberger LK, Nijmeh LJ, *et al.* Fetal pericardial teratoma: presentation of two cases and review of literature. *Am J Perinatol* 2006; 23: 53-8.

Berg C, Bender F, Soukup M, *et al.* Right aortic arch detected in fetal life. *Ultrasound Obstet Gynecol* 2006; 28: 882-9.

Bernasconi A, Azancot A, Simpson JM, *et al.* Fetal dextrocardia: diagnosis and outcome in two tertiary centres. *Heart* 2005; 91: 1590-4.

Bhat AH, Kehl DW, Tacy TA, *et al.* Diagnosis of tetralogy of Fallot and its variants in the late first and early second trimester: details of initial assessment and comparison with later fetal diagnosis. *Echocardiography* 2012; Sep 11: doi: 10.1111/j.1540-8175.2012.01798.x. [Epub ahead of print].

Bonnet D, Coltri A, Butera G, *et al.* Fetal detection of transposition of the great arteries reduces morbidity and mortality in newborn infants. *Circulation* 1999; 99: 916-8.

Borenstein M, Minekawa R, Zidere V, *et al.* Aberrant right subclavian artery at 16 to 23 + 6 weeks of gestation: a marker for chromosomal abnormality. *Ultrasound Obstet Gynecol* 2010; 36: 548-52.

Boudjemline Y, Fermont L, Le Bidois J, *et al.* Prevalence of 22q11 deletion in fetuses with conotruncal cardiac defects: a 6-year prospective study. *J Pediatr* 2001; 138: 520-4.

Boyd PA, Tonks AM, Rankin J, *et al*; BINOCAR Working Group. Monitoring the prenatal detection of structural fetal congenital anomalies in England and Wales: a register-based study. *J Med Screening* 2011; 18: 2-7.

British Congenital Cardiac Association: Fetal cardiology standards. www.bcs.com/documents/fetal_cardiology_standards_final_version_2012pdf.

Bull C, on behalf of British Paediatric Cardiac Association. Current and potential impact of fetal diagnosis on prevalence and spectrum of serious congenital heart disease at term in the UK. *Lancet* 1999; 354: 1242-7.

Burn J, Brennan P, Little J. Recurrence risks in offspring of adults with major heart defects: results from first cohort of British collaborative study. *Lancet* 1998; 351: 311-6.

Chaoui R, Heling KS, Sarioglu N, *et al.* Aberrant right subclavian artery as a new cardiac sign in second and third trimester fetuses with Down syndrome. *Am J Obstet Gynecol* 2005; 192: 257-63.

Cook AC, Allan LD, Anderson RH, *et al.* Atrioventricular septal defect in fetal life – a clinicopathological correlation. *Cardiol Young* 1991; 1: 334-43.

Cook AC, Fagg NLK, Ho SY, *et al.* Echocardiographic-anatomic correlations in aortico-left ventricular tunnel. *Br Heart J* 1995; 74: 443-8.

Crowe DA, Allan LD. Patterns of pulmonary venous flow in the fetus with disease of the left heart. *Cardiol Young* 2001; 11: 369-74.

Cuneo BF. Treatment of fetal tachycardia. *Heart Rhythm* 2008; 5: 1216-8.

Daubeney PEF, Sharland GK, Cook A, *et al.* Pulmonary atresia with intact ventricular septum: impact of fetal echocardiography on incidence at birth and postnatal outcome. *Circulation* 1998; 98: 562-6.

Dolk H, Loane M, Garne E; European Surveillance of Congenital Anomalies (EUROCAT) Working Group. Congenital heart defects in Europe: prevalence and perinatal mortality, 2000 to 2005. *Circulation* 2011; 123: 841-9.

Duke C, Sharland GK, Jones AMR, *et al.* Echocardiographic features and outcome of truncus arteriosus diagnosed during fetal life. *Am J Cardiol* 2001; 88: 1379-84.

Eliasson H, Sonesson SE, Sharland G, *et al*: Fetal Working Group of the European Association of Pediatric Cardiology. Isolated atrioventricular block in the fetus: a retrospective, multinational, multicenter study of 175 patients. *Circulation* 2011; 124: 1919-26.

Ettedgui J, Sharland GK, Chita SK, *et al*. Absent pulmonary valve syndrome and ventricular septal defect: role of the arterial duct. *Am J Cardiol* 1990; 66: 233-4.

Ferencz C, Rubin JD, McCarter RJ, *et al*. Congenital heart disease: prevalence at livebirth. The Baltimore-Washington Infant Study. *Am J Epidemiol* 1985; 121: 31-6.

Fetal Echocardiography Task Force; American Institute of Ultrasound in Medicine Clinical Standards Committee; American College of Obstetricians and Gynecologists; Society for Maternal-Fetal Medicine. AIUM practice guideline for the performance of fetal echocardiography. *J Ultrasound Med* 2011; 30: 127-36.

Fisher J. Termination of pregnancy for fetal abnormality: the perspective of a parent support organisation. *Reproductive Health Matters* 2008; 16 (31 Supplement): 57-65.

Fouron JC, Proulx F, Miró J, *et al*. Doppler and M-mode ultrasonography to time fetal atrial and ventricular contractions. *Obstet Gynecol* 2000; 96: 732-6.

Fuchs IB, Muller H, Abdul- Khaliq H, *et al*. Immediate and long-term outcomes in children with prenatal diagnosis of selected isolated congenital heart defects. *Ultrasound Obstet Gynecol* 2007; 29: 38-43.

Fyler DC, Buckley LP, Hellenbrand WE, *et al*. Report of the New England Regional Infant Care Programme. *Pediatrics* 1980; 65(suppl): 376-461.

Gardiner HM, Belmar C, Tulzer G, *et al*. Morphological and functional predictors of eventual circulation in the fetus with pulmonary atresia or critical pulmonary stenosis with intact septum. *J Am Coll Cardiol* 2008; 51: 1299-308.

Gembruch U, Smrcek JM. The prevalence and clinical significance of tricuspid valve regurgitation in normally grown fetuses and those with intrauterine growth retardation. *Ultrasound Obstet Gynecol* 1997; 9: 374-82.

Gill HR, Splitt M, Sharland GK, *et al*. Patterns of recurrence of congenital heart disease: an analysis of 6640 consecutive pregnancies evaluated by detailed fetal echocardiography. *J Am Coll Cardiol* 2003; 42: 923-9.

Groves AM, Allan LD, Rosenthal E. Outcome of isolated congenital complete heart block diagnosed in utero. *Heart* 1996; 75: 190-4.

Groves AM, Fagg NLK, Cook AC, *et al*. Cardiac tumours in intrauterine life. *Arch Dis Child* 1992; 67: 1189-92.

Head CE, Jowett VC, Sharland GK, *et al*. Timing of presentation and postnatal outcome of infants suspected of having coarctation of the aorta during fetal life. *Heart* 2005; 91: 1070-4.

Hoffman JI, Kaplan S. The incidence of congenital heart disease. *J Am Coll Cardiol* 2002; 39: 1890-900.

Holley DG, Martin GR, Brenner JI, *et al.* Diagnosis and management of fetal cardiac tumours: a multicentre experience and review of published reports. *J Am Coll Cardiol* 1995; 26: 516-20.

Hornberger LK, Sahn DJ, Kleinman C, *et al.* Antenatal diagnosis of coarctation of the aorta. A multicentre experience. *J Am Coll Cardiol* 1994; 23: 417-23.

Hornberger LK, Sanders SP, Rein AJ, *et al.* Left heart obstructive lesions and left ventricular growth in the midtrimester fetus. A longitudinal study. *Circulation* 1995; 92: 1531-8.

Hornberger LK, Sanders SP, Sahn DJ, *et al.* In utero pulmonary artery and aortic growth and potential for progression of pulmonary outflow tract obstruction in tetralogy of Fallot. *J Am Coll Cardiol* 1995; 25: 739-45.

Huggon IC, Cook AC, Smeeton NC, *et al.* Atrioventricular septal defects diagnosed in fetal life; associated cardiac and extracardiac abnormalities and outcome. *J Am Coll Cardiol* 2000; 36: 593-601.

Huggon IC, Ghi T, Cook AC, *et al.* Fetal cardiac abnormalities identified prior to 14 weeks' gestation. *Ultrasound Obstet Gynecol* 2002; 20: 22-9.

Huhta JC, Paul JJ. Doppler in fetal heart failure. *Clin Obstet Gynecol* 2010; 53: 915-29.

Hyett J, Perdu M, Sharland G, *et al.* Using fetal nuchal translucency to screen for major congenital cardiac defects at 10-14 weeks of gestation: population-based cohort study. *Br Med J* 1999; 318: 81-5.

ISUOG Education Committee. Cardiac screening examination of the fetus: guidelines for performing the 'basic' and 'extended basic' cardiac scan. *Ultrasound Obstet Gynecol* 2006; 27: 107-13.

Jaeggi ET, Carvalho JS, De Groot E, *et al.* Comparison of transplacental treatment of fetal supraventricular tachyarrhythmias with digoxin, flecainide, and sotalol: results of a nonrandomized multicenter study. *Circulation* 2011; 124: 1747-54.

Jaeggi E, Fouron JC, Fournier A, *et al.* Ventriculo-atrial time interval measured on M-mode echocardiography: a determining element in diagnosis, treatment, and prognosis of fetal supraventricular tachycardia. *Heart* 1998; 79: 582-7.

Jaeggi ET, Fouron JC, Silverman ED, *et al.* Transplacental fetal treatment improves the outcome of prenatally diagnosed complete atrioventricular block without structural heart disease. *Circulation* 2004; 110: 1542-8.

Jaeggi ET, Hornberger LK, Smallhorn JF, *et al*. Prenatal diagnosis of complete atrioventricular block associated with structural heart disease: combined experience of two tertiary care centres and review of the literature. *Ultrasound Obstet Gynecol* 2005; 26: 16-21.

Jaeggi ET, Scholler GF, Jones OD, *et al*. Comparative analysis of pattern, management and outcome of pre versus postnatally diagnosed major congenital heart disease: a population-based study. *Ultrasound Obstet Gynecol* 2001; 17: 380-5.

Jain S, Kleiner B, Moon-Grady A, *et al*. Prenatal diagnosis of vascular rings. *J Ultrasound Med* 2010; 29: 287-94.

Jouannic JM, Gavard L, Fermont L, *et al*. Sensitivity and specificity of prenatal features of physiological shunts to predict neonatal clinical status in transposition of the great arteries. *Circulation* 2004; 110: 1743-6.

Kaguelidou F, Fermont L, Boudjemline Y, *et al*. Foetal echocardiographic assessment of tetralogy of Fallot and post-natal outcome. *Eur Heart J* 2008; 29: 1432-8.

Karatza AA, Wolfenden JL, Taylor MJ, *et al*. Influence of twin-twin transfusion syndrome on fetal cardiovascular structure and function: prospective case-control study of 136 monochorionic twin pregnancies. *Heart* 202; 88: 271-7.

Khoshmood B, Lelong N, Houyet L, *et al*, on behalf of the EPICARD Study Group. Prevalence, timing of diagnosis and mortality of newborns with congenital heart disease: a population-based study. *Heart* 2012; Aug 11: doi: 10.1136/heartjnl-2012-302543 [Epub ahead of print].

Kipps AK, Feuille C, Azakie A, *et al*. Prenatal diagnosis of hypoplastic left heart syndrome in current era. *Am J Cardiol* 2011; 108: 421-7.

Kohl T, Sharland G, Allan LD, *et al*. World experience of percutaneous ultrasound-guided balloon valvuloplasty in human fetuses with severe aortic valve obstruction. *Am J Cardiol* 2000; 85: 1230-3.

Krapp M, Kohl T, Simpson JM, *et al*. Review of diagnosis, treatment, and outcome of fetal atrial flutter compared with supraventricular tachycardia. *Heart* 2003; 89: 913-7.

Lagopoulos ME, Manlhiot C, McCrindle BW, *et al*. Impact of prenatal diagnosis and anatomical subtype on outcome in double-outlet right ventricle. *Am Heart J* 2010; 160: 692-700.

Landis BJ, Levey A, Levasseur SM, *et al*. Prenatal diagnosis of congenital heart disease and birth outcomes. *Pediatr Cardiol* 2012; Oct 6: [Epub ahead of print].

Langford K, Sharland G, Simpson J. Relative risk of abnormal karyotype in fetuses found to have an atrioventricular septal defect (AVSD) on fetal echocardiography. *Prenat Diagn* 2005; 25: 137-9.

Laux D, Fermont L, Bajolle F, *et al*. Prenatal diagnosis of isolated total anomalous pulmonary venous connection: a series of ten cases. *Ultrasound Obstet Gynecol* 2012; May 17: doi: 10.1002/uog.11186 [Epub ahead of print].

Lee W, Allan L, Carvalho JS, *et al*. ISUOG Fetal Echocardiography Task Force. ISUOG consensus statement: what constitutes a fetal echocardiogram? *Ultrasound Obstet Gynecol* 2008; 32: 239-42.

Levey A, Glickstein JS, Kleinman CS, *et al*. The impact of prenatal diagnosis of complex congenital heart disease on neonatal outcomes. *Pediatr Cardiol* 2010; 31: 587-97.

Lim JS, McCrindle BW, Smallhorn JF, *et al*. Clinical features, management, and outcome of children with fetal and postnatal diagnoses of isomerism syndromes. *Circulation* 2005; 112: 2454-61.

Loughheed J, Sinclair BG, Fung Kee Fung K, *et al*. Acquired right ventricular outflow tract obstruction in the recipient twin in twin-twin transfusion syndrome. *J Am Coll Cardiol* 2001; 38: 1533-8.

Maeno YV, Boutin C, Hornberger LK, *et al*. Prenatal diagnosis of right ventricular outflow tract obstruction with intact ventricular septum, and detection of ventriculocoronary connections. *Heart* 1999; 81: 661-8.

Maeno YV, Kamenir SA, Sinclair B, *et al*. Prenatal features of ductus arteriosus constriction and restrictive foramen ovale in d-transposition of the great arteries. *Circulation* 1999; 99: 1209-14.

Makikallio K, McElhinney DB, Levine JC, *et al*. Fetal aortic valve stenosis and the evolution of hypoplastic left heart syndrome: patient selection for fetal intervention. *Circulation* 2006; 113: 1401-5.

Makrydimas G, Sotiriadis A, Huggon IC, *et al*. Nuchal translucency and fetal cardiac defects: a pooled analysis of major fetal echocardiography centres. *Am J Obstet Gynecol* 2005; 192: 89-95.

Marek J, Tomek V, Skovranek J, *et al*. Prenatal ultrasound screening of congenital heart disease in an unselected national population: a 21-year experience. *Heart* 2011; 97: 124-30.

Marijon E, Ou P, Fermont L, *et al*. Diagnosis and outcome in congenital ventricular diverticulum and aneurysm. *J Thorac Cardiovasc Surg* 2006; 131: 433-7.

Marino B, Diglio MC, Toscano A, *et al*. Anatomic patterns of conotruncal defects associated with deletion 22q11. *Genet Med* 2001; 3: 45-8.

Matsui H, Mellander M, Roughton M, *et al*. Morphological and physiological predictors of fetal aortic coarctation. *Circulation* 2008; 118: 1793-801.

Matta MJ, Cuneo BF. Doppler echocardiography for managing fetal cardiac arrhythmia. *Clin Obstet Gynecol* 2010; 53: 899-914.

McElhinney DB, Salvin JW, Colan SD, *et al*. Improving outcomes in fetuses and neonates with congenital displacement (Ebstein's malformation) or dysplasia of the tricuspid valve. *Am J Cardiol* 2005; 96: 582-6.

McElhinney DB, Tworetzky W, Lock JE. Current status of fetal cardiac intervention. *Circulation* 2010; 121: 1256-63.

Menon SC, O'Leary PW, Wright GB, *et al*. Fetal and neonatal presentation of noncompacted ventricular myocardium: expanding the clinical spectrum. *J Am Soc Echocardiogr* 2007; 20: 1344-50.

Meyer-Wittkopf M, Simpson JM, Sharland GK. Incidence of congenital heart defects in fetuses of diabetic mothers: a retrospective study of 326 cases. *Ultrasound Obstet Gynecol* 1996; 8: 8-10.

Michelfelder E, Gomez C, Border W, *et al*. Predictive value of fetal pulmonary venous flow patterns in identifying the need for atrial septoplasty in the newborn with hypoplastic left ventricle. *Circulation* 2005; 112: 2974.

Moon-Grady AJ, Tacy TA, Brook MM, *et al*. Value of clinical and echocardiographic features in predicting outcome in the fetus, infant and child with tetralogy of Fallot with absent pulmonary valve complex. *Am J Cardiol* 2001; 89: 1280-5.

National Institute for Health and Clinical Excellence. Antenatal Care – Routine Care for the Healthy Pregnant Woman. Clinical guideline, March 2008. London: NICE, 2008. www.nice.org.uk/cg62.

NHS Fetal Anomaly Screening Programme. http://fetalanomaly.screening.nhs.uk/ standardsandpolicies.

Oberhoffer R, Cook AC, Lang D, *et al*. Correlation between echocardiographic and morphologic investigations of lesions of the tricuspid valve diagnosed during fetal life. *Br Heart J* 1992; 68: 580-5.

Paladini D, Sglavo G, Pastore G, *et al*. Aberrant right subclavian artery: incidence and correlation with other markers of Down syndrome in second-trimester fetuses. *Ultrasound Obstet Gynecol* 2012; 39: 191-5.

Park JK, Taylor DK, Skeels M, *et al*. Dilated coronary sinus in the fetus: misinterpretation as an atrioventricular septal defect. *Ultrasound Obstet Gynecol* 1997; 10: 126-9.

Pascal CJ, Huggon I, Sharland GK, *et al*. An echocardiographic study of diagnostic accuracy, prediction of surgical approach, and outcome for fetuses diagnosed with discordant ventriculo-arterial connections. *Cardiol Young* 2007; 17: 528-34.

Pasquini L, Mellander M, Seale A, *et al*. Z-scores of the fetal aortic isthmus and duct: an aid to assessing arch hypoplasia. *Ultrasound Obstet Gynecol* 2007; 29: 628-33.

Pedra SR, Smallhorn JF, Ryan G, *et al*. Fetal cardiomyopathies: pathogenic mechanisms, hemodynamic findings, and clinical outcome. *Circulation* 2002; 106: 585-91.

Pepas LP, Savis A, Jones A, *et al*. An echocardiographic study of tetralogy of Fallot in the fetus and infant. *Cardiol Young* 2003; 13: 240-7.

Pepes S, Zidere V, Allan LD. Prenatal diagnosis of left atrial isomerism. *Heart* 2009; 95: 1974-7.

Persico N, Moratella J, Lombardi CM, *et al*. Fetal echocardiography at 11-13 weeks by transabdomainal high-frequency ultrasound. *Ultrasound Obstet Gynecol* 2011; 37: 296-301.

Pezard P, Bonnemains L, Boussion F, *et al*. Influence of ultrasonographers' training on prenatal diagnosis of congenital heart disease: a 12-year population-based study. *Prenat Diagn* 2008; 28: 1016-22.

Poon LC, Huggon IC, Zidere V, *et al*. Tetralogy of Fallot in the fetus in the current era. *Ultrasound Obstet Gynecol* 2007; 29: 625-7.

Punn R, Silverman NH. Fetal predictors of urgent balloon atrial septostomy in neonates with complete transposition. *J Am Soc Echocardiogr* 2011; 24: 425-30.

Quartermain MD, Glatz AC, Goldberg DJ, *et al*. Pulmonary outflow obstruction in the fetus with complex congenital heart disease: predicting the need for neonatal intervention. *Ultrasound Obstet Gynecol* 2012; May 17: doi: 10.1002/uog.11196 [Epub ahead of print].

Raymond FL, Simpson JM, Sharland GK, *et al*. Fetal echocardiography as a predictor of chromosomal abnormality. *Lancet* 1997; 350: 930.

Razavi RS, Sharland GK, Simpson JM. Prenatal diagnosis by echocardiogram and outcome of absent pulmonary valve syndrome. *Am J Cardiol* 2003; 91: 429-32.

Roman KS, Fuoron JC, Nii M, *et al*. Determinants of outcome of fetal pulmonary valve stenosis or atresia with intact ventricular septum. *Am J Cardiol* 2007; 99: 699-703.

Rona RJ, Smeeton NC, Barnett A, *et al.* Anxiety and depression in mothers related to severe malformation of the heart of the child and fetus. *Acta Paediatr* 1998; 87: 201-5.

Rosenberg KB, Monk C, Glickstein JS, *et al.* Referral for fetal echocardiography is associated with increased maternal anxiety. *J Psychosom Obstet Gynaecol* 2010; 31: 60-9.

Rychik J, Ayres N, Cuneo B, *et al.* American Society of Echocardiography guidelines and standards for performance of the fetal echocardiogram. *J Am Soc Echocardiogr* 2004; 17: 803-10.

Saada J, Hadj Rabia S, Fermont L, *et al.* Prenatal diagnosis of cardiac rhabdomyomas: incidence of associated cerebral lesions of tuberous sclerosis complex. *Ultrasound Obstet Gynecol* 2009; 34: 155-9.

Salvin JW, McElhinney DB, Colan SD, *et al.* Fetal tricuspid valve size and growth as predictors of outcome in pulmonary atresia with intact ventricular septum. *Pediatrics* 2006; 118: 415-20.

Sandor GG, Cook AC, Sharland GK, *et al.* Coronary arterial abnormalities in pulmonary atresia with intact ventricular septum diagnosed during fetal life. *Cardiol Young* 2002; 12: 436-44.

Sau A, Sharland G, Simpson J. Agenesis of the ductus venosus associated with direct umbilical venous return into the heart – case series and review of the literature. *Prenat Diagn* 2004; 24: 418-23.

Shah A, Moon-Grady A, Bhogal N, *et al.* Effectiveness of sotalol as first-line therapy for fetal supraventricular tachyarrhythmias. *Am J Cardiol* 2012; 109: 1614-8.

Sharland G. Echocardiographic features of common arterial trunk. *Progress in Pediatric Cardiology* 2002; 15: 33-40.

Sharland G. Routine fetal cardiac screening: what are we doing and what should we do? *Prenat Diagn* 2004; 24: 1123-9.

Sharland G. Fetal cardiac screening and variation in prenatal detection rates of congenital heart disease: why bother with screening at all? *Future Cardiol* 2012; 8: 189-202.

Sharland GK, Allan LD. Screening for congenital heart disease prenatally. Results of a 21/2-year study in the South East Thames Region. *Br J Obstet Gynaecol* 1992; 9: 220-5.

Sharland GK, Chan KY, Allan LD. Coarctation of the aorta: difficulties in prenatal diagnosis. *Br Heart J* 1994; 71: 70-5.

Sharland GK, Chita SK, Allan LD. The use of colour Doppler in fetal echocardiography. *Int J Cardiol* 1990; 28: 229-36.

Sharland GK, Chita SK, Allan LD. Tricuspid valve dysplasia or displacement in intrauterine life. *J Am Coll Cardiol* 1991; 17: 944-9.

Sharland GK, Chita SK, Fagg NLK, *et al.* Left ventricular dysfunction in the fetus: relationship to aortic valve anomalies and endocardial fibroelastosis. *Br Heart J* 1991; 66: 419-24.

Sharland GK, Lockhart SM, Chita SK, *et al.* Factors influencing the outcome of congenital heart disease detected prenatally. *Arch Dis Child* 1991; 66: 284-7.

Sharland G, Tingay R, Jones A, *et al.* Atrioventricular and ventriculoarterial discordance (congenitally corrected transposition of the great arteries): echocardiographic features, associations, and outcome in 34 fetuses. *Heart* 2005; 91: 1453-8.

Sharland GK, Tynan M, Qureshi SA. Prenatal detection and progression of right coronary artery to right ventricle fistula. *Heart* 1996; 76: 79-81.

Shipp TD, Bromley B, Hornberger LK, *et al.* Levorotation of the fetal cardiac axis: a clue for the presence of congenital heart disease. *Obstet Gynecol* 1995; 85: 97-102.

Simpson JM, Jones A, Callaghan N, *et al.* Accuracy and limitations of transabdominal fetal echocardiography at 12-15 weeks of gestation in a population at high risk for congenital heart disease. *Br J Obstet Gynecol* 2000; 107: 1492-7.

Simpson JM, Milburn A, Yates RW, *et al.* Outcome of intermittent tachyarrhythmias in the fetus. *Paed Cardiol* 1997; 18: 78-82.

Simpson JM, Sharland GK. The natural history and outcome of aortic stenosis diagnosed prenatally. *Heart* 1997; 77: 205-10.

Simpson JM, Sharland GK. Fetal tachycardias: management and outcome of 127 consecutive cases. *Heart* 1998; 79: 576-81.

Simpson JM, Yates RW, Sharland GK. Irregular heart rate in the fetus: not always benign. *Cardiol Young* 1996; 6: 28-31.

Sivasankaran S, Sharland GK, Simpson JM. Dilated cardiomyopathy presenting during fetal life. *Cardiol Young* 2005; 15: 409-6.

Skinner JR, Sharland G. Detection and management of life threatening arrhythmias in the perinatal period. *Early Human Development* 2008; 84: 161-72.

Smith RS, Comstock CH, Kirk JS, *et al.* Ultrasonographic left cardiac axis deviation: a marker for fetal anomalies. *Obstet Gynecol* 1995; 85: 187-91.

Song MS, Hu A, Dyamenahalli U, *et al.* Extracardiac lesions and chromosomal abnormalities associated with major fetal heart defects: comparison of intrauterine, postnatal and postmortem diagnoses. *Ultrasound Obstet Gynecol* 2009; 33: 552-9.

Taketazu M, Lougheed J, Yoo SJ, *et al.* Spectrum of cardiovascular disease, accuracy of diagnosis, and outcome in fetal heterotaxy syndrome. *Am J Cardiol* 2006; 97: 720-4.

Tegnander E, Eik-Nes S. The examiner's ultrasound experience has significant impact on the detection rate of congenital heart defects at the second-trimester fetal examination. *Ultrasound Obstet Gynecol* 2006; 28: 8-14.

Tham EB, Wald R, McElhinney DB, *et al.* Outcome of fetuses and infants with double-inlet single left ventricle. *Am J Cardiol* 2008; 101: 1652-6.

Tometzki AJ, Suda K, Khol T, *et al.* Accuracy of prenatal echocardiographic diagnosis and prognosis of fetuses with conotruncal abnormalities. *J Am Coll Cardiol* 1999; 33: 1696-701.

Tulzer G, Arzt W, Franklin RC, *et al.* Fetal pulmonary valvuloplasty for critical pulmonary stenosis or atresia with intact septum. *Lancet* 2002; 360: 1567-8.

Tworetzky W, Marshall AC. Fetal interventions for cardiac defects. *Pediatr Clin North Am* 2004; 51: 1503-13.

Tworetsky W, McElhinney DB, Reddy VM, *et al.* Improved surgical outcome after fetal diagnosis of hypoplastic left heart syndrome. *Circulation* 2001; 103: 1269-73.

Ultrasound Screening – Supplement to Ultrasound Screening for Fetal Abnormalities. London: Royal College of Obstetrics and Gynaecology, July 2000. www.rcog.org.uk/womens-health/clinical-guidance/ultrasound-screening.

Vesel S, Rollings S, Jones A, *et al.* Prenatally diagnosed pulmonary atresia with ventricular septal defect: echocardiography, genetics, associated anomalies and outcome. *Heart* 2006; 92: 1501-5.

Vida VL, Bacha EA, Larrazabal A, *et al.* Hypoplastic left heart syndrome with intact or highly restrictive atrial septum: surgical experience from a single centre. *Ann Thorac Surg* 2007; 84: 581-5.

Vogel M, Sharland GK, McElhinney DB, *et al.* Prevalence of increased nuchal translucency in fetuses with congenital cardiac disease and a normal karyotype. *Cardiol Young* 2009; 19: 441-5.

Vogel M, Vernon MM, McElhinney DB, *et al.* Fetal diagnosis of interrupted aortic arch. *Am J Cardiol* 2010; 105: 727-34.

Volpe P, De Robertis V, Campobasso G, *et al.* Diagnosis of congenital heart disease by early and second-trimester fetal echocardiography. *J Ultrasound Med* 2012; 31: 563-8.

Volpe P, Ubaldo P, Volpe N, *et al.* Fetal cardiac evaluation at 11-14 weeks by experienced obstetricians in a low-risk population. *Prenat Diagn* 2011; 31: 1054-61.

Wald RM, Tham EB, McCrindle BW, *et al.* Outcome after prenatal diagnosis of tricuspid atresia: a multicenter experience. *Am Heart J* 2007; 153: 772-8.

Wertaschnigg D, Jaeggi M, Chitayat D, *et al.* Prenatal diagnosis and outcome of absent pulmonary valve syndrome: contemporary single-center experience and review of the literature. *Ultrasound Obstet Gynecol* 2012; May 17: doi: 10.1002/uog.11193 [Epub ahead of print].

Williams IA, Shaw R, Kleinman CS, *et al.* Parental understanding of neonatal congenital heart disease. *Pediatr Cardiol* 2008; 29: 1059-65.

Wren C, Reinhardt Z, Khawaja K. Twenty-year trends in diagnosis of life-threatening neonatal cardiovascular malformations *Arch Dis Child – Fetal and Neonatal Edition* 2008; 93: F33-5.

Yamamoto Y, Hornberger LK. Progression of outflow tract obstruction in the fetus. *Early Hum Dev* 2012; 88: 279-85.

Yeager SB, Parness IA, Spevak PJ, *et al.* Prenatal echocardiographic diagnosis of pulmonary and systemic venous anomalies. *Am Heart J* 1994; 128: 397-405.

Yinon Y, Chitayat D, Blaser S, *et al.* Fetal cardiac tumors: a single-center experience of 40 cases. *Prenat Diagn* 2010; 30: 941-9.

Zidere V, Tsapakis EG, Huggon IC, *et al.* Right aortic arch in the fetus. *Ultrasound Obstet Gynecol* 2006; 28: 876-81.

Index

Page numbers given in blue and bold refer to figures